PRIMARY CARE
RHEUMATOLOGY

JOHN H KLIPPEL * **PAUL A DIEPPE** * **FRED F FERRI**

MD FACP
Arthritis Foundation,
Washington DC,
USA

BSc MD FRCP
MRC Health Services
Research Collaboration
University of Bristol
Bristol,
UK

MD FACP
Brown University
School of Medicine
Department of Community Health
St. Joseph's Health Services
Division of Internal Medicine
Providence,
USA

With contributions from

**PETER
HOLLINGWORTH**
Department of
Rheumatology
Southmead Hospital
Bristol, UK

SCOTT TODER
Division of
Rheumatology
Fatima Hospital
Providence,
USA

 Mosby

London St Louis Philadelphia Sydney Tokyo

MOSBY
An imprint of Elsevier Science Limited

M is a registered trademark of Elsevier Science Limited

© Mosby 1999
© Harcourt Publishers Limited 2000
© Elsevier Science Limited 2002. All rights reserved.

First published in 1999 by Mosby
  Reprinted 2000, 2002

ISBN 0 7234 3143 4

British Library Cataloguing in Publication Data
A catalogue record for this book is available from the British Library.

Library of Congress Cataloging-in-Publication Data has been applied for.

Printed in Spain by Grafos S.A. arte sobre papel, Barcelona, Spain

Publisher	Fiona Foley
Managing Editor	Sue Hodgson
Project Manager	Sarah Gray
	Susan Rana
Design	Pete Wilder
Cover Design	Greg Smith
Illustration	The EDI Partnership: Mark Willey,
	Lee Smith
	Lynda Payne
	Danny Pyne
	Mike Saiz
	Mick Ruddy
Proofreader	Roddy Crews
Copyeditor	John Ormiston
Production	Siobhan Egan
Index	Jan Ross

DRUG NOTICE
The contributors, the editors, and the publishers have made every effort to ensure the accuracy and appropriateness of the drug dosages presented in this textbook. The medications described do not necessarily have specific approval by the Food and Drug Administration for use in the diseases and dosages for which they are recommended. The package insert for each drug should be consulted for use and dosage as approved by the FDA. Because standards for usage change, it is advisable to keep abreast of revised recommendations, particularly those concerning new drugs.

CONTENTS

PREFACE

This book is for primary care physicians.

Musculoskeletal disorders account for between 10 and 20% of all visits to primary care physicians. The causes range from mild, self-limiting soft tissue injuries, to chronic, disabling arthropathies, to life-threatening systemic diseases. It is therefore essential that all primary care physicians have a good working knowledge and understanding of how to diagnose and treat disorders of the musculoskeletal system. This book has been specifically developed for just that purpose.

The first section of the book provides a general introduction to the principles and practice of diagnosis and therapy of the musculoskeletal system. The following sections, which form the main part of the book, cover all the common disorders of the system and are organized by presenting features (monoarticular pain, back pain, generalized pain, and so on) as well as by the conventional disease classification used in most books. Musculoskeletal problems present in different ways at the extremes of age, thus sections of the book are devoted to musculoskeletal disorders in children and in the elderly.

Information is only of use if it is accessible – the ways in which facts are presented are as important as the facts themselves. This book presents information in as user-friendly a way as possible. Each of the major chapters is preceded by a diagnostic algorithm which provides guidance to the key clinical features of differential diagnoses of the main disorders. We have also used standard templates for the main chapters, to make it easy for the reader to find information. The major rheumatic diseases are introduced by brief case vignettes followed by a boxed summary of the main features of each condition, diagnostic issues, treatment principles (including education, physical treatments, dietary issues and complementary techniques, as well as drugs and surgery) and indications for referral from primary care to specialist services (be they rheumatologists, orthopedists, physical therapists or others). In addition, the liberal use of beautiful illustrations and color make this book easy to the eye as well as easy to use.

We are proud of this book, and confident that it will be an essential and practical guide on the diagnosis and management of musculoskeletal disorders for primary care physicians.

This project has only been made possible as a result of the editors and authors responsible for the parent subspecialty book (*Rheumatology*) and, most importantly, the vision and leadership of Fiona Foley, and her wonderful team of editors and illustrators, particularly Sue Hodgson, to whom we are most grateful.

Jack Klippel and Paul Dieppe

INTRODUCTION

With the advent of managed care, primary care physicians are expected to provide a rapid and cost-effective approach to the diagnosis and treatment of a myriad medical problems. Rheumatology cases constitute a significant portion of visits to primary care physicians. In this era of high technology and increasing demand for sophisticated and expensive diagnostic and therapeutic modalities, the primary care physician is faced with the increasingly difficult tasks of controlling costs and delivering high quality care.

To facilitate the diagnosis and treatment of patients with disorders of the musculoskeletal system there are several books available. I strongly believe that our book stands alone in this crowded field. It clearly addresses the concerns of primary care physicians with its unique and outstanding features. It is written in a clear and concise style with emphasis on the practical aspects of diagnosis and care. 'Key Points' are presented in a box format to facilitate quick retrieval and recollection. The experienced primary care practitioner will welcome its emphasis on cost-effective quality care. Physicians new to private practice, medical students, and residents will appreciate its presentation of 'Typical Cases' in the form of clinical vignettes which describe real patients encountered in the daily practice of medicine. Everyone will enjoy the numerous beautiful illustrations, graphs, and charts used throughout the book to present various rheumatic disorders and enhance recollection of important points.

Another major challenge faced by primary care physicians is knowing when it is appropriate to refer a patient to a specialist. This book facilitates this task by providing 'recommendations for referral'. This practical feature offers much needed criteria and guidance to primary care physicians. As a practicing internist I am also well aware of the importance of patient education. This book contributes significantly to this crucial aspect of patient care by providing numerous 'self-help' pages which can be photocopied and given to our patients to complement information provided during the visit to the office or clinic.

In conclusion, *Primary Care Rheumatology* is a valuable reference for the office, the clinic or even the emergency room. As the title states, this text is directed mainly at primary care physicians – family and general practitioners, internists, and pediatricians, however its unique format and graphics make it an ideal reference for all physicians involved in the care of patients with disorders of the musculoskeletal system. It is without a doubt the standard rheumatology textbook for primary care physicians by which all others will be judged.

Fred F Ferri

ICD–9 CODES

Symbols and formats
The '#' sign indicates that the ICD-9 code is not to the ultimate specificity. The appropriate 4th or 5th digit menu will immediately follow the diagnoses.

The '0' in place of a code indicates that the code(s) for that particular description is listed under a synonym.

NEC = Not elsewhere classified.
NOS = Not otherwise specified.

E-CODES
An E-code is an ICD-9 code that provides supplementary information concerning the external cause of any injury.

Ankle
726.70	Enthesopathy
959.7	Injury
845.00	Separation (Rupture) (Tear) (Laceration)
845.00	Strain (Avulsion) (Hematosis)
726.70	Tendinitis or Bursitis
720.0	Ankylosing Spondylitis

Ankylosis
718.54	Finger
718.57	Foot
718.55	Hip
718.56	Knee
724.6	Lumbosacral (Nonvertebral) (Nondiscogenic)
724.6	Sacroiliac (Nonvertebral) (Nondiscogenic)
724.6	Sacrum (Nonvertebral) (Nondiscogenic)
724.9	Spine (Nonvertebral) (Nondiscogenic)
795.79	Antinuclear Antibodies Raised (Positive)
795.79	Antiphospholipid Antibody Syndrome

Arthritis
716.9#	NOS
274.0	Gout
253.0	Acromegalic [713.0]
277.3	Amyloid [713.7]
	Arthritis, Osteoarthritis *see* DJD
	Arthritis, Rheumatoid *see* Rheumatoid Arthritis
0.94.0	Charcot's
274.0	Crystal Induced – Gouty
	Crystal induced – Pseudogout *see* Chondrocalcinosis
098.50	Gonococcal
275.0	Hemochromatosis (due to) [713.0]
286.0	Hemophilia VIII Arthritis [713.2]
286.1	Hemophilia IX Arthritis [713.2]
287.0	Henoch Schonlein Pupura (Due to) [713.6]
252.0	Hyperparathyroid [713.0]
696.0	Psoriatic
099.3	Reiter's Disease [711.1#]
0.82.8	Rickettsial (Lone Star Fever) [711.8#]
135	Sarcoid
282.60	Sickle Cell Anemia Arthritis [713.2]
282.5	Sickle Cell Trait Arthritis
094.0	Syphilitic (Tabes Dorsalis) [713.5]
282.4	Thalassemia Arthritis [713.2]
079.99	Viral Arthritis

Back
307.89	Ache Psychogenic
724.6	Ache Sacroiliac
724.5	Ache Vertebrogenic (Postural)
724.5	Pain (Postural)
724.2	Pain (Low Back)
307.89	Pain Psychogenic
724.8	Stiff
847.9	Strain (Sprain) (Avulsion) (Hemarthrosis) Unspecified
724.8	Other Symptoms Referable to Back
307.89	Backache Psychogenic
724.6	Backache Sacroiliac
724.5	Backache Vertebrogenic (Postural)

Bone
733.9	Atrophy – NOS
733.99	Atrophy – Posttraumatic
733.90	Disorder (and Cartilage)
733.29	Disorder (and Cartilage) Fibrocystic
733.99	Hypertrophy
	Infection *see* Osteomyelitis

Bone Spur
726.91	NOS
726.73	Calcaneus
726.30	Elbow
726.73	Foot
726.4	Hand
726.73	Heel
726.5	Hip
726.60	Knee
726.91	Nose
726.33	Olecranon
726.69	Prepatellar or Subpatellar
726.4	Wrist
736.21	Boutonniere Deformity Finger (Acquired)
736.42	Bowleg Acquired
754.44	Bowleg Congenital
727.82	Bursa Calcification

Bursitis
727.3	NOS
726.71	Achilles
726.90	Adhesive Site Unspecified
726.79	Ankle
726.5	Buttock
726.79	Calcaneal
727.82	Calcification
726.19	Deltoid
726.33	Elbow
098.52	Gonococcal
726.4	Hand
726.5	Hip
726.69	Infrapatellar
726.60	Knee
726.33	Olecranon
726.61	Pes Anserinus
726.65	Prepatellar
727.3	Radiohumeral
726.19	Scapulohumeral
726.10	Shoulder
726.19	Subacromial
726.19	Subcoracoid
726.19	Subdeltoid
726.69	Subpatellar
095.7	Syphilitic
726.62	Tibial
726.62	Tibial Collateral Ligament
726.5	Trochanteric
354.0	Carpal Tunnel Syndrome
344.60	Cauda Equina Syndrome

Cervical
952.0#	Cord Injury
722.0	Disc Herniation (HNP)
722.71	Disc Herniation (HNP) With Myelopathy
722.0	Nerve Compression - Discogenic
722.71	Nerve Compression - Discogenic With Myelopathy
723.4	Nerve Compression - Root (By Scar Tissue) NEC
723.4	Radiculitis (Nondiscogenic)
756.2	Rib
353.0	Rib Syndrome (Nondiscogenic)
953.0	Root Injury (Nerve)

353.2	Root Lesions NEC (Nondiscogenic)
723.3	Spine Disorder (Nondiscogenic)
337.0	Sympathetic Dystrophy Or Paralysis Syndrome
954.0	Sympathetic Nerve Injury

Chondrocalcinosis
275.49	Crystal Deposition, dicalcium phosphate [712.1#]
275.49	Crystal Deposition, pyrophosphate crystals [712.2#]

5th digit: 712.1-3
1. Shoulder region
2. Upper arm
3. Forearm
4. Hand
6. Lower leg, knee
7. Ankle and/or foot
9. Multiple

Coccyx, Coccygeal
724.70	Disorder
724.71	Hypermobility
959.1	Injury NOS
724.79	Pain
847.4	Separation (Rupture) (Tear) (Laceration)
847.4	Strain (Sprain) (Avulsion) (Hemarthrosis)
710.9	Connective Tissue Disease

DJD (Degenerative Joint Disease)
715.90	Site Unspecified
715.97	Ankle and or Foot (Metatarsals) (Toes) (Tarsals)
715.93	Forearm (Radius) (Wrist) (Ulna)
715.94	Hand (Carpal) (Metacarpal) (Fingers)
715.96	Lower Leg (Fibula) (Knee) (Patella) (Tibia)
715.95	Pelvic Region And Thigh (Hip) (Buttock) (Femur)
715.91	Shoulder Region
721.90	Spine - NOS
721.0	Spine - Cervical
721.3	Spine - Lumbosacral
721.2	Spine - Thoracic
715.92	Upper Arm (Elbow) (Humerus)
715.98	Other Specified
277.3	Familial Mediterranean Fever
729.1	Fibromyalgia
729.1	Fibromyositis

Finger
755.59	Contraction Congenital
736.20	Deformity (Acquired)
718.94	Joint Ligament Relaxation
718.14	Joint Loose Body
446.5	Giant Cell Arteritis
274.0	Gout

Hallux
735.9	Deformity Acquired
735.0	Valgus Acquired
755.66	Valgus Congenital
735.1	Varus Acquired
755.66	Varus Congenital

735.4	Hammer Toe Acquired

Hand
726.4	Bone Spur
736.00	Deformity Acquired
842.10	Separation (Rupture) (Tear) (Laceration) Site NOS
842.10	Strain (Sprain) (Avulsion) (Hemarthrosis) Site NOS
719.1#	Hemarthrosis - Old (Nontraumatic)

5th Digit: 719.1
0. Site NOS
1. Shoulder Region
2. Upper Arm (Elbow) (Humerus)
3. Forearm (Radius) (Wrist) (Ulna)
4. Hand (Carpal) (Metacarpal) (Fingers)
5. Pelvic Region And Thigh (Hip) (Buttock) (Femur)
6. Lower Leg (Fibula) (Knee) (Patella) (Tibia)
7. Ankle and Foot (Metatarsals) (Toes) (Tarsals)
8. Other
9. Multiple

Hip
736.30	Deformity - Acquired
959.6	Injury
719.85	Joint Calcification
754.3#	Joint Disorder - Congenital Dislocation or Subluxation

5th Digit: 754.3
0. Dislocation Unilateral Or Unspecified
1. Dislocation Bilateral
2. Subluxation Unilateral
3. Subluxation Bilateral
5. Dislocation One Hip, Subluxation Other Hip

V82.3	Joint Disorder - Congenital Dislocation Or Subluxation Screening
711.05	Joint Disorder - Suppurative (Pyogenic)
718.85	Joint Instability (Old)
718.15	Joint Loose Body
718.95	Joint Ligament Relaxation
754.32	Preluxation Congenital

Hypermobility
718.8#	Joint (Acquired)

5th Digit: 718.8
0. Site
1. Shoulder Region
2. Upper Arm (Elbow) (Humerus)
3. Forearm (Radius) (Wrist) (Ulna)
4. Hand (Carpal) (Metacarpal) (Fingers)
5. Pelvic Region (Hip) (Buttock) (Femur)
6. Lower Leg (Fibula) (Knee) (Patella) (Tibia)
7. Ankle and/or Foot (Metatarsals) (Toes) (Tarsals)
8. Other
9. Multiple

252.0	Hyperparathyroidism

Lumbar

721.3`	Arthritis
722.93	Disc Calcification or Discitis
722.52	Disc Disease/Degeneration
722.73	Disc Disease/Degeneration - with Myelopathy
722.93	Disc Disorder
722.73	Disc Disorder with Myelopathy
722.10	Disc Displacement
722.73	Disc Displacement with Myelopathy
722.10	Disc Herniation
722.73	Disc Herniation with Myelopathy
722.73	Disc Syndrome
722.10	Nerve Compression - Discogenic
722.73	Nerve Compression - Discogenic with Myelopathy
724.4	Nerve Compression - Root (by Scar Tissue) Neg
722.83	Nerve Compression - Root Postoperative
721.3	Osteoarthritis
724.4	Radiculitis (Nonvertebral) (Nondiscogenic)
739.3	Region Segmental or Somatic Dysfunction
953.2	Root Injury (Nerve)
724.02	Stenosis
847.2	Strain (Sprain) (Avulsion) (Hemarthrosis)
721.3	Spondylarthritis
721.3	Spondylosis
721.42	Spondylosis with Myelopathy (Cord Compression)
724.4	Vertebral Syndrome

Lumbosacral

724.6	Ankylosis (Nonvertebral) (Nondiscogenic)
724.6	Disorder (Nonvertebral) (Nondiscogenic)
724.6	Instability (Nonvertebral) (Nondiscogenic)
721.3	Spondylosis
721.42	Spondylosis with Myelopathy (Cord Compression)
846.0	Strain (Sprain) (Avulsion) (Hemarthrosis)
724.6	Strain (Sprain) Chronic (Nonvertebral) (Nondiscogenic)

Lupus

695.4	Lupus, Discoid
710.0	Lupus erythematosus disseminated
088.81	Lyme Disease
354.5	Mononeuritis multiplex

Myopathy

277.3	Amyloid [359.6]
244.#	Hypothyroid [359.5]
710.0	Lupus [359.6]
446.0	Polyarteritis Nodosa [359.6]
714.0	Rheumatoid [359.6]
135	Sarcoid [359.6]
710.1	Scleroderma [359.6]
710.2	Sjorgen's [359.6]
255.0	With Cushing's Syndrome [359.5]

Myositis

729.1	Myositis
728.19	Ossificans Other
728.11	Ossificans Progressive
728.12	Ossificans Traumatic
729.1	Rheumatoid
095.6	Syphilitic
729.1	Traumatic Old

732.4	Osgood Slatter Disease (Tibia Tubercle)

Osteoarthritis (see DJD, Degenerative Joint Disease)

Osteochondritis

732.7	Dissecans
732.6	Juvenile

Osteochondrosis

732.6	Site NOS Juvenile
732.#	Specified Site (Juvenile) 4th Digit: 732
	0. Spine
	1. Hip and Pelvis
	3. Upper extremity
	4. Lower Extremity excluding foot
	5. Foot
	6. Other
732.8	Spine Adult
737.0	Spine Adolescent Postural Kyphosis
732.0	Spine Juvenile
090.0	Syphilitic
756.51	Osteogenesis Imperfecta
268.2	Osteomalacia Vitamin D Deficiency
275.3	Osteomalacia Vitamin D-Resistant

Osteomyelitis

730.2#	NOS
730.0#	Acute
730.1#	Chronic
5th Digit: 730.0-2	
	0. Site Unspecified
	1. Shoulder Region
	2. Upper Arm (Elbow) (Humerus)
	3. Forearm (Radius) (Wrist) (Ulna)
	4. Hand (Carpal) (Metacarpal) (Fingers)
	5. Pelvic Region and Thigh (Hip) (Buttock) (Femur)
	6. Lower Leg (Fibula) (Knee) (Patella) (Tibia)
	7. Ankle and/or Foot (Metatarsals) (Toes) (Tarsals)
	8. Other (Head) (Neck) (Rib) (Skull) (Trunk) (Vertebrae)
	9. Multiple (Tarsals)
733.90	Osteopenia

Osteoporosis

733.00	NOS
733.03	Disuse
733.09	Drug Induced
733.02	Idiopathic
733.01	Postmenopausal
733.01	Senile
733.00	Vertebra

Paget's Disease

731.0	Bone (Osteitis Deformans)
719.3#	Palindromic Rheumatism 5th Digit: 719.3
	0. Site Unspecified
	1. Shoulder Region
	2. Upper Arm (Elbow) (Humerus)
	3. Forearm (Radius) (Wrist) (Ulna)
	4. Hand (Carpal) (Metacarpal) (Fingers)

	5. Pelvic Region and Thigh (Hip) (Buttock) (Femur)
	6. Lower Leg (Fibula) (Knee) (Patella) (Tibia)
	7. Ankle and/or Foot (Metatarsals) (Toes) (Tarsals)
	8. Other
	9. Multiple
446.0	Polyarteritis Nodosa
446.0	Polyarteritis Nodosa Myopathy [359.6]

Polyarthritis

716.5#	NOS 5th Digit: 716.5
	0. Site NOS
	1. Shoulder Region
	2. Upper Arm (Elbow) (Humerus)
	3. Forearm (Radius) (Wrist) (Ulna)
	4. Hand (Carpal) (Metacarpal) (Fingers)
	5. Pelvic Region and Thigh (Hip) (Buttock) (Femur)
	6. Lower Leg (Fibula) (Knee) (Patella) (Tibia)
	7. Ankle and/or Foot (Metatarsals) (Toes) (Tarsals)
	8. Other (Head) (Neck) (Rib) (Skull) (Trunk) (Vertebrae)
	9. Multiple
714.0	Atrophic
714.9	Inflammatory
714.89	Inflammatory Neck
714.31	Juvenile Acute
714.30	Juvenile Chronic
725	Polymyalgia Rheumatica
710.4	Polymyositis

Pseudogout see Chondrocalcinosis

Psoriasis

696.1	NOS
696.0	Arthritic

Radiculitis

729.2	Radiculitis
723.4	Accessory Nerve
724.4	Anterior Crural
723.4	Brachial (Nondiscogenic)
723.4	Cervical
723.4	Cervical (Nondiscogenic)
724.4	Leg
724.4	Lumbar
724.4	Thoracic
443.0	Raynaud's Syndrome/Phenomenon (Paroxysmal Digital cyanosis)

Rheumatoid Arthritis

714.0	Adult
714.30	Juvenile Chronic or Unspecified
714.33	Juvenile Monoarticular
714.32	Juvenile Pauciarticular
714.31	Juvenile Polyarticular Acute
V82.1	Screening
720.0	Spine
714.2	With Visceral or Systemic Involvement

Rotator Cuff

727.61	Capsule Rupture Nontraumatic
840.4	Capsule Rupture Traumatic
727.61	Rupture Complete Nontraumatic
840.4	Rupture Traumatic
840.4	Separation (Rupture) (Tear) (Laceration)
840.4	Sprain

840.4	Strain (Sprain) (Avulsion) (Hemarthrosis)
726.10	Syndrome NOS

Rubella

056.71	Arthritis

Sarcoid, Sarcoidosis

135	Any site or unspecified
135	Myopathy [359.6]
Polyneuropathy [357.4]	

Sciatica

722.10	Discogenic
722.73	Discogenic with Myelopathy
355.0	Due to Specified Lesion
724.3	Nonvertebral (Nondiscogenic)

Scleroderma

710.1	NOS
701.0	Circumscribed
701.0	Circumscribed or Localized

Scoliosis

737.30	And Kyphoscoliosis Idiopathic
737.43	Associated with other conditions
844.9	Shin Splints

Shoulder

337.9	Arm Syndrome
718.31	Dislocation Recurrent
337.9	Hand Syndrome
726.2	Impingement Syndrome
959.2	Injury
718.81	Joint Instability
718.91	Joint Ligament Relaxation
719.81	Joint (Region) Calcification
718.11	Joint (Region) Loose Body
V43.61	Joint replacement status
726.19	Ligament or Muscle instability sites
710.2	Sicca Syndrome (Keratoconjunctivitis)
710.2	Sjogren's Disease
736.22	Swan Neck Deformity Finger Acquired

Swelling

719.0#	Joint 5th Digit: 719.0
	0. Site NOS
	1. Shoulder Region
	2. Upper Arm (Elbow) (Humerus)
	3. Forearm (Radius) (Wrist) (Ulna)
	4. Hand (Carpal) (Metacarpal) (Fingers)
	5. Pelvic Region and Thigh (Hip) (Buttock) (Femur)
	6. Lower Leg (Fibula) (Knee) (Patella) (Tibia)
	7. Ankle and/or Foot (Metatarsals) (Toes) (Tarsals)
	8. Other
	9. Multiple
355.5	Tarsal Tunnel Syndrome
446.5	Temporal Arteritis
524.6#	Temporomandibular Joint Disorder or Syndrome 5th Digit: 524.6
	0. Unspecified
	1. Adhesions and Ankylosis
	2. Arthralgia

ICD-9 CODES continued

3. Articular disc disorder
(reducing or non-reducing)
9. Other specified Joint disorder
(Malocclusion)

Tendinitis
726.90	Site NOS
726.71	Achilles
726.70	Ankle and Tarsus
726.12	Biciptal
727.82	Calcific
726.30	Elbow
726.64	Patellar
726.61	Pes Anserinus
726.11	Shoulder (Calcific)
726.72	Tibialis
726.5	Trochanteric

Tendon
727.82	Calcification
727.81	Contracture (Achilles)
726.10	Disorder Shoulder Region
726.90	Inflammation Nec
726.67	Rupture - Achilles Nontraumatic
727.62	Rupture - Biceps (Long Head) Nontraumatic
727.68	Rupture - Foot and Ankle Nontraumatic
727.66	Rupture - Patellar nontraumatic
727.65	Rupture - Quadriceps Nontraumatic
727.61	Rupture - Rotator Cuff Nontraumatic
727.63	Rupture - Wrist and Hand Extensor Nontraumatic

727.64	Rupture - Wrist and Hand Flexor Nontraumatic
727.60	Rupture - Nontraumatic
727.69	Rupture - Nontraumatic Nec
727.42	Sheath Ganglion (any)
756.89	Shortening Congenital
726.32	Tennis Elbow

Tenosynovitis
726.90	Adhesive
727.06	Ankle
727.09	Elbow
727.05	Finger
727.06	Foot and Ankle
727.05	Hand and Wrist
727.09	Hip

727.09	Knee
727.04	Radial Styloid
726.10	Shoulder
720.1	Spine
726.10	Supraspinatus
727.06	Toe
727.05	Wrist

Vasculitis
447.6	NOS
287.0	Allergic
273.2	Cryoglobulinemic
446.29	Leukoclastic (Leukocytoclastic)

GUIDE TO CASE PRESENTATIONS

USER GUIDE

Four types of colored boxes appear in *Primary Care Rheumatology*:

 Green boxes are key points or summary boxes.

 Red boxes give recommendations for patient referral.

 Brown boxes contain information on general aspects or features of disorders.

Purple boxes contain information on differential diagnosis.

Two types of symbol appear throughout the book:

 Marks important points to look out for.

 Marks a section of the book dealing with disease management.

PRINCIPLES OF DIAGNOSIS AND MANAGEMENT

PRINCIPLES OF DIAGNOSIS AND MANAGEMENT

INTRODUCTION TO DISORDERS OF THE MUSCULOSKELETAL SYSTEM

Disorders of the musculoskeletal system are common. They range from mild regional problems, such as a tennis elbow or trigger finger, to severe life-threatening, multisystem disorders, such as systemic lupus erythematosus or vasculitis. Most rheumatic diseases are initiated by the interaction of complex genetic predisposition with a variety of environmental factors, which include trauma and infection. Their pathogenesis involves disturbances of connective tissue turnover, changes in immune surveillance, inflammation, crystal deposition, and many other disease processes. The many possible outcomes of a rheumatic disease include pain, physical disability, and psychosocial problems. Rheumatology is therefore an exciting

PRAGMATIC CLASSIFICATION OF THE MAJOR MUSCULOSKELETAL DISORDERS	
Musculoskeletal class	**Rheumatic disorder**
Back pain	• mechanical (including periarticular problems around the spine) • inflammatory (e.g. ankylosing spondylitis) • neurogenic (involving irritation of nerve roots or spinal cord) 'sinister' (infection or neoplasm) • other types/causes of back pain
Periarticular Also called 'soft tissue' or regional disorders of the musculoskeletal system	• bursitis, tendon problems, and enthesopathies • other regional pain syndromes • generalized nonarthric pain syndromes such as fibromyalgia
Osteoarthritis Includes idiopathic and secondary forms of osteoarthritis and related diseases	• secondary osteoarthritis (e.g. post-traumatic) • idiopathic monoarticular osteoarthritis • ideopathic polyarticular (generalized) osteoarthritis
Inflammatory arthropathies	• rheumatoid arthritis • juvenile chronic arthritis • seronegative spondyloarthritides • diffuse connective tissue disorders • crystal-related arthropathies • infectious arthritis • metabolic, endocrine, and other systemic arthropathies
Bone diseases Includes developmental and acquired skeletal abnormalities	• osteopenia (osteoporosis and osteomalacia) • osteonecrosis • Paget's disease • other forms of bone disease
Connective tissue diseases	• systemic lupus erythematosus • scleroderma • inflammatory myopathy • Sjögren's syndrome

KEY POINTS

- Musculoskeletal disorders are extremely common causes of pain and disability, but uncommon causes of death.
- The different disorders can be classified into six categories – back pain, periarticular or regional soft tissue disorders, osteoarthritis and related conditions, inflammatory arthropathies, bone disorders, and connective tissue diseases.
- The consequences of rheumatic disorders include pain and functional impairment which can lead to severe restriction of activities and participation.
- Therapeutic options can be divided into five categories – education, empowerment, and self-help; physical and other nonpharmacologic interventions; drugs; surgery; diet and complementary techniques.

Fig. 1.1 Pragmatic classification of the major musculoskeletal disorders.

subspeciality of medicine, which must encompass multidisciplinary areas of medical science, as well as the art of managing patients with chronic disease.

CLASSIFICATION OF THE RHEUMATIC DISEASES

Disorders of the musculoskeletal system are divided into six main classes: back pain, periarticular disorders, osteoarthritis, inflammatory arthropathies, connective tissue disease, and disorders of bone. These classes of musculoskeletal disorders can be further subdivided to include the main categories of rheumatic disorders (Fig. 1.1).

PREVALENCE ESTIMATES FOR SELECTED RHEUMATIC DISORDERS		
Disorder	Part affected	Estimated prevalence (%)
Back pain and peri-articular disorders (both)		>20
Osteoporosis	Spine, hip, or wrist fracture	5
Osteoarthritis	Radiographic (all sites)	25
	Knee disease	3.8
	Hip disease	1.3
Inflammatory arthropathies (total):		2.5
Rheumatoid arthritis		1.0
Crystal arthropathies		1.0
Ankylosing spondylitis		0.1
Psoriatic arthritis		0.1
Arthritis in children (<16 years)		0.06
Systemic lupus erythematosus		0.02

Fig. 1.2 Prevalence estimates for selected rheumatic disorders.

FREQUENCY OF THE MAJOR RHEUMATIC DISEASES

A rough guide to the frequency of the rheumatic diseases is provided in Figure 1.2. Back pain and periarticular disorders are extremely common, both affecting well over 20% of the population. The major bone disorder is osteoporosis, which is very common in elderly females. Radiographic evidence of osteoarthritis is also present in a large proportion of the older population, but the overall prevalence of significant hip or knee disease is nearer 5%. Inflammatory arthropathies are less common, but more severe, and affect about 2% of the population. Most forms of rheumatic disease rise in prevalence with increasing age, in particular back and periarticular disorders, osteoporosis and osteoarthritis.

In older people, the expression of the diseases can be different from that seen in other age groups, and treatment presents special difficulties; therefore, a special chapter is included on musculoskeletal problems in older people (Section 8). Similarly, rheumatic diseases in childhood are a special category of disorders, and they are dealt with separately in Section 7.

IMPACT OF RHEUMATIC DISEASE

A summary of the impact of the rheumatic diseases is shown in Figure 1.3. The overall prevalence is very high (30% with some symptoms), but mortality is low (0.02%). The main impact is through the very high prevalence of disability, which is usually combined with pain. Rheumatic diseases also cause a huge economic burden, and have been estimated to cost the USA about 1% of its GNP through a combination of lost wages and health costs.

TREATMENT OF RHEUMATIC DISEASES

Good management of the rheumatic diseases involves the co-ordination of five different modalities of care (Fig. 1.4) – where possible the management of diseases is presented in this book under five headings that correspond to these methodologies, with additional notes on the management of complications and reasons for referral. Specific, effective therapy is available for

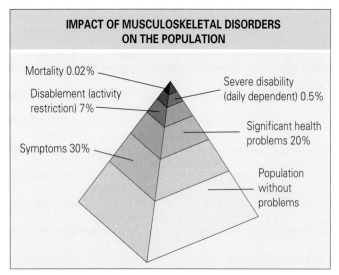

IMPACT OF MUSCULOSKELETAL DISORDERS ON THE POPULATION

Mortality 0.02%

Disablement (activity restriction) 7%

Symptoms 30%

Severe disability (daily dependent) 0.5%

Significant health problems 20%

Population without problems

Fig. 1.3 Summary of the impact of musculoskeletal diseases on the population. Although the prevalence of significant health problems is very high (20%), mortality from these diseases is very low (0.02%).

**MAIN MODALITIES OF TREATMENT
FOR RHEUMATIC DISORDERS**

- Patient education, including self-empowerment and joint protection techniques

- Physical therapies and other nonpharmacologic interventions, including exercise therapy, manipulation and hydrotherapy, and adaptive aids and devices

- Drug therapy, including both disease-modifying and symptomatic therapy, and both systemic and local therapy

- Surgery, including joint replacement

- Dietary and complementary techniques

Fig. 1.4 Main modalities of treatment for rheumatic disorders.

some disorders such as gout, and interesting developments in our understanding of the disease processes in rheumatology are resulting in the introduction of exciting new biologic agents, which may control many of the inflammatory arthropathies. However, in many cases there is, as yet, no totally effective way of controlling the disease process. In these instances, and where a disease has caused severe joint damage, a multidisciplinary approach to care is needed, with modalities such as patient education (including the empowerment of self-help) and physical and occupational therapy being of paramount importance. It is also necessary to use a framework that extends beyond the narrow medical approach to many illnesses. One such framework is shown in Figure 1.5, which emphasizes the interaction of rheumatic diseases with psychosocial factors.

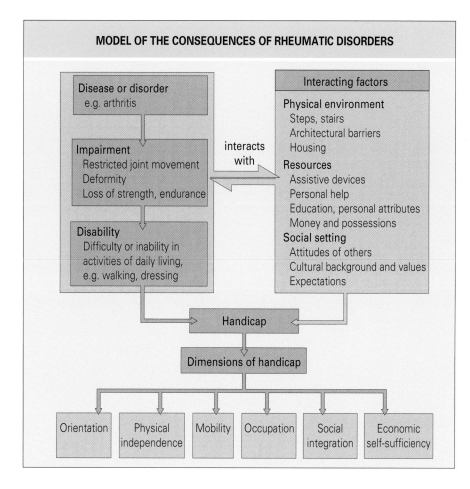

MODEL OF THE CONSEQUENCES OF RHEUMATIC DISORDERS

Fig. 1.5 A framework for approaching the consequences of rheumatic disorders. This is based on the WHO international classification of impairments, disabilities, and handicaps. It is often helpful when constructing a management plan with a patient to differentiate the impairment (restriction in movement, for example) from disability (restriction in activities that results from impairments) and handicap (disadvantage or restriction in participation) that result from an interaction of disability with a variety of environmental and psychosocial factors.

PRINCIPLES OF DIAGNOSIS AND MANAGEMENT

2

THE RHEUMATOLOGIC HISTORY AND EXAMINATION – THE 'GALS' SCREEN FOR MUSCULOSKELETAL DISEASES

Patients frequently attend doctors' offices with musculoskeletal complaints, most of which can be diagnosed through a good history and examination, without recourse to investigations. However, an exhaustive history and extensive examination is not always either necessary or practical. As with other systems, a brief screening procedure to identify common problems is often more appropriate. If abnormalities are found in a specific region, a fuller examination of that region is warranted (the examination of individual joints is covered in Section 2).

The screening history and examination presented here detects most abnormalities and allow the diagnosis of most disorders of the musculoskeletal system. They concentrate on abnormalities that are of functional significance to the patient.

THE SCREENING HISTORY

Pain and stiffness are the most common symptoms of musculoskeletal disorders, and functional impairment is the most important consequence. Hence the three suggested screening questions in Figure 2.1.

Consideration of dressing/undressing capability permits the initial assessment of both upper and lower limb function, while the ability to go up and down stairs unaided is a sensitive measure of any significant lower limb abnormality. If the answer to all three screening questions is no, a rheumatic disorder is unlikely; a positive answer may require further enquiry into medical history.

THE SCREENING EXAMINATION

The 'GALS' system describes the four key elements of the examination – gait, arms, legs, and spine; in practice, it is usually more convenient to examine gait and the spine first, with the patient standing, followed by the upper limb examination with the patient sitting on the side of the examining table and the lower limb examination with the patient lying on the examining table.

The patient is stripped to underclothes for the examination during which, particularly when joints are being moved, it is important to watch the patient's face for evidence of discomfort.

The basis of this quick, simple screening examination is inspection at rest and inspection during selected, functionally important movements that are sensitive tests of any musculoskeletal disease. In addition, palpation for tenderness across the metacarpophalangeal and metatarsophalangeal joints is recommended, as they

KEY POINTS

- The history and physical examination leads to the diagnosis of most musculoskeletal disorders, without the need for any investigations.
- A full history and complete examination of the musculoskeletal system are very time consuming.
- As with other systems, a simple screening history and examination allows most abnormalities of the musculoskeletal system to be detected quickly and efficiently.
- The examination concentrates on detecting abnormalities of functional significance to the patient, and on simple questions and maneuvers that are most sensitive to the presence of a disorder of the musculoskeletal system.
- The 'GALS' acronym refers to the four elements of the examination – gait, arms, legs, and spine.

NORMAL JOINTS SHOULD

- Look normal, and be bilaterally symmetric.
- Assume a normal resting position.
- Move smoothly and painlessly through the full range of motion.

THREE SCREENING QUESTIONS TO DETECT ABNORMALITIES OF THE MUSCULOSKELETAL SYSTEM

- 'Have you any pain or stiffness in your muscles, joints, neck or back?'
- 'Can you dress yourself completely without any difficulty?'
- 'Can you walk up and down stairs without any difficulty?'

Fig. 2.1 Three screening questions to detect abnormalities of the musculoskeletal system.

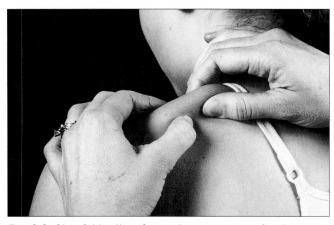

Fig. 2.2 Skin-fold rolling for tenderness as a test for the presence of fibromyalgia. In fibromyalgia, a number of muscular sites are abnormally tender, of which the supraspinatus is one of the most commonly and severely affected sites. Applied pressure over the midpoint of the supraspinatus, or skin-fold rolling, as shown here, usually produces severe tenderness, which may be followed by the development of erythema at the site.

are frequent sites of early inflammatory arthritis, which may not be apparent without these test procedures. A single check for the tenderness of fibromyalgia can be included, by skin-fold rolling of the skin that overlies the supraspinatus (Fig. 2.2).

GAIT
Inspect the patient as they walk across the room, turn, and walk back. Look for any lack of smooth flowing movements, difficulty with movement, or deformity (Fig. 2.3).

SPINE
The spine is also best examined with the patient standing and stripped to underwear. Look from behind for symmetry and a straight spine (check particularly for the presence of any scoliosis or leg-length asymmetry). Next, examine from the side to look for any lordosis or kyphosis, and also ask the patient to bend down and touch the toes (Fig. 2.4) while you

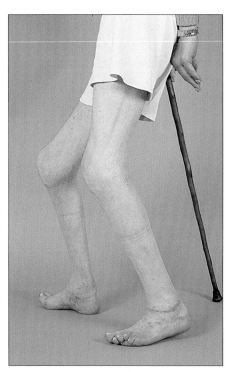

Fig. 2.3 Examination of the gait is an essential part of the musculoskeletal examination. Walking time (e.g. the time taken to walk 50 feet/50 meters) is sometimes used as a measure of change in response to treatment. This patient with rheumatoid arthritis is using a stick and has flexion deformities of his knees – his main deformities and functional problems were apparent as soon as he was asked to walk.

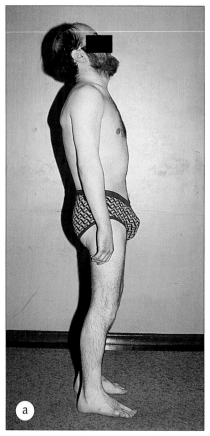

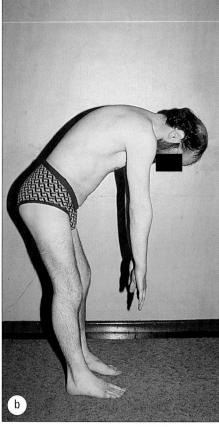

Fig. 2.4 Movement of the lumbar spine is best examined from the side, and by asking the patient to bend forward to touch the toes. This man with ankylosing spondylitis has very limited movement of the lumbar spine – most of his forward flexion comes from the hips. In addition, he has had to bend his knees to obtain forward flexion.

place your fingers over the posterior spinous processes to check for a good range of smooth, painless movement. Finally, inspect from in front, and ask the patient to place the left ear on the left shoulder, and to do the same on the right side, to check for painless, good lateral flexion of the cervical spine (lateral spinal flexion is generally the most sensitive test for cervical spine disease).

ARMS

The patient should be seated. First, inspect the hands with palms down, after which ask the patient to turn them over, and then inspect the palmar side (most hand abnormalities can be seen by simple inspection, and the movement checks supination and wrist or elbow problems). Second, ask the patient to make a fist and to pinch the index finger and thumb together (this assesses the two key functional movements of the hand – power grip and pinch grip) (Fig. 2.5). Next, ask the patient to straighten the arms out fully as you check for flexion deformities of the elbow, and then to put their hands behind the head, a complex movement which adequately screens for any significant shoulder disease. Finally, perform the metacarpophalangeal squeeze test (Fig. 2.6) and the skin-fold rolling test for fibromyalgia (see Fig. 2.2).

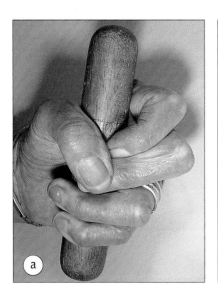
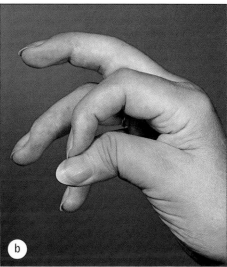

Fig. 2.5 **Power grip and pinch grip are the two most important functional movements of the hand.** In this patient with established rheumatoid arthritis, lack of flexion of the fingers means that a full power grip is impossible (a) and instability of the interphalangeal joint of the thumb prevents a stable pinch grip (b).

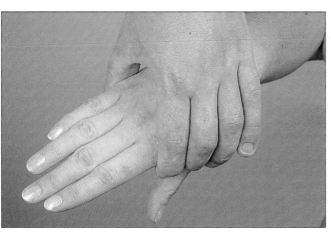

Fig. 2.6 **The metacarpophalangeal squeeze test.** Inflammation of the metacarpophalangeal joints is an early feature of many forms of inflammatory arthritis, especially rheumatoid disease. Nothing abnormal may be seen on inspection, but if the knuckles are squeezed together as shown, great tenderness may result from the pressure on the joints and associated bursae.

LEGS

The patient should be lying on the examining table. Hip disease can be screened for by flexing both hip and knee to 90°, and then internally rotating the hip – this movement is the first to be painful and restricted in most hip disorders (Fig. 2.7). Knees are inspected for swelling or quadriceps wasting and palpated for crepitus during movement. Inspect the feet, particularly the soles, for deformity and any evidence of abnormal weight bearing (such as callus), and then perform the metatarsophalangeal squeeze test (Fig. 2.8).

With practice these screening questions and examination can be carried out extremely quickly, and they are very sensitive to abnormalities, which enables you to screen for problems in joints other than those of which the patient may complain. The system is very helpful in pattern recognition of arthritic disorders, which often affect many sites (see Chapter 3), and in directing your attention to sites of a single regional abnormality that may require a fuller examination of the types outlined in Section 2.

SUMMARY OF THE 'GALS' SCREENING EXAMINATION

Gait – examine the patient walking away, turning, and walking back.

Arms – inspect dorsum of hands, observe supination, and inspect palmar side of hands, then check power grip and pinch grip; check full extension of elbow, and ask the patient to put their hands behind the head; apply the metacarpophalangeal squeeze test, and supraspinatus skin-fold rolling test.

Legs – internal rotation of the hip with knee–hip flexion, inspection of the knee for swelling or quadriceps wasting; feel knee during flexion for crepitus, inspect soles of feet; metatarsophalangeal squeeze test.

Spine – examine from behind for scoliosis and leg-length inequality, examine from the side for kyphosis and lordosis, and ask the patient to touch their toes; examine from in front and ask the patient to put their ear on each shoulder.

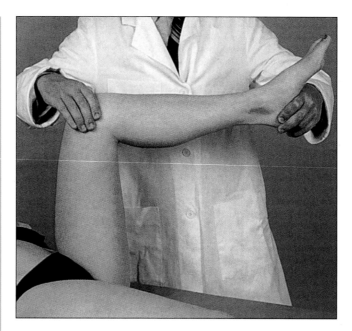

Fig. 2.7 Testing for hip disease by flexing both hip and knee to 90° and then internally rotating the hip. In any form of hip disorder, this is uncomfortable and/or restricted in range in comparison with the normal side.

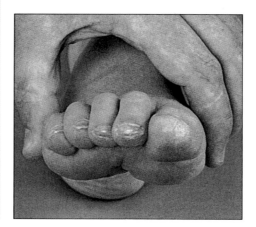

Fig. 2.8 The metatarsophalangeal squeeze test. Pressure is applied across the heads of the metatarsals (while you watch the patient's face for signs of tenderness) to elicit signs of early inflammation.

PRINCIPLES OF DIAGNOSIS AND MANAGEMENT

3

PATTERN RECOGNITION IN ARTHRITIS

Pattern recognition is the key to diagnosis of the rheumatic disorders; the central questions that need to be asked are:
- Is there a locomotor problem or a disease of another system?
- Is the condition articular or periarticular?
- Is the condition mechanical or inflammatory?
- Does the condition affect appendicular or axial structures, or both?

These questions can be answered by reference to two areas:
- History – the mode of onset, sequence of development of different features, and the duration and pattern of the symptoms.
- Examination – the number, distribution, and pattern of the affected joints or periarticular structures, and the nature of any systemic involvement.

KEY POINTS

- Most rheumatic diseases can be diagnosed by clinical pattern recognition alone.
- Key features in the history include the speed and mode of onset, and the pattern of joint symptoms (additive, migratory, or intermittent).
- Key features on examination include the pattern of joint involvement, arthritis falling into four main categories – monoarticular, polyarticular, arthritis with axial involvement, and isolated back pain.

INTRODUCTION

The history and physical examination are the two most important components of the diagnostic process for patients who complain of musculoskeletal pain or stiffness, or other rheumatic symptoms. Clinical judgment in interpretation of the findings elicited from the history and physical examination should allow the physician to answer several key questions:
- Is the disorder a monoarticular, periarticular, or articular process (i.e. which structures in or around the joint are giving rise to pain, see Fig. 3.1)?
- Is there evidence of other organ involvement (e.g. systemic connective tissue disorders) or does the disorder appear to be restricted to the musculoskeletal system (e.g. osteoarthritis [OA])?
- Is the articular problem inflammatory, degenerative, or something else?

Once the physician establishes that the disorder originates in the joints, several other aspects of the history and physical examination help to delineate a diagnostic pattern of arthropathy (Fig. 3.2).

MODE OF ONSET AND DURATION OF SYMPTOMS

Some arthropathies typically present with an acute onset of pain, with the peak intensity reached within hours or a few days, whereas in others maximum severity is reached gradually (over several weeks or months). Examples of an acute onset include bacterial and viral arthritis (e.g. parvovirus B19 and rubella), rheumatic fever, reactive arthritis, palindromic rheumatism, and crystal-induced arthritis (the best example is nocturnal attacks of gout). An insidious pattern is common in osteoarthritis (OA), mycobacterial and fungal arthritis, and most cases of neuropathic arthropathy (Charcot's joints). Variations may occur and the same disorder may have a sudden onset in some patients and be gradual in others. Rheumatoid

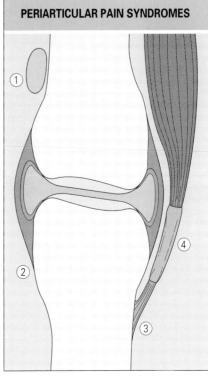

PERIARTICULAR PAIN SYNDROMES

Fig. 3.1 Anatomic structures that can give rise to painful periarticular syndromes.
(1) Bursitis is characterized by localized pain and swelling. (2) Capsular or ligament tears are characterized by pain on movements that stretch or produce tension of the affected ligament. (3) Tendon insertion (enthesis) problems are characterized by pain induced on isometric contraction of the muscle acting through the affected tendon. (4) Tendon sheath inflammation is characterized by pain and movement of the affected ligament.

PRINCIPLES OF DIAGNOSIS AND MANAGEMENT

MAJOR DIAGNOSTIC FEATURES OF JOINT DISORDERS

Mode of onset
  Acute
  Insidious
Duration of symptoms
  Self-limiting
  Chronic
Number of affected joints
  Monoarthritis
  Oligoarthritis (2–4 joints)
  Polyarthritis
Distribution of joint involvement
  Symmetric
  Asymmetric
Localization of affected joints
  Axial
  Appendicular
  Both
Patterns of involvement
  Additive
  Migratory
  Intermittent
Local pattern of involvement
(in individual joints)

Fig. 3.2 Major diagnostic features of joint disorders.

arthritis (RA), for instance, may present as an acute polyarthritis (especially in the elderly) and psoriatic arthropathy as an acute monoarthritis that resembles gout, whereas in most cases both disorders begin insidiously.

Arthritic disorders that last <4–6 weeks are considered to be self-limiting in practical terms, while those that last longer are considered chronic. In self-limiting arthritic disorders, the duration of symptoms and signs may be a valuable discriminating feature. Early episodes of monoarticular gout tend to subside spontaneously after 3–10 days and resolution is complete; acute or subacute pseudogout attacks of calcium pyrophosphate dihydrate crystal deposition disease (CPDD) may last from 2 or 3 days to 3–4 weeks; most articular or periarticular episodes of palindromic rheumatism disappear within hours to several days, with no articular sequelae. A steady inflammation in an individual joint for more than a few days or a week in children is highly unlikely to be caused by rheumatic fever.

PATTERNS OF JOINT INVOLVEMENT

Clinical involvement of joints may follow three major patterns – additive, migratory, and intermittent (Fig. 3.3):
- additive pattern refers to the involvement of more joints while the previous joints remain symptomatic;
- migratory pattern means that the process ceases or abates in one joint while simultaneously or immediately after starts in a previously normal joint;
- in the intermittent rheumatic disorders, complete remission of symptoms and signs occurs until the next recurrence in the same or other joints – no evidence of active disease or residual signs can be detected during intervals.

MONOARTICULAR SYMPTOMS

THE THREE COMMON PATTERNS OF JOINT DISEASE IN ARTHRITIS	
Pattern	Joint disease
Additive	Generalized osteoarthritis (see Chapter 42) Reactive arthritis (see Chapter 22) Rheumatoid arthritis (see Chapter 19)
Migratory	Gonococcal arthritis (see Chapter 23) Rheumatic fever (see Chapter 39)
Intermittent	Gout (see Chapter 16) Pseudogout (see Chapter 44) Systemic lupus erythematosus (see Chapter 29) Adult onset Still's disease (see Chapter 33) Familial Mediterranean fever (see Chapter 40) Palindromic rheumatism (see Chapter 23)

Fig. 3.3 The three common patterns of joint disease in arthritis.

Most patients who present with musculoskeletal complaints have pain restricted to one region. The first matter to resolve in these cases is whether the pain is referred from another region, periarticular, or articular. A full coverage of the regional disorders of peripheral joints is given in Section 2.

Although almost any individual arthropathy may begin as monoarthritis, the initial pattern of some disorders is characteristically monoarticular inflammatory arthritis, regardless of the subsequent course. Monoarticular arthritis can be categorized into acute (<10 days) and chronic types. Patients who have an acute, painful synovitis of a single joint and varying degrees of overlying redness require prompt evaluation, as they could have septic arthritis. Although redness may occur in any acute arthritis regardless of the cause, its presence usually evokes a restricted number of possible diagnoses, the most common being crystal-induced synovitis (including acute calcific periarthritis), bacterial infectious arthritis (Fig. 3.4), and traumatic conditions.

Chronic monoarthritis is often the presenting manifestation of a variety of joint disorders, the most important of which are chronic infections; histologic elucidation may be necessary to make the correct diagnosis. In a substantial number of patients the cause remains undetermined.

POLYARTICULAR SYMPTOMS

A wide variety of inflammatory and noninflammatory disorders, both common and uncommon, may present as polyarthritis; these disorders are covered in more detail in Section 3.

To determine whether the polyarthritis is symmetric or asymmetric helps in the differential diagnosis of polyarticular conditions, with RA being the classic example of symmetric arthritis. Symmetry is not necessarily strict in the hands; the same metacarpophalangeal (MCP) or proximal interphalangeal (PIP) joint may not be equally affected in both extremities of RA patients. Erosive inflammatory OA, parvovirus arthritis, and many cases of systemic lupus erythematosus (SLE) may resemble RA, whereas reactive arthritis, psoriatic arthropathy, and poly-articular gout usually present with asymmetric involvement of appendicular joints.

This feature of the articular pattern has obvious limitations; every patient who has a symmetric disorder may have an initial asymmetric phase. Figure 3.5 lists a number of polyarticular conditions classified according to the most characteristic pattern.

ARTHRITIS WITH AXIAL SYMPTOMS

Axial structures include, apart from the spine, centrally located joints such as the sacroiliac, sternoclavicular, and manubriosternal, and the rest of the chest wall. Sometimes these joints are involved in patients who have peripheral arthritis, most notably in ankylosing spondylitis (AS) and related disorders, covered in Section 4.

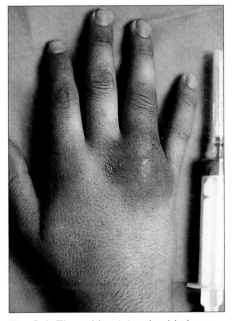

Fig. 3.4 **The red-hot joint should always raise suspicion of sepsis.** In this case, the ring finger metacarpophalangeal joint is swollen with intense redness of the overlying skin, and the syringe shows the pus that was aspirated from this infected joint. In such cases, aspiration, such that synovial fluid can be examined to culture the responsible organism, is required .

DISTRIBUTION OF OLIGO- AND POLYARTHRITIS		
	Symmetric	**Asymmetric***
Inflammatory	RA; JCA (systemic and polyarticular types) Adult onset Still's disease Systemic lupus erythematosus Mixed connective tissue disease Polymyalgia rheumatica Rheumatic fever (adult onset) Jaccoud's arthritis	Ankylosing spondylitis Reactive arthritis Psoriatic arthropathy (oligoarticular type) Enteropathic arthritis Undifferentiated spondyloarthropathy JCA (pauciarticular types) Palindromic rheumatism
Degenerative/ crystal induced	OA (primary generalized, erosive and nodal types) CPPD (pseudo-RA type) 'Milwaukee shoulder' Hemochromatosis arthropathy	Gout (especially oligoarthritis) CPPD (pseudogout type)
Infectious	Viral arthritis Lyme disease	Bacterial arthritis Bacterial endocarditis
Miscellaneous	Hypertrophic osteoarthropathy Amyloid arthropathy Myxedematous arthropathy Sarcoid arthritis (acute type)	

*Most asymmetric arthritides may be or are characteristically initially monoarticular.
JCA = Juvenile chronic arthritis; CPPD = Calcium pyrophosphate dihydrate crystal deposition disease

Fig. 3.5 Distribution of selected oligo- and polyarthritis.

CHRONIC ARTHROPATHIES WITH PERIPHERAL AND AXIAL INVOLVEMENT
Inflammatory

Spondyloarthropathies
  Ankylosing spondylitis
  Reactive arthritis
  Psoriatic arthropathy (a subset of patients)
  Enteropathic arthritis
  Undifferentiated
Juvenile chronic arthritis
  Systemic and polyarticular onset
Adult onset Still's disease
Syndrome of SAPHO (synovitis, acne, pustulosis, hyperostosis and osteitis)

Noninflammatory
OA Diffuse idiopathic skeletal hyperostosis Acromegaly Ochronosis Spondyloepiphyseal dysplasia

Fig. 3.6 Chronic arthropathies with peripheral and axial involvement.

While some rheumatic conditions rarely affect the axial segments (e.g. gout, SLE, systemic vasculitis), a combined pattern is often seen in others (Fig. 3.6). Often, OA of the spine coexists with appendicular involvement. Patients who have AS, psoriatic arthropathy, reactive arthritis (both following enteric and sexually transmitted infection), and arthritis accompanying inflammatory bowel disease may also exhibit varying degrees of combined axial and peripheral involvement. Polyarticular and systemic onset juvenile chronic arthritis (JCA), as well as adult onset Still's disease, commonly affect the apophyseal joints of the cervical spine in addition to peripheral joints.

Involvement of the cervical spine structures is frequent in RA patients, whereas the dorsal and lumbar segments are spared. Persistent pain in these areas should lead to other diagnoses (e.g. insufficiency fractures of the spine, sacrum, or iliac bones).

BACK PAIN

Pain in the back and neck is also covered in Section 4. Most acute low back pain is self-limited and related to postural problems or strain and not to a systemic rheumatic illness. The practical task is to differentiate the benign and self-limited cases of back pain from the serious or chronic cases, and to recognize when the pain is a symptom of other problems. Radiographic examinations of the lumbo-sacral spine, the major expense in an uncritical approach to the diagnosis of low back pain, are insensitive and nonspecific. Many spinal lesions, including disease of the disc (which may cause back pain), are not detected by radiography. Radiographic findings of osteophytes, narrowed disc space, lumbarization, sacralization, mild scoliosis, facet arthrosis, subluxation, and spina bifida occulta are found equally in symptomatic and asymptomatic individuals. Magnetic resonance imaging and computerized axial tomography are far more useful for imaging all the structures of the spine, but are also more costly and sensitive to anatomic changes of unproved significance.

When the history and physical examination are compatible with a benign disease, radiographs have limited clinical utility. Radiographs of the spine are indicated in a few situations (Fig. 3.7).

If a lumbar nerve root is compressed, the earliest clinical sign is loss or diminution of deep tendon reflexes. After 3–6 weeks of compression, objective muscle wasting or diminished strength may be evident.

To separate patients with mechanical causes from all the other patients and to not miss causes of back pain that require prompt treatment, therefore, can be done by a directed history and examination to identify atypical clinical features (Fig. 3.8) that suggest diagnoses other than mechanical causes. If the history and physical examination are typical for a mechanical origin, conservative treatment is indicated. The patient should be followed to ensure adequate pain control and first seen again after 3 weeks to ensure resolution of the problem and to reinforce back care instructions and specific exercise therapy.

MUSCULOSKELETAL DISORDERS IN YOUNG AND OLD PATIENTS

At the extremes of age, rheumatic patterns and expression of rheumatic disorders are quite different, because a number of diseases are specific to the very young or the very old, and because the expression of others depends on age. Special coverage of pediatric rheumatology is given in Section 7, and of rheumatic disorders of the elderly in Section 8.

INDICATIONS FOR RADIOGRAPHS IN LOW BACK PAIN
• New onset of back pain without antecedent trauma <15 years or >50 years of age. • Back pain after significant trauma. • Pain not significantly relieved by lying flat with knees flexed. • History of prolonged corticosteroid usage. • Known cancer. • Fevers or weight loss. • Drug abuse.

Fig. 3.7 Indications for radiographs in low back pain.

PEDIATRIC PROBLEMS

Spontaneous joint or musculoskeletal disorders in young patients usually arise from trauma, but special features must be kept in mind. The history that is so helpful in identifying disorders in adults is less helpful in young patients. Although not always true, disorders in young subjects are usually minimized or attributed to trivial causes. Arthritis may present as a limp, delayed growth and development (failure to achieve normal developmental milestones), local growth disturbance, or a systemic febrile illness. A variety of important diagnoses occur with greater frequency in youth and can lead to disability and pain. These diagnoses include osteochondritis, primary bone tumors, growth disturbances, and spontaneous infectious arthritis.

The physician must try to make a diagnosis before attributing disorders to growing pains. When the symptoms and/or signs are confusing or conflicting, the functional consequences of the symptoms should be considered and the family asked how they react when the youth or child complains. Signs or symptoms that do not make sense may be an indication of school or family stress, or sometimes are behavior learned from parents or siblings or used by the child to attract attention.

On physical examination, if the patient has constitutional symptoms or looks sick, a full physical examination is required. If clear evidence is found of a soft-tissue lesion (tendinitis, bursitis, or localized muscle tenderness), further evaluation is usually not needed. However, if joint inflammation is present or the symptom cannot be produced or explained, a radiograph is mandatory. Radiographs are useful because congenital disorders, growth disturbances, and tumors occur at a greater frequency in the young and may present with vague symptoms and a normal physical examination. Trauma severe enough to result in soft-tissue swelling may be forceful enough to cause a fracture to the epiphyseal plate or a slipped epiphysis, either of which may lead to future problems if not treated properly.

The term 'growing pains' is used most accurately as a description rather than as a diagnosis, and is a diagnosis of exclusion. True growing pains are typically seen in children under 8 years of age in whom leg pain that occurs between joints is not associated with growth spurts, aspirin-responsive symptoms, or a family history of the same.

RHEUMATIC PROBLEMS IN THE ELDERLY

In older people, diagnostic and management problems abound. Diagnosis can be complicated by the high prevalence of an elevated erythrocyte sedimentation rate (ESR) or of autoantibodies in older people. Osteoarthritis and osteoporosis are particularly common in older people, and some rheumatic diseases, including polymyalgia rheumatica and pseudogout, have their onset virtually confined to those over 60 years of age. In addition, the expression of disorders such as RA and SLE is different in older people and a variety of other conditions, such as hypothyroidism and depression, may mimic a rheumatic disease.

Management is complicated by a high prevalence of comorbidities, such as renal or hepatic disease (which make drug usage hazardous), by the dangers associated with excessive rest in this age group, and by complicating psychosocial issues.

'RED FLAGS' FOR BACK PAIN – FEATURES OF THE HISTORY THAT INDICATE A SERIOUS CAUSE	
History	Possible diagnosis
Pain and stiffness worst in the morning	Ankylosing spondylitis
Pain made worse by walking and by hyperextension of the spine	Spinal stenosis
Acute severe pain	Abdominal aneurysm Compression fracture Disc herniation
Pain radiating below the knee, made worse by coughing or sneezing, and described as shooting or burning	Nerve root compression
Radiation of pain into both legs	Central disc herniation Tumor
First episode of severe pain <30 or >50 years of age	Infection Tumor Metabolic disease
Fever, weight loss, or other systemic features	Infection Tumor
Bowel or bladder problems	Spinal stenosis Cauda equina syndrome Tumor
Recent severe trauma	Fracture Spondylolisthesis
Prolonged corticosteroid usage	Compression fracture
Drug abuse	Infection
Pain not relieved by lying with legs flexed or persistent pain for >2 months	Infection Tumor

Fig. 3.8 'Red flags' for back pain – features of the history that should alert the physician to a serious cause.

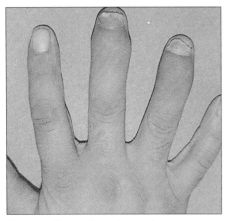

Fig. 3.9 Psoriatic arthropathy causes swelling of two distal interphalangeal joints with associated nail lesions of psoriasis.

COMMON PATTERNS OF COMMON JOINT DISEASES

Some joint disease patterns are closely associated with the early phases of a selected group of diseases. Consequently, their involvement often facilitates the diagnostic process. Common examples seen in clinical rheumatology include the following:

- bilateral and symmetric involvement of small and large joints, typical of RA;
- exclusive inflammatory distal interphalangeal (DIP) joint involvement of the fingers, an important clue in the diagnosis of psoriatic arthropathy (Fig. 3.9);
- the metatarsophalangeal (MTP) joint of the big toe, typically affected in acute gouty attacks (Fig. 3.10);
- pain in the muscle girdles (neck, shoulders, lower back, buttocks) in an appropriate clinical setting is highly indicative of polymyalgia rheumatica;
- juxta-articular pain and tenderness (symptoms of inflammatory enthesopathies) may dominate the clinical picture in some patients affected by seronegative spondyloarthropathies;
- acute involvement of a sternoclavicular joint (rarely affected by arthritis) suggests septic arthritis in intravenous drug abusers;
- bilateral and symmetric bony enlargement of the DIP and PIP joints (Heberden's and Bouchard's nodes respectively) (Fig. 3.11), typical of generalized osteoarthritis.

The MCP and PIP joints of the fingers, wrists, and knees, as well as MTP joints, are commonly affected bilaterally or symmetrically, with a striking absence of DIP joint disease. Patients who have SLE or other systemic rheumatic diseases may occasionally present with a 'rheumatoid' pattern of disease. Nodal OA (Heberden's nodes) is by far the most frequently encountered polyarticular disorder to affect the DIP joint. Crystalline disorders, such as CPDD, as well as OA, psoriatic arthropathy, and a wide variety of conditions, may mimic the podagra of gout. The occurrence of 'pseudopodagra' is one of the best examples of how the specific site of the index joint, although helpful, can only suggest the diagnosis.

An enthesopathy is a pathologic process at the sites of tendinous, ligamentous, or articular capsule attachment to the bone and can be inflammatory, degenerative, crystalline, or metabolic. Achilles' tendon and plantar fascia insertions into the calcaneum (heel pain) are principally involved. The costosternal areas, iliac crests, ischial tuberosities, greater trochanters, and manubriosternal joint may be also affected.

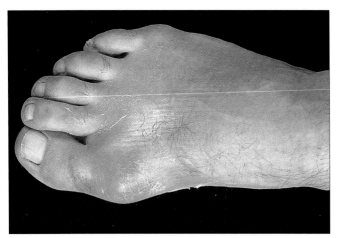

Fig. 3.10 The metatarsophalangeal joint of the big toe is the most common site of gout. In acute attacks, severe pain, swelling, and often redness of the overlying skin occurs; as the attack subsides, the skin may desquamate, as in the case illustrated.

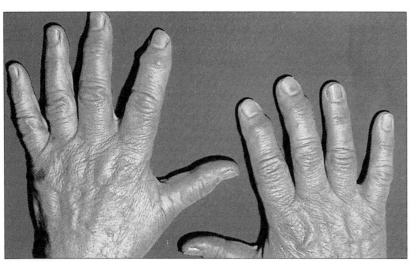

Fig. 3.11 Swelling of the distal interphalangeal joints in generalized osteoarthritis (Heberden's nodes).

The presence of inflammatory tarsal involvement and enthesopathy in pediatric patients (<16 years of age) may be a discriminating feature in differentiating AS and JCA (except late-onset, pauciarticular JCA) in the absence of axial disease. The finding of an enthesopathic digit or dactylitis (sausage finger) (Fig. 3.12) strongly suggests psoriatic arthropathy (more common in the hands) or reactive arthritis (more common in the feet).

A diffusely painful, swollen hand or foot may indicate reflex sympathetic dystrophy syndrome in that extremity. Bilateral, symmetric, puffy swelling of hands and fingers (and sometimes the feet) may be seen in the early phases of systemic sclerosis and other connective tissue diseases.

A number of rarer disorders also have characteristic patterns of joint involvement, which help the rheumatologist toward a diagnosis.

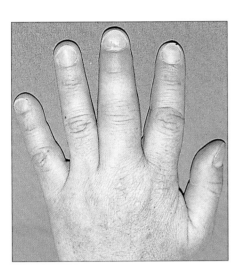

Fig. 3.12 Psoriatic arthropathy resulting in a 'sausage finger'. This swelling of the long finger is caused by a combination of tendinitis and arthritis along the length of the finger. A similar phenomenon can happen in the toes, particularly in reactive arthritis.

4

PRINCIPLES OF DIAGNOSIS AND MANAGEMENT

ARTHRITIS WITH GENERALIZED SIGNS AND SYMPTOMS

In this chapter three forms of presentation (other than pattern recognition, Chapter 3) of rheumatic diseases are dealt with:
- Generalized symptoms – such as diffuse aches and pains, myalgia and fatigue, in which case the challenge is to differentiate a rheumatic complaint from some other nonmusculoskeletal cause, such as depression.
- Arthritis presenting with systemic signs and symptoms – such as fever and weight loss, in which case a serious underlying illness should be suspected.
- Arthritis accompanied by problems in specific organ systems – such as the skin, genitourinary tract, heart, lungs, and kidneys, which can provide important clues to the diagnosis of specific rheumatic diseases.

PRESENTATIONS WITH GENERALIZED SYMPTOMS

DIFFUSE ACHES AND PAINS
The majority of patients who suffer diffuse aches and pains have a benign, self-limited syndrome associated with various infectious diseases, primarily viral. In addition, patients with systemic rheumatic or serious conditions can also present with aches and pains (Fig. 4.1).

A history, physical examination, and (in some cases) limited laboratory evaluation suffice to sort out such complaints. The history is directed toward identifying precipitating factors, such as a prodromal illness or associated constitutional symptoms or repetitive tasks. Some associated symptoms in the

> **KEY POINTS**
>
> - Musculoskeletal disorders may present with generalized signs and symptoms rather than regional pain.
> - Some patients present with diffuse aches or pains, myalgia, or fatigue, in which case the diagnostic challenge is to differentiate a rheumatic disease from some nonmusculoskeletal cause.
> - Other patients present with fever or weight loss, in which cases severe illnesses, such as infection or neoplasia, must be considered.
> - A number of rheumatic diseases affect other organ systems, such as the skin, eyes, or genitourinary tract, in addition to the joints, and the patterns of involvement in these cases provide clues to the diagnosis.

DIFFERENTIAL DIAGNOSIS OF DIFFUSE ACHES AND PAINS
Postviral arthralgias/myalgias
Bilateral soft tissue rheumatism
Overuse syndromes
Fibromyalgia
Hypothyroidism
Metabolic bone disease
Paraneoplastic syndrome
Myopathy (polymyositis, dermatomyositis)
Rheumatoid arthritis
Sjögren's syndrome
Polymyalgia rheumatica with or without temporal arteritis
Hypermobility
Benign arthralgias/myalgias
Chronic fatigue syndrome
Hypophosphatemia

Fig. 4.1 Differential diagnosis of diffuse aches and pains.

DIFFUSE ACHES AND PAINS – 'RED FLAGS'	
Clinical feature	Significance
Age >50 years	Polymalgia rheumatica, paraneoplastic syndrome
Constitutional symptoms	Inflammatory disease Vasculitis, sepsis, malignancy
Weakness	Myopathy, endocrinopathy
Gelling	Inflammatory rheumatic disorder
New headache Claudication Visual symptoms Tender, nodular, thickened or reddened temporal artery	Temporal arteritis
Bilateral symptoms	Systemic or metabolic cause

Fig. 4.2 Diffuse aches and pains – 'red flags'.

patient who has diffuse aches and pains are 'red flags' for systemic or metabolic diseases (Fig. 4.2). Gelling or morning stiffness that lasts longer than 30 minutes is such a symptom and can be seen in polymyalgia rheumatica (PMR), rheumatoid arthritis (RA), systemic lupus erythematosus (SLE), and some inflammatory muscle diseases. Diffuse aches and pains with no localizing physical findings may also occur in the myopathies associated with endocrine disorders and metabolic bone disease (particularly osteomalacia).

When the patient has diffuse aches with no systemic symptoms or abnormal laboratory evaluation, fibromyalgia may be the diagnosis. The typical patient is otherwise healthy and complains of sleep disturbance and diffuse aches and pains that do not correspond to any specific anatomic site and has, as the only physical finding, tender points in characteristic locations. Such patients are a tremendous challenge and require great patience in management; although no physical dysfunction is evident, patients may show a persistent course of disease for many years.

Important inflammatory diseases in the elderly patient who has aches and pains are PMR and giant cell arteritis (GCA). They should always be considered in a patient over the age of 50 years who develops aches and pains of the shoulder and hip girdle muscles. PMR is a myalgia with no findings of muscle tenderness or weakness. Occasionally, synovitis of small joints may be seen, which makes it difficult to differentiate from an inflammatory polyarthritis. By definition, an elevated Westergren erythrocyte sedimentation rate (ESR) >50mm/h is part of the syndrome. The symptoms and ESR are dramatically sensitive to low-dose corticosteroids (i.e. prednisone <20mg/day); the symptoms usually improve within 24–48 hours and the ESR within a week of starting corticosteroids. However, once an elevated ESR is identified in a patient who has aches and pains, other systemic diseases need to be considered; for example, early RA, SLE, polymyositis, vasculitis, myeloma, and paraneoplastic syndrome.

In about 10–30% of cases, PMR overlaps with GCA, but unless the patient has abnormalities of the temporal arteries or its branches, such as redness, nodularity, or pain, or has headache, visual disturbance, ischemia, or claudication of the masseter muscles or tongue, or systemic symptoms, the general recommendation is to not biopsy the temporal arteries. Careful examination of the temporal artery can be useful in targeting an artery for biopsy and for making a presumptive diagnosis of GCA. A clinically reddened and tender artery occurs in <10% of the cases now seen. The findings of a potentially involved artery are the lack of a pulse, tenderness, nodularity, or a cord. Both branches and both sides should be palpated through their course, as skip lesions occur. If GCA is suspected, prednisone should be started and a biopsy of the temporal artery obtained. Blindness, the major complication, can occur with devastating rapidity. Once an eye is involved the contralateral eye is also at considerable risk.

CRAMPS, WEAKNESS AND MYALGIAS

The most common complaints referable to the muscles are cramps, weakness, myalgias, and (occasionally) isolated muscle enzyme elevation. These problems (Fig. 4.3) can be sorted out effectively with a good history and examination for signs of abnormal muscle function, and being alert to atypical features.

MUSCLE SYNDROMES
Generalized weakness: subacute or chronic

Usually with atrophy
  Progressive muscular dystrophy
    Duchenne type
    Fascioscapulohumeral type
    Limb girdle types
  Polymyositis
  Inclusion body myositis
  Endocrine myopathies
  Chronic, slowly progressive polymyopathies,
    (i.e. central core disease, glycogen storage disease)

Episodic weakness
Familial (hypokalemic) periodic paralysis Normokalemic or hyperkalemic familial periodic paralysis Acute thyrotoxic myopathy
Exertional stiffness or cramps or spasms

Leg cramps
Metabolic defects of muscle metabolism
  McArdle's disease
  Phosphofructokinase deficiency
  Carnitine palmitoyl transferase deficiency
  Debranching enzyme deficiency
  Myoadenylate deaminase deficiency
Defects of electron transport
  Congenital myotonia, paramyotonia congenita,
    and myotonic dystrophy
  Hypothyroidism with pseudomyotonia

Fig. 4.3 Muscle syndromes.

Patients can be categorized by finding the answer to these questions:
- Are symptoms periodic, constant, or progressive?
- Are symptoms proximal, distal, or general?
- Are symptoms use related?
- Is weakness, asthenia, or general lassitude present?

Constant weakness and loss of muscle power unchanged from day to day, week to week, and within a day suggest a neurologic cause, such as peripheral neuropathy, cord lesion, or stroke. In the patient who complains of constant weakness without objective findings of weakness, a functional cause should be sought. Weaknesses from primary muscle disorders or from metabolic causes (i.e. myasthenia gravis) are variable and often related to ambient temperature (heat makes almost all forms of myopathies worse) or to repeated use of the specific muscles. The location and distribution of weakness can suggest specific syndromes. An asymmetric, peripheral weakness is usually neurologic. Symmetric proximal weakness is typical of both primary and secondary myopathies. Symmetric proximal and distal myopathy is seen in inclusion body myositis. Both polymyositis and dermatomyositis are rarely associated with malignancy and routine screening studies (Fig. 4.4) are essential in most patients.

Bulbar weakness that involves muscles of the eye and swallowing is suggestive of myasthenia. When asymmetric bulbar musculature is involved, cranial neuropathies and brainstem lesions are considered. Weakness that is symmetric, distal, and bulbar suggests amyotrophic lateral sclerosis.

The regional distribution of cramps can be diagnostic. Nearly all benign cramps are asymmetric and distal (the common nocturnal calf cramp or foot cramp).

Cramps in other muscle groups (abdominal or upper arm) in the absence of overuse or unusual use suggest primary or secondary myopathy. Cramps in specific muscle groups after strenuous exercise suggest myopathies with rare, specific enzyme deficiencies that usually involve the oxidative phosphorylation of adenosine triphosphate.

True loss of muscle power needs to be differentiated from asthenia and easy fatigability. Weakness comes from loss of muscle power, but patients who have generalized weakness may interpret this symptom as not feeling well (asthenia) or as decreased stamina or endurance, or fatigability. In a given individual the history may not be decisive and the issue is best resolved by formal muscle testing. People who have primary myopathies have fatigability of strength – repetitive use of the muscle groups should induce fatigability. Some muscle disorders are differentiated by an abnormal reaction to repetitive electrical stimulation or repetitive use in which, paradoxically, the contractions become more intense after repetition. These are the myotonias (congenital myotonia, myotonia dystrophica, and paramyotonia).

Muscle strength examination is subjective and the clinician who needs to follow muscle strength accurately should attempt to quantitate it more finely (Fig. 4.5). Maneuvers to quantitate strength include isometric strength measurement, measurement of grip strength, and using a weak muscle in some standardized activity to see how many repetitions a patient can carry out (e.g. the number of times one can rise from a chair in 30 seconds). Respiratory muscles might be investigated by pulmonary function testing.

Tenderness on palpation of muscles is unusual even in inflammatory myopathies (polymyositis, dermatomyositis). Rather, patients complain of muscle pain and myalgias at rest and with use of the muscles. Muscle tenderness on palpation

TESTS TO SCREEN FOR MALIGNANCY IN PATIENTS WITH INFLAMMATORY MYOSITIS	
First level	Second level
Chest radiograph	Upper and lower GI barium studies OR Upper endoscopy and colonoscopy
Stool for occult blood	
Liver function profile	Abdominal CT scan
Prostate-specific antigen (♂)	Chest CT scan
Mammogram (♀)	Pelvic culposcopy (♀)
CA-125 (♀)	
Gynecologic examination (♀)	

Fig. 4.4 Recommended tests to screen for the presence of malignancy in patients with inflammatory myositis.

MANUAL MUSCLE STRENGTH TESTING GRADES	
0	No muscle contraction
1 (trace)	Palpable contraction, little or no motion
2 (poor)	Motion possible but not against gravity
3 (fair)	Motion against gravity possible
4 (good)	Motion possible against manual resistance
5 (normal)	Motion possible against considerable manual resistance

Fig. 4.5 Manual muscle strength testing grades.

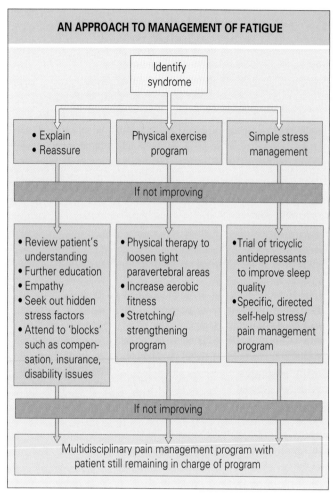

AN APPROACH TO MANAGEMENT OF FATIGUE

Identify syndrome

- Explain
- Reassure

Physical exercise program

Simple stress management

If not improving

- Review patient's understanding
- Further education
- Empathy
- Seek out hidden stress factors
- Attend to 'blocks' such as compensation, insurance, disability issues

- Physical therapy to loosen tight paravertebral areas
- Increase aerobic fitness
- Stretching/ strengthening program

- Trial of tricyclic antidepressants to improve sleep quality
- Specific, directed self-help stress/ pain management program

If not improving

Multidisciplinary pain management program with patient still remaining in charge of program

Fig. 4.6 An approach to management of fatigue.

raises the possibility of *Trichinella* infections of the muscle (myonecrosis), or rhabdomyolysis and compartment syndromes.

Fasciculations or muscle twitches during rest combined with muscle weakness and atrophy usually signify motor neuron disease (amyotrophic lateral sclerosis, progressive bulbar palsy), but may also be seen in other disorders of the gray matter of the spinal cord, including syringomyelia or tumor, lesions of the anterior horn, ruptured disc, or peripheral neuropathy. Syndromes of benign fasciculations may be seen either sporadically or with rippling and twitching sensations in muscles, but without weakness or atrophy – these are common and benign, and require no action.

FATIGUE

Fatigue is reported by most patients who have rheumatic disorders and is often a very disabling symptom. Management of fatigue is a complex task (Fig. 4.6). Very little is known about the cause of fatigue, although increased production of cytokines and sleep disturbances are thought to contribute to the problem. The major clinical challenge is to differentiate fatigue caused by the rheumatic diseases from that secondary to underlying depression.

Most patients who suffer fibromyalgia report profound fatigue. It is often notable when arising from sleep, but is also marked in the mid-afternoon. Seemingly minor activities aggravate the pain and fatigue, although prolonged inactivity also heightens the symptoms. Patients are stiff in the morning and feel unrefreshed, even if they have slept 8–10 hours. Many patients do not report sleep disturbances, since they interpret sleep problems in terms of insomnia. Nevertheless, they usually recognize that they sleep 'lightly', waking frequently during early morning and having difficulty returning to sleep.

Fig. 4.7 Example of the typical fever curve seen in systemic onset juvenile chronic arthritis.

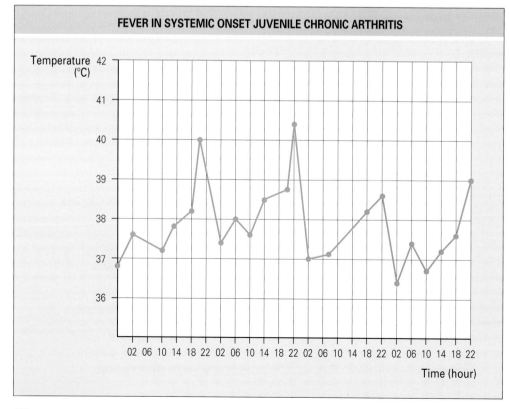

FEVER IN SYSTEMIC ONSET JUVENILE CHRONIC ARTHRITIS

Temperature (°C)

Time (hour)

Fatigue is common in both SLE and RA, and is often a major and over-whelmingly disabling symptom.

ARTHRITIS PRESENTING WITH SYSTEMIC SIGNS

FEVER

All febrile patients who have arthritis should first be evaluated for infection with blood cultures, chest radiography, urinalysis and culture, and other tests as appropriate. The most immediate concern is septic arthritis, and careful screening studies for a red, hot joint should be carried out early.

Fever may be seen in a number of rheumatic diseases – it is surprisingly common in RA and typically occurs in association with extra-articular involvement, such as serositis or vasculitis. Fever is a major feature of juvenile chronic arthritis. One or sometimes two temperature peaks above 101.8°F (38.8°C) can occur on a daily basis, and fevers as high as 104.9°F (40.5°C) occur occasionally (Fig. 4.7). Fever is a prominent feature of SLE and always requires a careful search for the co-existence of infection in lupus patients.

WEIGHT LOSS

Weight loss is feature of most diffuse, inflammatory rheumatic syndromes. However, the association of weight loss and arthritis does not always imply the presence of a defined rheumatic disease, and the clinician must be able to identify other potential causes, such as hyperthyroidism, and infectious and neoplastic causes. Weight loss in association with arthritis may require a systematic investigation, which includes a careful search for occult infection, endocrine abnormalities, and malignancy (Fig. 4.8). Routine chest radiography, complete blood count, skin test for tuberculosis, investigation of stool for occult blood, breast examination, mammography, and pelvic examination should be included in this setting.

CAUSES OF ARTHRITIS AND FEVER

Septic arthritis
Rheumatoid arthritis
Juvenile chronic arthritis
Reactive arthritis
Systemic lupus erythematosus
Subacute bacterial endocarditis
Gout
Lyme disease

CAUSES OF ARTHRITIS AND WEIGHT LOSS

Rheumatoid arthritis
Ankylosing spondylitis
Reactive arthritis
Enteropathic arthritis
Whipple's disease
Systemic lupus erythematosus
Scleroderma

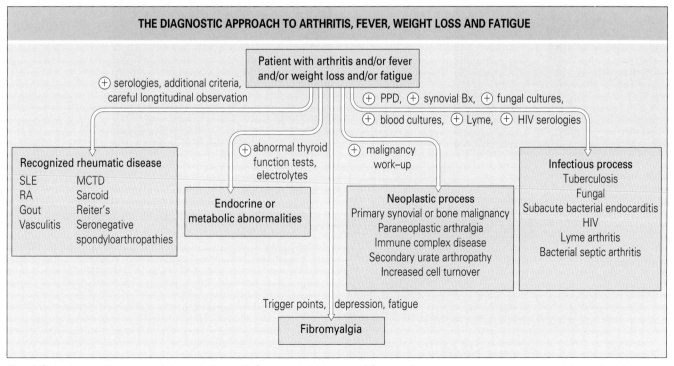

THE DIAGNOSTIC APPROACH TO ARTHRITIS, FEVER, WEIGHT LOSS AND FATIGUE

Patient with arthritis and/or fever and/or weight loss and/or fatigue

(+) serologies, additional criteria, careful longtitudinal observation

(+) PPD, (+) synovial Bx, (+) fungal cultures, (+) blood cultures, (+) Lyme, (+) HIV serologies

(+) abnormal thyroid function tests, electrolytes

(+) malignancy work–up

Recognized rheumatic disease
SLE   MCTD
RA   Sarcoid
Gout   Reiter's
Vasculitis Seronegative
           spondyloarthropathies

Endocrine or metabolic abnormalities

Neoplastic process
Primary synovial or bone malignancy
Paraneoplastic arthralgia
Immune complex disease
Secondary urate arthropathy
Increased cell turnover

Infectious process
Tuberculosis
Fungal
Subacute bacterial endocarditis
HIV
Lyme arthritis
Bacterial septic arthritis

Trigger points, depression, fatigue

Fibromyalgia

Fig. 4.8 A diagnostic approach to arthritis with fever, weight loss, and fatigue. The diagnosis may be apparent from the history and examination alone, and from a knowledge of what is most likely according to age and circumstances. However, in some cases a fairly full laboratory work-up is necessary to exclude serious causes, as outlined in this flow chart. PPD = purified protein derivative; SBE = subacute bacterial endocarditis; MCTD = mixed connective tissue disease.

ARTHRITIS AND DISORDERS OF OTHER SYSTEMS

ARTHRITIS AND SKIN RASHES

Skin rashes provide valuable diagnostic clues for a number of rheumatic diseases. Pattern recognition of skin lesions is based on type, distribution, and evolution of the lesions. The principal types of skin pathology that occur with rheumatic disorders include psoriasiform lesions (Figs 4.9 and 4.10), facial lesions (Fig. 4.11), pustules (Fig. 4.12), ulcerations (Fig. 4.13), and petechia or purpura (Fig. 4.14).

ARTHRITIS AND CARDIOPULMONARY SYMPTOMS

Cardiac and pulmonary complications can be a feature of most of the systemic rheumatic disorders, and are particularly likely to occur in the connective tissue diseases, such as SLE, scleroderma, or myositis. The two most common clinical presentations are pleuritic pain from pleuritis or pericarditis, progressive dyspnea, interstitial lung disease, and cough.

ARTHRITIS AND GASTROINTESTINAL SYMPTOMS

Gastrointestinal complaints occur with many drugs used to treat arthritis. By far, gastropathy induced by nonsteroidal anti-inflammatory drugs is the most common and potentially the most serious. In addition, however, abdominal complaints, which include pain, diarrhea, and blood loss, may be a feature of a number of

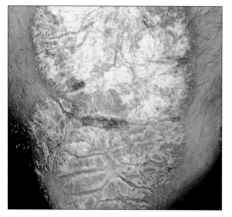

Fig. 4.9 Psoriatic plaque on an elbow.

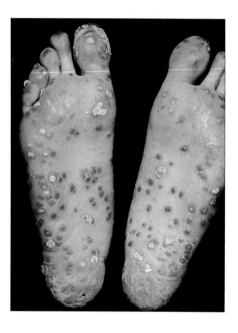

Fig. 4.10 Keratoderma blennorrhagicum on the soles of a patient who has Reiter's syndrome.

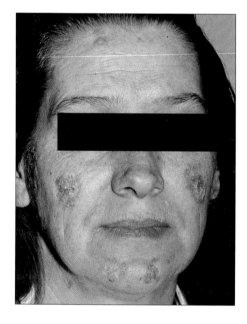

Fig. 4.11 The facial lesion of discoid lupus.

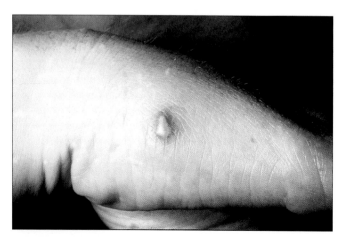

Fig. 4.12 In gonococcemia and gonococcal arthritis, pustules are often found on the hands and feet. (Reproduced with permission from McKee PH, Pathology of the Skin, 2E, London: Mosby–Wolfe, 1996, and by courtesy of Dr RN Thin, St Thomas's Hospital, London, UK.)

arthritis syndromes, particularly the forms of arthritis associated with Crohn's disease and ulcerative colitis, and enteropathic reactive arthritis.

ARTHRITIS WITH EYE DISEASE

Inflammation of different structures within the eye is a common feature of many of the inflammatory rheumatic diseases (the lining layers of the eye share many features with the synovium). The two common presentations are the painful red eye, caused by conjunctivitis, uveitis or scleritis, and the dry gritty eye that results from keratoconjunctivitis sicca.

Conjunctivitis is a major feature of reactive arthritis, and the combination of a lower limb arthritis with conjunctivitis, often accompanied by urethritis, is diagnostic of Reiter's syndrome (Fig. 4.15).

Uveitis occurs particularly in association with ankylosing spondylitis and other seronegative spondyloarthropathies associated with the HLA-B27 haplotype, and in some forms of juvenile chronic arthritis where it may be silent (painless). In adults, recurrent attacks of a painful red eye, which require prompt treatment, is a usual finding (Fig. 4.16).

Scleritis and episcleritis can occur in RA and other inflammatory arthropathies, generally presenting as a painful red eye, but it may take many forms, and can lead to necrosis (Fig. 4.17).

Corneal ulceration can also result from RA (one of its most common causes)

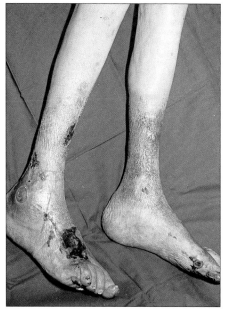

Fig. 4.13 Rheumatoid vasculitic ulceration in various stages of evolution. (Reproduced from the Revised Clinical Slide Collection on the Rheumatic Diseases, 1981. Used by permission of the American College of Rheumatology.)

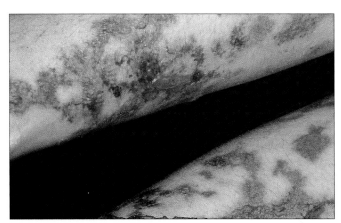

Fig. 4.14 Polyarteritis nodosa with irregular purpura and necrosis. (Reproduced with permission of the American Academy of Dermatology. All rights reserved.)

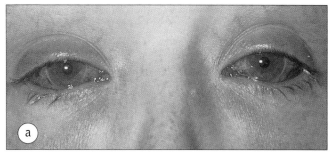

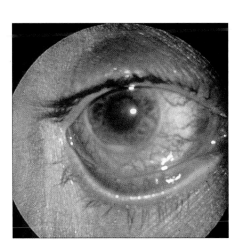

Fig. 4.16 Recurrent bouts of severe uveitis can occur in ankylosing spondylitis. In this case, much inflammation is seen, with considerable conjunctival injection and a hypopyon.

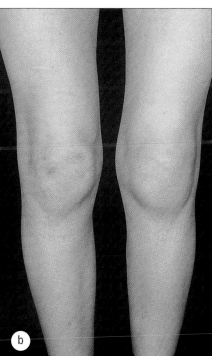

Fig. 4.15 The combination of lower limb arthritis and conjunctivitis is strongly suggestive of a reactive arthritis, such as Reiter's syndrome.
(a) Conjunctivitis.
(b) Knee arthritis.

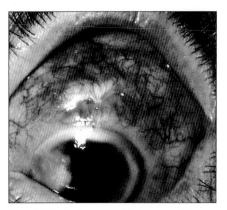

Fig. 4.17 Active necrotizing scleritis of the eye in rheumatoid arthritis, associated with sclerosing keratitis (white corneal lesion).

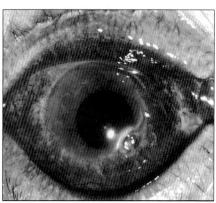

Fig. 4.18 Active corneal ulceration in rheumatoid arthritis, showing an obvious ulcer associated with conjunctival injection.

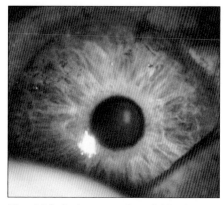

Fig. 4.19 In keratoconjunctivitis sicca (dry eye syndrome), patients complain of dry, gritty eyes, but they usually appear normal on inspection. However, it does result in corneal ulcers, which can be seen with Rose Bengal stain in the eye, as in this case.

Corneal ulceration can also result from RA (one of its most common causes) and from any form of systemic rheumatic disease associated with vasculitis (Fig. 4.18).

Keratoconjunctivitis sicca (dry eye syndrome) is the classic and perhaps most common ocular complication of rheumatic diseases. It occurs in many patients who have RA and connective tissue diseases, and also occurs as a part of Sjögren's disease in the absence of another rheumatic complaint. Lymphocytic infiltration of the lacrimal and salivary glands leads to reduced secretions, dry gritty eyes, and a dry mouth. Clinically, the eyes appear normal, but with staining keratitis can be demonstrated (Fig. 4.19), and a Schirmer's test can be used to demonstrate reduced secretions.

ARTHRITIS AND RENAL DISEASE

With the exception of the development of edema, few clinical clues suggest kidney disease – abnormalities are first detected on chemistry and urine studies only. Typical laboratory findings suggestive of renal involvement include proteinuria or an abnormal cellular sediment in the urinalysis, and evidence of impairment of renal function with elevations of the blood urea nitrogen or serum creatinine. In patients who have edema or the nephrotic syndrome, depressions of serum albumin and hyperlipidemia are found.

Kidney disease may be seen with a number of systemic rheumatic diseases; the most serious forms of kidney disease occur in patients who have autoimmune disorders such as SLE and various vasculitides.

5

PRINCIPLES OF DIAGNOSIS AND MANAGEMENT

LABORATORY TESTS IN RHEUMATOLOGY

INTRODUCTION

The five major sources of data that are used to arrive at a diagnosis of a rheumatic disease are:
- history;
- physical examination;
- radiographs and other imaging procedures;
- laboratory tests;
- synovial fluid analysis.

For most rheumatic diseases, laboratory testing has limited utility for diagnosis, although it is very useful for the monitoring of diseases and their treatment. Relevant diagnostic information for the major rheumatic diseases is summarized in Figure 5.1. This emphasizes the areas in which specific investigations are cost-effective: for example, in rheumatoid arthritis (RA), the diagnosis may be best established from the history and physical examination; for systemic lupus erythematosus (SLE), from a laboratory test, the antinuclear antibody (ANA); for gout (if there is significant diagnostic uncertainty), from a synovial fluid examination; and for ankylosing spondylitis (AS), from a radiograph. For common diseases like osteoarthritis (OA) or fibromyalgia, there is essentially no role for laboratory tests except to exclude other possible diagnoses.

The common practice to order a battery of laboratory tests rarely leads to a definitive diagnosis, and often introduces considerable 'false-positive' information and unnecessary costs into the diagnosis of rheumatic disease.

KEY POINTS

- Laboratory tests are of more value in monitoring the progress of chronic inflammatory rheumatic diseases, and assessing response to therapy, than they are in diagnosis.
- False-positive and false-negative results from laboratory investigations are frequent and can lead to major problems in practice.
- Common examples of false-positive results include rheumatoid factor without rheumatoid arthritis, a high uric acid without gout, and positive antinuclear antibodies without systemic lupus erythematosus.
- The three major categories of laboratory tests used in rheumatologic practice are: acute phase reactants (including erythrocyte sedimentation rate), autoantibodies and related investigations, and uric acid.
- HLA haplotyping is a research investigation of no value in clinical practice.
- Additional standard investigations, such as metabolic tests and renal and hepatic function tests, may be required in the diagnosis and monitoring of patients who have rheumatic disorders.

PROBLEMS OF INTERPRETING LABORATORY TESTS IN RHEUMATOLOGY

The problems of interpreting the results of laboratory testing generally involve one of four major areas:
- false-positive results,
- false-negative results,
- measurement error, and
- differences in groups of patients compared with individual patients.

FALSE-POSITIVE RESULTS

Inflammatory musculoskeletal diseases, for which patients are often 'screened' with laboratory tests, are seen in about 1% of the population, perhaps 2% if gout is included. However, even a small false-positive rate of serologic tests for RA or lupus, for example, results in many people being 'labeled' as having RA or SLE on the basis of laboratory findings alone, without clinical evidence of the disease. The three most important tests that frequently produce false-positive results are those for rheumatoid factor (RF), elevated serum uric acid, and ANAs:

DIAGNOSIS OF RHEUMATIC DISEASES				
Diagnosis	History and physical examination	Blood tests	Radiographs	Synovial fluid
RA	Symmetric polyarthritis Morning stiffness	RF+ in ~80% Elevated ESR in 50–60%	Demineralization Erosions Joint space narrowing	Inflammation WBC >10,000
SLE	Multisystem disease	ANA+ in >99% DNA antibodies in 60–75%	Generally nondestructive	Mild inflammation
AS	Back pain Axial involvement	HLA-B27 in ~90%	**Sacroiliitis** **Vertebral squaring**	Inflammation WBC 5–20,000
Gout	Recurrent attacks	Uric acid elevated in 75–90%	Erosions, cysts	**Negatively birefringent crystals**
OA	Pain, crepitus ± swelling ± limited motion	Nonspecific abnormalities	Joint space narrowing Osteophytes	Noninflammatory WBC <10,000
Fibromyalgia	Chronic pain 'all over' No swollen joints Muscle spasm	No abnormalities ANA+ in 2–5% Uric acid >8.0 in 2–5%	No severe abnormalities (may have cervical OA)	None
Scleroderma	Skin tightness dorsum of hand Facial skin tightening	ANA+ in >90% with Hep-2 cells	± Pulmonary fibrosis ± Esophageal dysmotility ± Calcinosis	Not specific
Polymyositis	Muscle weakness ± pain	CPK elevated in 80% ANA+ in 33%	Not helpful	Not specific

Fig. 5.1 Diagnosis of rheumatic diseases. The most important test for the diagnosis of individual rheumatic diseases is highlighted in bold text.

- Rheumatoid factor is present in about 4% of the normal population; and in 80% of people who have established RA, but is frequently negative in the early phases of the disease, it is therefore a poor test for the diagnosis of RA, and false-positives often lead to unnecessary worry.
- Gout is often misdiagnosed on the basis of an elevated serum uric acid, rather than on the finding of urate crystals in synovial fluid. Most people with elevated uric acid do not have gout, and need not be treated for hyperuricemia.
- False-positive results of ANA testing constitute one of the primary reasons for rheumatology consultations; however, whereas SLE occurs in 1/2000 of the population, positive ANA tests occur in 1–5% of normal individuals, and musculoskeletal symptoms are seen in about 15% of the population.

FALSE-NEGATIVE RESULTS

False-negative problems are more unusual, but may have serious consequences. Patients who have early RA, a negative RF test, and/or normal erythrocyte sedimentation rate (ESR) may suffer joint destruction while treatment is deferred on the basis of 'normal' laboratory values. Similarly, patients who have vasculitis and other life-threatening rheumatic diseases may develop irreversible end-organ renal failure or stroke, or even die, while undergoing extensive laboratory evaluation (and elaborate imaging studies), despite classic physical findings such as palpable purpura and foot drop, which make a clear diagnosis at presentation. In addition, acute gout can occur when people have a normal serum uric acid, cuasing potential diagnostic confusion.

MEASUREMENT ERROR

Whenever a laboratory value does not agree with clinical observation, the clinician should always consider laboratory error as an explanation of the findings. Measurement error is considerably more common than is generally acknowledged.

DIFFERENCES IN GROUPS OF PATIENTS COMPARED WITH INDIVIDUALS

An important example of this problem is the observation that the human leukocyte antigen (HLA) haplotype B27 is found in 90% of patients who have AS compared with 8% of the normal population. This observation may be interpreted to suggest that HLA typing has a clinical role in helping to identify patients who have AS. However, 10% of patients who have AS are HLA-B27 negative. This group may experience disease of equal severity to those who are HLA-B27 positive. Further, only about 1 in 20 people who have HLA-B27 have AS, and only 1 in 3 people who have back pain and HLA-B27 have AS. Therefore, HLA typing is rarely indicated in the diagnosis of patients with AS.

LABORATORY TESTS USED IN RHEUMATOLOGY

The main tests used can be split into four categories – acute phase reactants, autoantibodies and related tests, HLA haplotyping, and uric acid (Fig. 5.2).

ACUTE PHASE REACTANTS

Nonspecific laboratory indicators of the presence of inflammation include a raised ESR, high levels of acute phase reactants such as C-reactive protein (CRP), and changes in the blood count such as a normochromic, normocytic anemia.

There are two main indications for use of these tests:
- Screening for the presence of inflammation as the cause of a musculoskeletal complaint (such as polymyalgia rheumatica or the presence of infection or rheumatoid arthritis)
- Monitoring the activity and progression of systemic inflammatory diseases such as rheumatoid arthritis.

There is generally no need to use more than one test when looking for the presence or activity of inflammation. In many countries the ESR is the standard test, others use CRP preferentially, and this is generally regarded as the better test with which to monitor the progression of rheumatoid arthritis.

The use and interpretation of the ESR is generally the key question in primary care. In general the ESR is raised in inflammatory diseases, including all the inflammatory arthropathies, connective tissue and systemic disease (with the exception of SLE, when the ESR is generally normal), polymyalgia and in sepsis and neoplastic diseases. However, caution needs to be exercised when using the test as a diagnostic screen: the upper limit of normal for the ESR may increase with age: values up to 40mm/hr Westergren ESR are not uncommon in elderly people. Similarly, an elevated ESR may occasionally be seen in normal individuals and in patients with noninflammatory rheumatic diseases such as osteoarthritis and fibromyalgia, so this investigation, like any other, must be used and interpreted with care.

In spite of these reservations, the ESR is a useful investigation to consider first when you are not sure whether a musculoskeletal complaint represents a noninflammatory condition or the early phase of an inflammatory disorder. Similarly, ESR, or CRP, is a useful test to provide an indication of how active an established inflammatory rheumatic diseases is.

COMMON FALSE-POSITIVE TESTS IN RHEUMATOLOGY

- Rheumatoid factor – this is a poor test for rheumatoid arthritis.
- Elevated uric acid – this is a poor test for gout.
- Positive antinuclear antibody – false positives are frequent.

Fig. 5.2 Common false-positive tests in rheumatology.

AUTOANTIBODIES

Most autoantibodies are not specific for a clinical syndrome, but may be detected in people with markedly different clinical features, as well as in some normal individuals. Furthermore, autoantibodies may not be detected in many individuals who have clinical findings similar to patients in whom serum autoantibodies are usually detected, and treatment is similar for both groups. Therefore, while research into autoantibodies has yielded considerable information about pathogenetic mechanisms, serologic testing for autoantibodies in clinical practice remains generally more an adjunct to diagnosis and management rather than a precise clinical guide.

RHEUMATOID FACTOR

About 70–90% of patients who have RA are positive for RF, and the presence of this factor has often been misinterpreted as being diagnostic for the disease. However, in serologic surveys RF has been found in at least 1% of the normal population. Thus, since RA occurs in 0.5–1% of the population, there are at least as many individuals who have RF with no RA as RF-positive individuals that do have the disease. Furthermore, a false-positive RF (i.e. a positive result in a patient who does not have RA) is found in many diseases, including sarcoidosis, leprosy, tuberculosis, pulmonary fibrosis, liver disease, and syphilis. Moreover, in many of these diseases musculoskeletal symptoms may be seen in patients, which adds further to the diagnostic confusion with RA.

ANTINUCLEAR ANTIBODIES

A wide variety of antibodies to antigens within the cell nucleus occur, particularly in people who have systemic connective tissue disorders such as SLE, Sjögren's syndrome, polymyositis, scleroderma, and vasculitis. However, these same antibodies can be detected in some normal people, and may be elevated in a number of other diseases.

These specialized tests are of more use in monitoring established multisystem diseases than in routine diagnosis (Fig. 5.3). The main antibodies detected by ANA testing are summarized in Figure 5.4.

OTHER IMMUNOLOGIC TESTS

In patients who suffer acute rheumatic fever, the antistreptolysin O titer (ASOT) shows an acute rise, which reflects the presence of an active streptococcal infection. A simple elevated ASOT in itself is not diagnostic.

In clinical practice, if a history of antecedent 'strep throat' plus clinical features suggest acute rheumatic fever, paired sera should be drawn acutely and after 10–14 days tested to determine changes in ASOT.

In view of the low prevalence of Lyme disease versus the high prevalence of positive Lyme borreliosis *Borrelia burgdorferi* titers, probably fewer than 1 in 100 people with a positive test have Lyme disease. Therefore, it is recommended that a Lyme titer only be

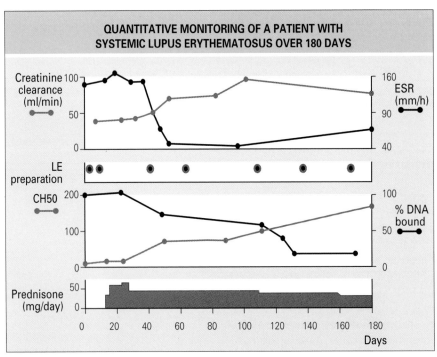

Fig. 5.3 Special investigations in rheumatology. These are often of more valuable to the clinician in monitoring the course of a severe inflammatory rheumatic disease, and its response to therapy, than in the initial diagnosis. The charted course (over a 6-month period) of a 14-year-old who had systemic lupus erythematosus shows the relationship between laboratory and clinical variables. LE = lupus erythematosus.

obtained in patients who show clinical evidence of Lyme disease, most notably the erythema chronicum migrans rash. The presence of musculoskeletal pain with a history of a tick bite is not generally an indication for a Lyme antibody test unless you are in an area where the disease is endemic.

HLA HAPLOTYPE TYPING

The association of several rheumatic diseases with the major histocompatibility complex, HLA, may provide important advances in our understanding of the pathogenesis of rheumatic diseases. For example, HLA-B27 is found in 90% of patients who have AS (versus 8% in the normal population), and HLA-DR4, now termed DRB1*04, in 67% of Caucasian people affected by RA (versus 30% in the normal population). These findings confer a relative risk of 80–100 for AS in individuals who have HLA-B27, and of 5–7 for RA in individuals who have HLA-DRB1*04, compared with the general population.

These observations have been interpreted to suggest that HLA typing may be useful clinically in helping to identify disease. However, this is not the case, for several reasons. A significant proportion of patients who have HLA-associated diseases do not bear the HLA marker (i.e. 10% of patients who suffer AS are HLA-B27 negative and 33% of patients who have RA are HLA-DR4 negative). Disease in these patients may have equally severe consequences, and requires a diagnosis based on other criteria. Conversely, most people with HLA-B27 or -DR4 do not have AS or RA.

URIC ACID

Uric acid measurement is included in the evaluation of patients who show musculoskeletal symptoms, as elevated uric acid is seen in 90% of people who have gout, either through overproduction or underexcretion. However, elevated uric acid levels are common in the general population, particularly in patients who take diuretics for hypertension and other conditions, as well as in 3–5% of normal individuals. Overdiagnosis of gout is associated with at least one potentially disastrous complication - allopurinol vasculitis. The diagnosis of gout is established definitively in the laboratory through identification of urate crystals in synovial fluid.

MUSCLE DISEASE

Inflammation or damage to muscles results in the release of enzymes, resulting in elevated levels of creatinine phosphokinase (CPK) and other muscle-derived enzymes in the serum. If you suspect myositis, this can be a useful screening test, although false-negative results sometimes occur.

THRYOID FUNCTION

Thyroid disease, particularly hypothyroidism, frequently results in musculoskeletal complaints. The most appropriate screening test if you suspect this diagnosis is the serum TSH level.

SCREENING FOR DRUG TOXICITY

Many drugs used for the treatment of rheumatic diseases can result in damage to the kidneys or liver, which can be detected by changes in renal or liver function tests.

THE MAIN ANTIBODIES FOUND IN ANTINUCLEAR ANTIBODY TESTING

- Antinuclear antibody test – a sensitive but very nonspecific test for SLE, with a very high false-positive rate.

- Antibodies to double-stranded DNA – less sensitive but much more specific test for SLE than is the ANA test; levels correlate with lupus nephritis and are used to monitor disease as well as in diagnosis.

- Extractable nuclear antigens – antibodies to extracts of nuclear material are common in many connective tissue diseases, particularly SLE.

- Antibodies to Ro (SSA) and La (SSB) – these antibodies are elevated in Sjögren's syndrome and SLE; Ro antibodies have been associated with congenital heart block in infants born to mothers who have SLE, and this test may have some utility in screening pregnant SLE patients.

- Antibodies to histones – these antibodies have particularly been associated with drug-induced SLE.

- Anticentromere and anti Scl-70 – these antibodies are found in most patients who have the CREST variant of scleroderma, and may have some value (along with other clinical evaluations) in screening people with 'primary' Raynaud's phenomenon.

- Antiphospholipid antibodies – the antiphospholipid antibody syndrome is characterized by thrombosis, recurrent fetal loss, livedo reticularis and thrombocytopenia.

- Antineutrophil cytoplasmic antibodies (ANCA) – these antibodies are strongly associated with vasculitic disorders, particularly Wegener's granulomatosis.

Fig. 5.4 The main antibodies found in antinuclear antibody testing.

PRINCIPLES OF DIAGNOSIS AND MANAGEMENT

6

IMAGING OF THE MUSCULOSKELETAL SYSTEM

A wide variety of imaging procedures are available to help visualize the anatomy of the musculoskeletal system. Of these, plain radiography is easily the most important, and the different modalities available are briefly discussed in this chapter.

PLAIN RADIOGRAPHY

Plain radiography is the most important imaging modality in rheumatology. However, plain radiographs are widely misused in this setting; the fact that they are cheap, easily available, and that much is known about the findings has led to vast overuse. Although films of peripheral sites, such as the hands and feet, confer very little radiation risk, more central radiographs of spinal and other structures do result in a radiation-exposure risk, and their use in particular should be minimized.

It is important to consider what outcome from a plain radiograph might alter decision making before the investigation is ordered. The physician must remember that plain radiographs have almost no role to play in either back pain or osteoarthritis (see Chapters 24 and 42, respectively), and that in most of the inflammatory rheumatic diseases the plain radiograph is normal in the early stages.

Plain radiographs are much more important in following disease progression and in helping to diagnose complications of rheumatic diseases than they are in the initial diagnosis. This is partly because they image bone best, and it takes many weeks or months for the effects on bone structure of any rheumatic disease to appear on a radiograph.

Examples of the value of plain radiography are shown in the Figures 6.1 and 6.2. In addition, plain radiographs are clearly of pivotal importance in the diagnosis of fractures, bone tumors, and a number of other bone conditions.

KEY POINTS

- Several techniques exist to help image the anatomy of the musculoskeletal system.
- Of these, plain radiography remains the most important.
- Plain radiographs are overused in primary-care rheumatology practice; they are of little help in the diagnosis of most disorders, and it is rarely cost-effective to investigate the cause of a musculoskeletal problem with plain radiography.
- Plain radiographs can be of value in following the progression of a chronic rheumatic disease, and in diagnosing complications or rare disorders.
- In complex situations in secondary care, particularly in suspected neoplasia or severe spinal disease, sophisticated imaging techniques, such as scintigraphy, computed tomography, and magnetic resonance imaging, are essential to show anatomic lesions and to plan surgery.

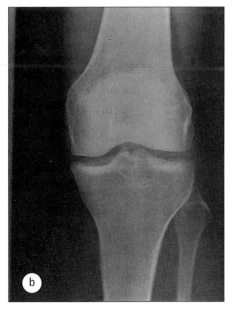

Fig. 6.1 Lateral and anteroposterior plain radiographs of the knee joint, illustrating the types of abnormality that can be detected with plain radiographs of good film quality. (a) On the lateral view the soft-tissue definition is sufficient to show the large effusion above the patella in the suprapatellar pouch. (b) On the anteroposterior view the calcification of the meniscal cartilage (chondrocalcinosis) can be seen in the lateral tibiofemoral compartment of the knee joint.

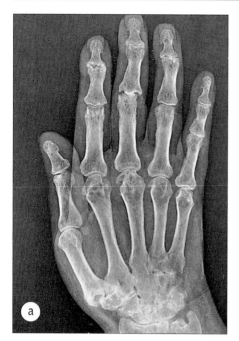

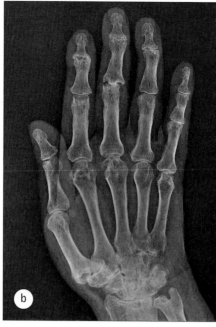

Fig. 6.2 One of the main values of plain radiography is to follow the structural progression of rheumatic diseases such as rheumatoid arthritis. In this patient, paired films 3 years apart [(a) early film, (b) later film] are shown, and it is apparent that, in spite of therapy, new erosions have developed at the metacarpophalangeal joints and that collapse of the carpal bones has occurred.

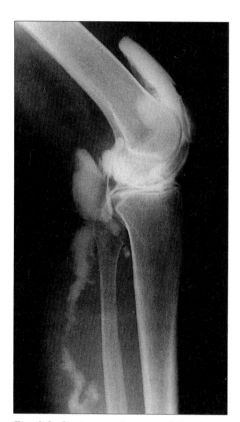

Fig. 6.3 Contrast arthrogram following acute synovial rupture of the knee joint. Acute rupture of the knee joint results in signs and symptoms similar to those of a deep vein thrombosis in the calf. One way of confirming the diagnosis of a ruptured Baker's cyst is through this imaging technique, in which contrast medium is injected into the knee and leakage of this material from the posterior Baker's cyst into the calf is clearly apparent.

OTHER IMAGING MODALITIES

ARTHROGRAPHY

Arthrography involves the injection of an iodine-containing contrast agent into the joint followed by radiography. Knee arthrography can confirm the diagnosis of a popliteal cyst and delineate the extent of rupture (Fig. 6.3). In addition, arthrography is useful for the assessment of menisci in patients who are claustrophobic or whose size precludes magnetic resonance imaging. Wrist arthrography is excellent for evaluating the integrity of ligaments within the wrist.

ULTRASOUND

Ultrasound produces images based on the location of acoustic interfaces in articular tissues. Resolution is limited by the depth of tissue being studied, and is much higher for superficial structures. Ultrasound is excellent for assessing size and location of fluid collections, such as joint effusions, popliteal cysts, and ganglion cysts, and can therefore be used to guide fluid aspiration. Superficial tendons such as the Achilles' tendon and patellar tendon (Fig. 6.4) can be studied for tears, and ultrasound may be useful in the detection of rotator cuff tears. Ultrasound is excellent for differentiating thrombophlebitis from pseudothrombophlebitis.

SCINTIGRAPHY

Scintigraphy following intravenous administration of radioactively labeled isotopes is useful for evaluating a variety of musculoskeletal disorders. The most commonly used radionuclide, technetium-99m methylene diphosphonate (^{99m}Tc MDP), accumulates in areas of high bone formation, calcium deposition, and high blood flow. The ^{99m}Tc MDP triple-phase bone scan is widely used for early detection of osteomyelitis; bone scans can also be used to detect stress injuries such as shin splints or stress fractures, tendon avulsions, and both primary or metastatic neoplastic lesions in bone (Fig. 6.5).

COMPUTED TOMOGRAPHY

Computed tomography (CT) scanning is particularly useful to evaluate the spine where the spatial anatomy is complex. In CT, cross-sectional images are created of the internal structure of the spine at various levels and, with reformatting, sagittal and coronal images can be created. The CT scan is the best technique for assessing the bony architecture of the spinal column, including the sacroiliac joints, before changes are noted on plain radiographs. In addition, the structural relationships of soft tissues (ligaments, nerve roots, fat, intervertebral discs) can be evaluated as they relate to their bony environment. An excellent technique for identifying mechanical disorders of the spine, which include spinal stenosis (Fig. 6.6), spondylosis, spondylolisthesis, trauma, and congenital abnormalities, CT can also visualize cortical bone destruction, calcified tumor matrix, and soft-tissue extension of tumors that affect the spine.

In addition, CT may be useful for the evaluation of other musculoskeletal structures with complex anatomy in which overlying structures obscure the view on conventional radiographs.

MAGNETIC RESONANCE IMAGING

Today, MRI is the procedure of choice for the imaging of abnormalities that affect soft-tissue structures of the joint, which includes cartilage (Fig. 6.7). It is of particular value in the assessment of disorders that affect the axial skeleton, including herniated intervertebral discs (Fig. 6.8), spinal stenosis, disorders that affect vertebral bone marrow, and disorders of the atlantoaxial joint in rheumatoid arthritis (Fig. 6.9). Joint effusions, popliteal cysts, ganglion cysts, meniscal and cruciate tears of the knee, tears of the rotator cuff, and bursitis are clearly imaged and the integrity of tendons can be assessed. Also, MRI is the study of choice for the diagnosis of early osteonecrosis, in which plain radiographs are normal. However, cost consideration obviously limits its usage.

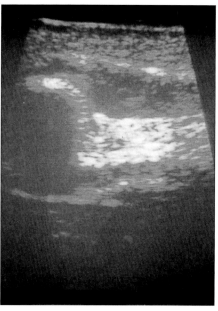

Fig. 6.4 Ultrasonography of the patellar tendon showing enlargement and reduced echogenicity of the tendon because of overuse injury to it.

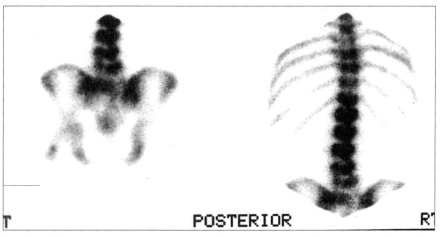

Fig. 6.5 This technetium bone scan shows heavy retention of isotope throughout the axial skeleton, caused in this case by extensive metastatic prostate cancer.

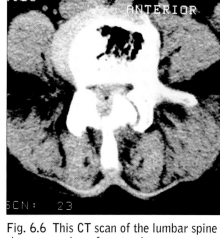

Fig. 6.6 This CT scan of the lumbar spine shows a number of anatomic abnormalities. These include: a thickened ligamentum flavum, facet joint hypertrophy, and posterior disc bulging, with absence of epidural fat; and a trefoil deformity of the lumbar spinal canal, a defect typical of lumbar stenosis. Computed tomography is particularly valuable in the assessment of spinal anatomic abnormalities such as spinal stenosis.

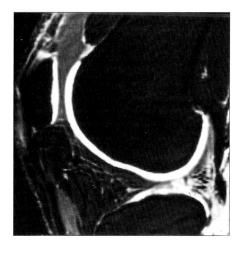

Fig. 6.7 Magnetic resonance imaging of the knee joint. A special technique of fat suppression was used here to increase the contrast between the cartilage (white band), bone (black), and synovial fluid (gray), illustrating the high level of soft-tissue imaging quality that can be achieved with modern musculoskeletal MRI.

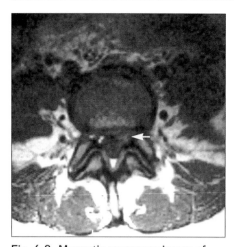

Fig. 6.8 Magnetic resonance image of the lumbar spine showing a herniated disc (arrowhead) which is blocking the right neural foramen.

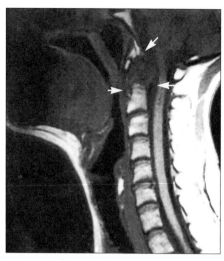

Fig. 6.9 Magnetic resonance image of the cervical spine in a patient who has advanced rheumatoid arthritis. Replacement of the odontoid peg with soft tissue is shown, compatible with rheumatoid pannus (arrows) and which is difficult to image in any other way. Stenosis of the canal and compression of the spinal cord are also apparent.

BONE DENSITOMETRY

Bone densitometry is used primarily for the evaluation of osteoporosis. The most widely available techniques used are dual-energy X-ray absorptiometry (DEXA) and quantitative computed tomography (QCT). The former is relatively inexpensive and delivers little radiation to the patient. The lumbar spine and proximal femur are most commonly studied and age-reference, standard values are available for comparison (Fig. 6.10). The latter technique scans several lumbar vertebrae while simultaneously scanning a phantom containing bone-equivalent material of different concentrations. One advantage of this technique in comparison to DEXA is that cancellous bone in the middle of the vertebrae can be evaluated, since overlying cortical bone and posterior elements of the vertebrae are not measured. Cancellous bone has tremendous surface area and is more rapidly affected during bone loss than cortical bone.

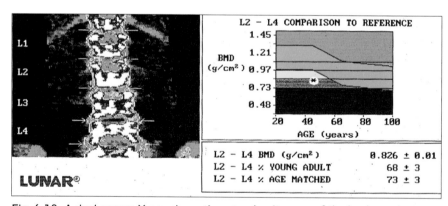

Fig. 6.10 A dual-energy X-ray absorptiometry density scan of the lumbar spine showing reduced bone density. The image (left) is accompanied by a recording of the age-adjusted expected bone density (normal range in the blue band) and this patient's bone mineral density is recorded by the white asterisk – this shows that bone density is well below the expected normal value, indicative of marked osteoporosis.

7

PRINCIPLES OF DIAGNOSIS AND MANAGEMENT

SYNOVIAL FLUID ANALYSIS

INTRODUCTION

Variation in the volume and composition of synovial fluid (SF) reflects pathologic processes within the joint. As a result of the unusual relationship between the tissues within the joint, chemically mediated events (such as inflammation and enzyme-mediated degradation within the synovium and cartilage) are reflected in changes in the chemical composition of SF. These changes include the production of factors responsible for the accumulation cells of different types within the fluid. In terms of their diagnostic utility, both chemical and cytologic changes in the SF have been studied.

By far the most important two investigations of SF are the bacteriologic examination and culture of samples in cases of suspected septic arthritis, and the examination by polarized-light microscopy to identify urate or pyrophosphate crystals in cases of gout or pseudogout, respectively.

SYNOVIAL FLUID ANALYSIS

Fluid should be examined for color, clarity, and viscosity.

COLOR
Normally, SF is pale yellow. In hemarthroses it is red or orange, and in inflammatory arthropathies cream or white. In septic arthritis it may be colored yellow or green by bacterial chromogens.

CLARITY
Normal SF is clear, but with increasing numbers of particles and/or cells it becomes cloudier.

VISCOSITY
Synovial fluid is viscid because of the complex saccharides it contains. In inflammatory joint disease the viscosity of SF falls as a result of enzymatic digestion and altered saccharide synthesis. This is easily demonstrated at the bedside by simply dripping the drawn-off SF from the end of the syringe immediately after aspiration. In cases of inflammatory joint disease, the low-viscosity SF forms individual droplets, whereas in noninflammatory arthropathies with more viscid fluid, a 'stringing' effect is seen (Fig. 7.1).

NUCLEATED CELL COUNT
The nucleated cell count may be performed manually or automatically. For convenience, the nucleated cell count of SF is expressed as cells/mm^3. Normal SF contains <200 cells/mm^3 (<0.2×10^9/l). In inflammatory joint disease the cell count is greater than 1000 cells/mm^3 (1×10^9/l) and in noninflammatory arthropathies it is lower. Cell counts in excess of

KEY POINTS

- In joint disease the synovial fluid increases in volume and can be aspirated.
- Changes in the composition of synovial fluid reflect the pathogenesis of the arthropathy.
- Synovial fluid analysis is a simple, cheap, and accurate test that yields information of diagnostic and prognostic significance.
- The two most important tests are bacteriologic examination and polarized-light microscopy for crystals, to diagnose septic arthritis and crystal-induced arthritis, respectively.

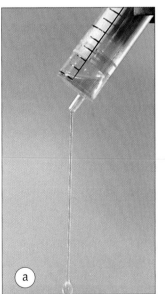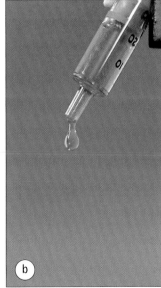

Fig. 7.1 Viscosity in synovial fluids. (a) This is normally high, which results in a stringing effect when fluid is dripped from a syringe. (b) However, in inflammatory arthritis the viscosity is lower, such that fluid falls from the syringe as normal droplets.

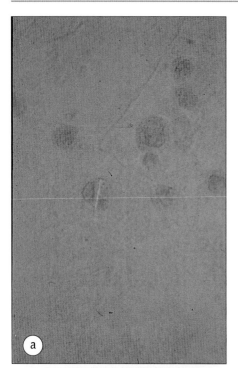

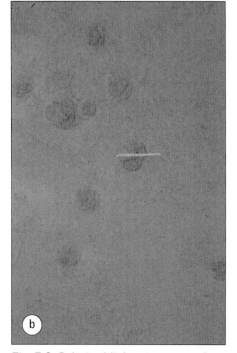

Fig. 7.2 Polarized-light microscopy of urate crystals seen in gout. These needle-shaped crystals are highly birefringent, and often seen attached to synovial fluid cells, as in this case. Their color in polarized-light is characteristic because of their negative birefringency, which makes them easy to differentiate from other crystals – hence the blue (a) or yellow (b) coloration, depending on the orientation of the particle.

25,000 cells/mm^3 (25×10^9/l) are found in three clinical conditions – rheumatoid arthritis (RA), septic arthritis, and reactive arthritis.

'WET PREPARATION' FOR CRYSTALS AND OTHER PARTICLES

Synovial fluid aspirates often contain visible particles. In making the 'wet preparation', the specimen is agitated and a small aliquot, that contains as many of these particles as possible is placed on a microscope slide. It is then gently squeezed flat beneath a cover slip and viewed unstained through a conventional microscope. For optimal results the condenser diaphragm is closed to produce diffuse light, in which the unstained cells and particles are more clearly seen. This preparation is examined for cell types, and by ordinary- or polarized-light microscopy for the several different classes of noncellular particulate material.

CLASSES OF CRYSTALLINE MATERIAL

Several classes of crystalline materials are found in the joints. Monosodium urate monohydrate crystals (the gout culprit) are needle-shaped, 5–30µm in length, and highly birefringent (Fig. 7.2). They can be differentiated from other crystals as they are negatively birefringent when viewed in polarized light with an interposed quarter-wave plate. These crystals, especially when intraleukocytic, are diagnostic of gout. If found within the background of SF with a high cell count, their presence usually signifies acute gout, but even if the cell count is low the diagnosis is confirmed.

Calcium pyrophosphate dihydrate crystals (Fig. 7.3) accumulate within joints with advancing age. In elderly patients, they can therefore be regarded as a normal finding, a condition known as chondrocalcinosis. Sometimes the crystals are associated with a high nucleated cell count, as in an acute monoarthritis, which is the typical presentation of pseudogout. The presence of calcium pyrophosphate crystals in association with otherwise typical features of osteoarthritis (OA) characterizes hypertrophic OA.

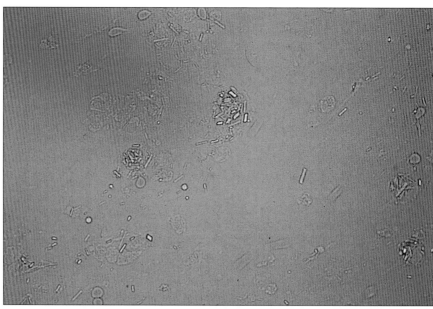

Fig. 7.3 Polarized-light microscopy of pyrophosphate crystals from a case of pseudogout. These crystals are weakly positively birefringent and have a quite different morphology from the urate crystals, most being rhomboids or rods, which helps to differentiate them from other particles.

Hydroxyapatite within SF indicates damage to calcified cartilage or underlying subarticular bone. Loss of cartilage, sufficient to expose these structures, is seen most commonly in OA and RA. The crystals are too small and amorphous to be seen with the light microscope, but staining with alizarin red produces a birefringent red product that is easily visualized (Fig. 7.4). A specific arthropathy, 'Milwaukee shoulder', is associated with larger apatite microspherules.

Lipids enter SF in inflammatory joint disease, in fracture of juxta-articular bone, and in hemarthrosis. They can be differentiated from one another by their shape and varying solubility in hydrocarbon solvents. Following intra-articular injection of depot corticosteroids, the crystalloid remains within the joint for up to 10 weeks and may mislead the unwary if they are not recognized for what they are if 'seen'.

BACTERIOLOGIC EXAMINATION AND CULTURE OF SYNOVIAL FLUIDS

An essential part in the investigation of any arthropathy is the submission of specimens of SF to culture for microorganisms (Fig. 7.5). As well as cases of suspected infective arthritis, unsuspected infections may be identified by this means. In addition to common bacterial joint pathogens (*Staphylococcus*, *Streptococcus*, etc.), *Neisseria*, *Salmonella*, *Mycobacterium tuberculosis*, and fungi that require special culture methods should also be considered.

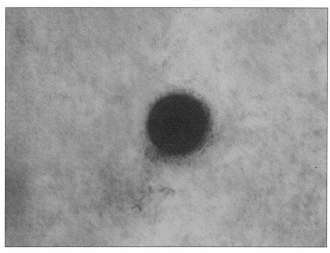

Fig. 7.4 Particles that contain masses of apatite crystals derived from bone or cartilage are commonly found in joint fluids. However, they have little diagnostic or prognostic significance. They cannot be seen in ordinary- or polarized-light microscopy, and require stains, such as the alizarin-red S stain used here, or special techniques.

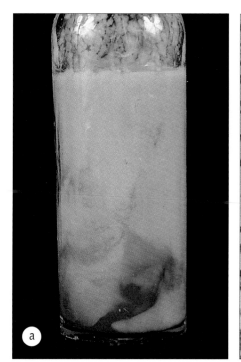
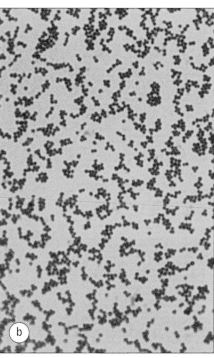

Fig. 7.5 Synovial fluid from a case of staphylococcal septic arthritis. (a) The fluid can look like frank pus, and may be blood stained. (b) Examination by Gram stain shows the massive numbers of Gram-positive cocci, and culture confirmed the nature of the organism and its antibiotic sensitivity.

SUMMARY

Synovial fluid analysis is of greatest value in differentiating inflammatory and noninflammatory arthropathies (Fig. 7.6), and in identifying specific disorders within these two groups. It is also very valuable in the rapid diagnosis of joint disease, in particular suspected cases of septic arthritis for which prognosis is inversely related to the delay in diagnosis, and crystal arthropathies, which are often misdiagnosed because SF crystals are not sought.

SYNOVIAL FLUID FINDINGS				
	Normal	Osteoarthritis	Rheumatoid and other inflammatory arthritides	Septic arthritis
Gross appearance	Clear	Clear	Opaque	Opaque
Volume (ml)	0–1	1–10	5–50	5–50
Viscosity	High	High	Low	Low
Total white cell count/mm^3	<200	200–10,000	5000–75,000	>50,000
% Polymorphonuclear cells	<25%	<50%	>50%	>75%

Fig. 7.6 Knee joint synovial fluid findings in common forms of arthritis.

PRINCIPLES OF DIAGNOSIS AND MANAGEMENT

8

PRINCIPLES OF MANAGEMENT OF MUSCULOSKELETAL DISORDERS

INTRODUCTION

Management of patients who have rheumatic disease remains a significant challenge and one that requires careful consideration and judgment, and an adherence to the principles of evidence-based medicine. Some rheumatic diseases are acute and settle completely with early and appropriate treatment (e.g. infectious arthritis and gout), but in many instances the disorder is a chronic one that requires careful management over a long time period.

COMPLEXITIES IN THE MANAGEMENT OF CHRONIC ARTHRITIS

The process of management of rheumatic disease is complex, for several reasons.

COORDINATION OF MULTIDISCIPLINARY MANAGEMENT

The doctor who provides rheumatologic management must coordinate specialist input in a variety of areas and must be knowledgeable about management options and their application, and their risks and benefits. To orchestrate these various approaches and to monitor their efficacy requires knowledge of what each offers, but, as importantly, requires the doctor to think in terms of the influence of life stages on disease and treatment and how they may relate to disease expression and modulation (e.g. the effect of aging on drug metabolism and toxicity). Of great importance here is the establishment of realistic goals for the various treatments. Although doctors can give patients information on the likely outcomes of treatment, the final decision on a particular therapy should be made in consultation with the patient. It is generally recognized that the goals of the patient and the physician are often different, which must be acknowledged by the treating 'team'. The ability to communicate with patients is extremely important when caring for any patient who has a chronic disease, particularly a rheumatic condition.

HOLISTIC USE OF MULTIPLE TREATMENT MODALITIES

Pharmacologic interventions and rehabilitation, and the use of orthoses and other devices, nonpharmacologic modalities, and surgery should acknowledged as influencing both disease and the patient, and a mutual interdependency obtains. These approaches cannot be seen as isolated intervention points in a disease process because they may significantly alter the course of the disease and affect the patient – sometimes permanently. Other life issues that are very important and have to be considered in treatment include the changes with age and development, be they those of childhood or adolescence, and the influence of activities such as school attendance, work, and home tasks. Rheumatic diseases are often chronic and are characterized by unpredictable remissions and relapses. The course of these diseases can be influenced by many factors, which include biologic processes, family and societal interactions, education, and treatment. Good management requires knowledge of all and attention to most of these. It is critical to remember that expectations for what a therapy will or will not do may differ substantially between the treating health-care professional and the patient. Great

KEY POINTS

Management of rheumatic diseases:
- Diagnosis should include the assessment of activity, prognosis, and goal setting.
- Treatment is adjusted in the light of evaluation of the response.
- Coordination of a multidisciplinary approach and re-evaluation of the disease is essential.

Therapeutic issues of particular importance:
- Which drugs should be used and when?
- Which surgical procedures should be used and when?
- Which physical therapies are appropriate?
- Continual re-evaluation of the patient's disease status, disability, expectations, and requirements is essential.

THERAPEUTIC STRATEGIES IN RHEUMATIC DISEASES

Pharmacotherapy	Nonpharmacologic
Analgesics NSAIDs Antirheumatic drugs Corticosteroids Immunosuppressive agents Biologic modifiers Specific antigout preparations Radiotherapy • Direct • Radiopharmaceutical	Rehabilitation
	Education Knowledge • General • Specific Behavioral modification • Relaxation techniques • Stress management
Surgery	Physical therapy Exercise • General preventive • Specific therapeutic Rest Light • Ultraviolet • Laser Heat/cold Hydrotherapy Electricity • Transcutaneous • Nerve stimulation Ultrasound Mobilization/manipulation Devices • Splints • Orthoses • Household modifications • Home/work/walking devices
Reconstruction • Tendon • Ligament Arthroplasty Arthrodesis Synovectomy Osteotomy Joint debridement Decompression • Spinal cord • Peripheral nerve	

Fig. 8.1 Classification of some of the therapeutic interventions available for the treatment of musculoskeletal disorders.

PRINCIPLES OF SELF-HELP

• Understand the condition that you have.
• Find out what you can do to help yourself.
• Find ways of taking control of the condition, rather than letting it control you.
• Learn how to protect your joints from unnecessary pain or stress.
• Learn how to conserve energy.
• Find out about the many simple tricks or techniques that can make everyday tasks easier.

care must be taken to inform patients of the benefits and risks of various therapies and to respect their ultimate treatment choices.

UNDERSTANDING PATIENT EXPERIENCES AND EXPECTATIONS

The difficulty of the problem of involving the patient in therapeutic decisions lies in the very different experiences of the doctor and the patient. The doctor can appreciate the long-term disability that is likely to result if the disease is not treated immediately, whereas the patient has little understanding of what is likely to occur in 10 or 20 years. The patient is much more likely to be influenced by the potential for immediate adverse consequences of a therapy (e.g. an adverse drug reaction, risks of surgery or anesthetic) than by a 'potential' reduction of disability (e.g. decreased pain or joint erosion) 10 years later. The optimal management of patients increasingly involves them in making decisions regarding risk factors such as weight and a range of lifestyle modifications.

THE DIFFERENT MODALITIES

The major therapeutic strategies in rheumatic diseases are shown in Figure 8.1. Very rare in chronic rheumatic diseases are these interventions used singly, so a critical issue in good management is the timing of each of the interventions. This is particularly so with drug therapy and with surgery, where a decision to use one modality may preclude others.

The various modes of intervention available are outlined in this chapter, following the order in which they are covered within the disease chapters of this book in Sections 2–8 (education and self-help, physical therapy and related non-phamacologic modalities, drug therapy, surgery, other treatment modalities, diet, and complementary techniques). In Chapter 9 further detail on the drugs used to treat rheumatic diseases is provided.

Rheumatic disease management needs to be problem oriented through a combination of techniques, as outlined in the examples shown in Figure 8.2.

EDUCATION, SELF-HELP, AND EMPOWERMENT

Education of patients and their carers is an essential part of the treatment of any musculoskeletal disorder, but of particular importance in chronic diseases and those diseases that can cause long-standing pain and disability. In such circumstances, it is particularly important to understand the context and meaning of the illness to individual patients, as well as the expectations that they and those who care for and support them have of the disease and its treatment. It has been shown that even brief attention to patient education at all clinic visits can have a positive impact, some of the main benefits being improved behavioral skills, self-help, patient empowerment, and enhanced psychologic outcomes. Patient education goals for physicians include improved communication, and increased understanding of the nature of the condition and the reasons for adherence to therapeutic advice (Fig. 8.3).

PROBLEM-ORIENTED TREATMENT OF IMPAIRMENTS

Impairment	Examples of underlying pathologies and other causes	Treatment options	
Acute inflammation of the joint and/or periarticular structures	Crystal arthropathy, inflammatory OA, reactive arthritis, RA, overuse, trauma	Relieve intra-articular pressure Relieve pain; reduce inflammation Maintain joint function	Aspiration of joints Immobilization, local cooling, iontophoresis (topical NSAID), NSAID, corticosteroids Active or active-assisted ROM exercise Static (isometric) muscle strengthening
Chronic inflammation of the joint and/or periarticular structures	RA, psoriatic arthritis, and other spondyloarthropathies, crystal deposition disease	Maintain joint function Joint protection Correct deformities Muscle relaxation Cardiovascular fitness	Active ROM exercise Dynamic (low load) muscle strengthening Cautious stretching Education Functional immobilization: splints Aids and devices Modify physical environment Splints and orthotics Heat (moist packs) Hydrotherapy Controlled physical activity Aerobic exercise Adapted recreational and sports activities
Joint hypermobility	Constitutional tendon and ligament laxity, pregnancy, Marfan's syndrome, Ehler–Danlos syndrome, ligament injury	Stabilization Functional immobilization	Dynamic, concentric, and eccentric exercise Corrective splinting Selective: preventive taping Nonselective: brace, abdominal binder or corset, collar
Joint hypomobility	Intra-articular problems: meniscus lesion, effusion, hemarthrosis, chondromatosis, loose body; reduced ROM due to muscle shortening, capsule retraction, osteophytes	Eliminate intra-articular obstruction Restore transversal gliding of surfaces	Aspirate effusion, hemarthrosis Arthroscopic removal of meniscus, loose body Transversal mobilization Consider impulse mobilization
Muscle dysfunction (strength, endurance, flexibility)	Unbalanced exercise, deconditioning, repetitive movements at work or with sports activities, joint pathologies	Restore muscle balance (include antagonists) Muscle relaxation	Stretching Strength and endurance exercises Heat Hydrotherapy
Acute sensorimotor loss	Radicular or nerve compression, e.g. acute disc herniation	Relieve pain; reduce inflammation Muscle relaxation Mobilization	Analgesics, NSAIDs Cold or galvanization therapy along irradiation (e.g. leg) Rest (limit to few days) Functional immobilization (e.g. hip flexion to reduce ischiadic tension) Muscle relaxants Hydrotherapy Local cooling or heat Start without gravity (pool exercise)
Chronic sensorimotor loss	Carpal or tarsal entrapment, disc herniation, spinal stenosis	Address inflammatory component to reduce edema Restore muscle balance General fitness	Local corticosteroid injection or oral corticosteroid therapy NSAIDs Immobilization (e.g. wrist splint, abdominal binder) Coordinated strengthening and stretching exercises Musculoskeletal and aerobic exercise

Fig. 8.2 Treatment of rheumatic diseases needs to be problem oriented and to combine pharmacologic, nonpharmacologic, and other treatments; some examples are listed here. (ROM = range of movement.)

IMPROVING COMMUNICATIONS IN PATIENT EDUCATION PRACTICE	
Key strategy	**Principles for clinical practice**
Address patient concerns	Listening to patient; doctor to write down concerns with patient
Set patient goals	Set realistic priorities and goals for the patient (based on above), and develop management plan for each
Inform patient of treatment options	Explain all therapies, their risks, benefits and costs; identify and discuss patient preferences
Adherence-enhancing strategies	Identify individual barriers to adherence, including time, cost, convenience, memory; develop simple strategies (written instructions, medication dosettes, etc.) for each patient to overcome potential problems with adherence
Integrate clinical practice with multidisciplinary patient education	Identify allied health personnel, specific professionalswho may help the patient, local structured group patient education programs, community resources and agencies

Fig. 8.3 Some issues that need to be addressed as part of improving communication in patient education practice.

PRINCIPLES OF JOINT PROTECTION IN PATIENTS WITH ARTHRITIS
To do
Use the strongest and largest joints available for a specific task Carry objects close to the body Spread the weight of objects over many joints Slide objects using both hands Plan work areas so that the most frequently used equipment is reached easily Use appropriate aids and devices
To avoid
Prolonged static positions Force in the direction of flexion and ulnar deviation of hands and fingers Lateral deviating pressures on the hand and the wrist Pressure against the volar surface of the fingers Activities involving tight grasp Force and constant pressure against the pad of the thumb

Fig. 8.4 Principles of joint protection in patients who have arthritis.

Joint protection and energy conservation are specific educational interventions that help patients to use their joints in the most comfortable way, and thus reduce pain and conserve energy. Energy conservation also involves splints and other aids. Central to the question of whether behavioral change results in improved symptoms is the question of which educational method is most effective in changing and maintaining optimum behavioral change. A large, controlled study documented a significant improvement in many aspects of joint protection and function in a 6-week trial. Principles of joint protection with a focus on the wrist and hand are listed in Figure 8.4.

Self-help is of great importance to patients, and included in several sections are some simple guides to self-help for different disorders to help practitioners in the education and empowerment of their patients.

PHYSICAL THERAPY AND OTHER NONPHARMACOLOGIC TREATMENTS

Physical and nonpharmacologic treatments vary in their sophistication, from massage of a painful area in soft-tissue rheumatism to careful mobilization of a lumbar apophyseal joint by a well-trained, physical therapist. Exercises may be specific for particular muscles or muscle groups, or they may be generalized. The importance of low-impact general exercise programs is seen throughout life; even the elderly can benefit in terms of musculoskeletal symptoms from a general aerobic exercise program. A variety of devices for patients afflicted by musculo-skeletal disease assist in performing activities of daily living, ranging from turning on faucets, getting on and off a toilet, and opening jars to remaining mobile.

REST

Bed rest or immobilization of joints with splints is used for treating joint inflammation arising from injury or from inflammatory, crystalline, degenerative, or metabolic arthropathies. The dilemma with rest is that, if prolonged, it causes adverse systemic and local effects, which include osteoporosis, muscle weakness, and reduced strength of tendons, ligaments, and other periarticular tissues. Therefore, immobilization is used as little as possible.

REST

- General bed rest reduces the activity of systemic inflammatory arthritis.
- Local rest relieves pain and inflammation of single joints.
- Splints can aid rest.
- Prolonged rest can lead to stiffness and loss of joint motion, as well as muscle wasting and osteoporosis.

REMEDIAL EXERCISES

There are three main forms of exercise therapy used by physiotherapists: range of movement exercises, strengthening exercises and endurance training. Maintaining or improving the range of motion of joints is a key objective in the management of all forms of arthritis, as restricted motion leads to impairment and disability, and can also accelerate joint damage and increase pain. Exercises to improve the range of motion can be passive, active or assisted: passive exercise is generally of least value, and active or assisted exercise programs are used for most patients where possible. Musculoskeletal pain and arthritis quickly lead to loss of bulk and strength of the muscles of the affected areas. Muscle strength is critical not only for normal function, but in the stabilization of joints, and to aid the shock-absorbing function of muscles. Strong muscles, therefore, protect joints from damage. Exercises to increase muscle strength can be isometric (no movement), or isokinetic (constant velocity) and these two approaches are generally used hand-in-hand. Improved endurance for activities is important for people with musculoskeletal diseases as it increases the sense of well being and reduces pain, as well as aiding rehabilitation and the reduction of any disability. Endurance exercises can be combined with the general physical exercise programs outlined below, and can include graded training exercise programs designed to gradually increase the duration of activities.

A number of other modalities are often used in conjunction with exercise therapy, to help minimize pain and relax muscles. These include heat or cold, and hydrotherapy. Warm water is a particularly valuable aid to exercises, either at home or in a physiotherapy department. At home a warm bath or shower may aid exercises, as well as the use of warm packs on affected joints (see below), and physiotherapists make good use of warm hydrotherapy pools, particularly to aid improved range of motion exercises and to re-educate patients towards more normal function. The combination of reduced gravitational resistance and relaxing warm water is of particularly great value to disabled patients undergoing rehabilitation programs.

HEAT AND COLD

HEAT

Heat is prescribed for muscle relaxation, to reduce stiffness, and to improve local circulation, each of which may contribute to pain relief. Muscle relaxation is achieved through reflexive relaxation and a direct effect. Heat can be delivered by radiation (light), conduction (hot pack, paraffin, water), or conversion (diathermy, ultrasound). Radiant and conductive heat sources are means of delivering local or superficial heat; short wave and microwave diathermy and ultrasound are means of delivering deep heat.

Deep heat is used to treat chronically, irritated structures with a low metabolic activity such as tendons. Ultrasound is used to manage adhesive capsulitis, but its effectiveness has not been confirmed for either pain relief or increased motion. In controlled trials, ultrasound was no better than placebo in an exercise program for osteoarthritis (OA) of the knee.

Unclear is whether heat can, and if so, should be applied to inflamed joints. There is agreement that heat is contra-indicated in acute arthritis (e.g. gout), because it produces increased and sustained inflammation and pain. However, heat might enhance pain reduction and muscle relaxation in patients who have moderate joint inflammation. Many patients who have rheumatoid arthritis (RA) find mild heat with moisture helpful. For degenerative joint diseases and soft-tissue syndromes that do not have prominent inflammation,

---

REMEDIAL EXERCISES (PHYSIOTHERAPY)

There are three main forms of exercise therapy:

- Exercises can improve the range of joint motion.
- Exercises can strengthen muscles, which are the main stabilizers and shock absorbers for joints.
- Exercises can improve endurance, aiding general fitness and rehabilitation.

- A combination of these three forms of exercise can improve or restore impaired function as part of a rehabilitation program.
- Physiotherapists can use exercise therapy to aid pain relief.
- Physiotherapists can also facilitate early recovery from local periarticular problems including sprains and strains, by use of local heat (see later) as well as exercises.

HEAT AND COLD

- Heat can relieve pain and induce muscle relaxation.
- Hot baths, showers and warm pools (including hydrotherapy pools) can provide general heat and relaxation, and aid remedial exercises and rehabilitation.
- Local heat can be produced by local applications, light, diathermy or ultrasound.
- Local applications and light produce superficial heat only.
- Diathermy and ultrasound can heat deeper structures such as capsules and tendons.
- Local cooling can reduce pain, inflammation and swelling, in both acute situations (such as trauma) and in chronic arthritis.
- All applications, be they hot or cold, need to be used with caution to avoid skin damage and excessive temperature alterations.
- Different people prefer and respond to different types of application (some obtaining pain relief with heat, others with cooling), so a pragmatic approach is needed.

modalities for delivering more intense heat are usually well tolerated. Similarly, patients who suffer spondyloarthropathies seem to prefer intense heat to mild heat.

The selection of a modality needs to include the personal preferences of the patient. While some patients feel comfortable and perceive an effect only with hot mud packs, others react to this regimen with anxiety and discomfort, and prefer mild heat from moisture packs or infrared lamps. When prescribing or applying heat, a pragmatic approach based on trial and error is preferable to strict adherence to standard 'cookbook' recipes.

LOCAL COOLING

The major physiologic effects of local cooling are vasoconstriction in both superficial and intra-articular tissues, reduction of local metabolic rate, and slowed nerve conduction and nerve-firing rates. Cooling has a local analgesic effect and reduces inflammatory responses to tissue trauma. Cold is applied by cold packs, ice massage, immersion, or vapocoolant sprays. No data show that any one type of cold application consistently produces superior results.

Cold therapy needs to be applied with caution – cold packs out of the freezer that have temperatures below 0°C may cause serious burns if applied directly to the skin. It is advisable to cover the pack with a towel.

Cooling with ice massage or ice packs empirically is a highly effective analgesic therapy (e.g. in acute shoulder periarthritis). Cold appears to be effective and well tolerated by patients who have many different forms of arthritis, especially with acute inflammation. It reduces edema and pain. However, in chronic mild inflammation (for instance, in patients who suffer RA), mild, moist heat, which reduces pain through muscle relaxation, is often preferred. In knee OA, cold provides significant pain relief more quickly than does heat.

MASSAGE

Massage is a technique commonly used to relieve muscle spasm, pain, and stiffness. It can boost blood flow in muscles, increase lymph flow, relax muscles, and decrease blood pressure. In many situations massage is used after the application of heat and cold to augment the effect on muscle relaxation and to decrease pain before stretching or strengthening exercises.

PHYSICAL FITNESS AND RECREATIONAL ACTIVITIES
PHYSICAL FITNESS

All patients affected by chronic musculoskeletal conditions should have a comprehensive training program to maintain and improve general and musculoskeletal fitness. The components include flexibility [range of movement (ROM) exercises], muscle balance (static and/or dynamic strengthening exercises and stretching exercises), musculoskeletal endurance, and training of coordination (e.g. play and modified sports activities), as well as cardiovascular training to maintain or improve aerobic capacity and prevent deconditioning.

For patients with normal aerobic capacity, exercise maintains fitness. For patients with low aerobic capacity, training may improve it. Physical training in patients who have systemic rheumatic disorders requires supervision, since patients may suffer coexisting conditions, such as lung disease, that require modification of the program. Studies have shown that rheumatic patients can perform aerobic exercises without negative effects.

Supervised aerobic training may improve symptoms, function, and work capacity, and reduce fatigue in a host of rheumatic conditions, which include fibromyalgia, OA of the knee, systemic lupus erythematosus, and RA. Regular aerobic exercise is also an important adjunct to the treatment of myofascial pain and chronic pain states. Aside from improving cardiovascular fitness, aerobic training aids in weight control and improves the patient's sense of well-being.

For cardiovascular fitness, the American College of Sports Medicine recommends aerobic exercise using large muscle groups that causes an elevation of training heart rate to 60–90% of the maximum heart rate or reaches 50–85% of

---

PHYSICAL FITNESS AND RECREATIONAL ACTIVITIES

- All patients with a chronic musculoskeletal condition should have a comprehensive training program. Such programs reduce pain and fatigue, and improve function.
- The components of the program should include flexibility, balance and coordination, endurance and cardiovascular fitness.
- Care needs to be taken in those patients with concomitant cardiovascular or respiratory problems, but no age or musculoskeletal problem is a barrier.
- Recreational activities are a valuable adjunct to general exercise, they may be more fun, and can provide a social function as well as a rehabilitative one.
- Low-impact activities are preferable, and some sports, such as swimming, are particularly well suited to those with musculoskeletal diseases.
- Chinese techniques such as t'ai chi can be helpful.
- High-impact activities (such as jogging) and contact sports are best avoided, and some modifications may be needed to other sports to accommodate an impairment.

Vo$_2$max for 20–60 minutes three to five times per week. Training heart rate is calculated by taking 60–90% of predicted maximum heart rate, which is approximately 220 minus age (in years). An endurance training program should start with low-intensity sessions to allow the exercise novice to maintain an appropriate training heart rate for the minimal length of time required for cardiovascular adaptation.

RECREATIONAL ACTIVITIES

Recreational activities are useful for improving neuromuscular functioning. They may contribute to body perception, expand skills, aid general conditioning, and recruit social supports. Also, they are more enjoyable than repetitive therapeutic exercises. For instance, the traditional Chinese technique t'ai chi ch'uan is an enjoyable alternative to traditional exercises for improving strength in patients who have knee OA. Training of hand and finger muscles or strengthening of shoulder or hip muscles can be facilitated with loom weaving. Some sports activities are particularly suited to musculoskeletal rehabilitation – examples include volleyball and swimming (particularly the crawl stroke) for patients who have spondyloarthropathies. Activities like walking, golf, low-impact aerobics, and cross-country skiing can be done by many patients who have musculoskeletal conditions. Jogging places a high impact upon the joints in the lower extremities and should be avoided in patients affected by arthropathies of weight-bearing joints, but walking can be done safely in mild-to-moderate disease. Contact sports such as basketball, football or soccer should be avoided.

Some general precautions should be given with respect to sports. The difficulty level is defined in the way that movement of individual joints and execution of complex functions is controlled. For instance, in sports like skiing, unexpected, demanding terrain may force uncontrolled movements that could damage joints. Certain sports need to be modified to accommodate functional limitations in patients who suffer particular conditions (e.g. avoid serving overhead in volleyball for patients who have spondyloarthropathies).

SPLINTS, ORTHOSES, WALKING AIDS AND OTHER AIDS
BRACES

Braces are external devices that aid simple or complex body functions. Splints and orthotics support or stabilize a body part, while prosthetics replace a body part. Splints and orthotics are used for a variety of reasons.

Progressive splinting is sometimes used as an alternative to surgery to reduce a severe joint contracture. Splints and orthotics can be fixed, or dynamic to accept some movement in the joint. Splints and orthotic devices need to be tested empirically on the individual – no method predicts those patients who will benefit.

Few braces and indications have been evaluated critically, but their use is considered best practice. Most studies have been conducted with RA patients, and have examined the effect of wrist and hand splinting on reducing inflammation. Splints reduce inflammation, increase motion and hand function, improve grip and pinch strength, decrease both day and night pain, and increase the ability to carry out daily activities.

WALKING AIDS

For limitations in walking, ambulation aids (namely canes, crutches, and walkers) are the most commonly used devices – several different types are available. They serve to lessen the weight of painful or damaged joints, often to a much greater extent than might be expected (via the application of limited force through a lever arm). Padded or custom handles can be provided for those who have hand deformities, but severe wrist and hand deformities may require a platform crutch or walker. For those in cold climates, attachments to ambulation aids and metal-studded, pull-on shoe rubbers improve the safety of walking on slippery surfaces. For those whose walking is limited by a limited field of view (e.g. patients who have severe kyphotic deformities because of ankylosing spondylitis), key holders

SPLINTS, ORTHOSES, WALKING AIDS AND OTHER AIDS

- Splints can be used to help immobilize and rest an inflamed joint.
- Splints or orthoses can be used to correct a malalignment or deformity that may be inducing symptoms (e.g. a foot orthosis can correct valgus stress on the medial side of the knee).
- Splints can be used as an interim measure to help the patient and doctor assess whether surgical fusion might be useful.
- A number of walking aids are available, including canes, crutches and walkers; they can reduce pain on locomotion, as well as improving function.
- Other aids available to those who have difficulty with standing or walking include raised toilet seats, special chairs, stair rails and wheelchairs.
- Great attention to detail is needed to get the most out of walking aids.
- A number of other simple devices are available to help compensate for a specific functional problem, such as key holders, faucet turners, brush and comb extensions and dressing sticks.

may allow the patient to open doors more easily (Figure 5.2a).

Standing and walking are sufficiently related to be considered together. For individuals who have limited standing tolerance, high stools or chairs in strategic locations may be used to help accomplish whatever otherwise may have been accomplished in the standing position. When aided walking is limited, wheeled mobility aids are helpful, such as simple stools with casters or office chairs that can be propelled with the feet, as well as wheelchairs and scooters. Upper extremity deformities limit the usefulness of manually propelled wheelchairs (unless propelled by someone else using the push handles). For such individuals, an electrically powered wheelchair or scooter is more appropriate. Wheeled mobility aids are available in a large number of modes, with a variety of options (e.g. brake extenders to increase the leverage), but are expensive.

For limited stair-climbing abilities, the addition or modification of hand rails may be all that is required. The stair rise (height of each step) may be excessive, so it is sometimes useful to use a half rise – indeed, a small platform attached to a cane-like device can be moved up and down the stairs, one at a time, by the patient. For more severe limitations to stair climbing, motorized devices on which the patient can sit transport them up and down the stairs safely. However, these are expensive and sometimes difficult to install in older homes. Installation of an elevator or moving to a home in which there are no stairs may be the only options. In other cases, modifying a downstairs room to make it unnecessary for the patient to climb stairs may be more appropriate. For stairs outside the home, a ramp may be installed. Ramps should not exceed a 5° grade, periodically have level rest platforms, be covered in nonslip material, and have a lip and a hand rail on each side.

OTHER AIDS TO FUNCTION

A number of other simple aids are available to compensate for specific functional problems. For example, if opening doors is a problem, the use of a modified key holder may help and door-knob extensions may help. For a patient in a wheelchair, offset door hinges can add to the width of the door without requiring any change to the door frame. Other simple examples of aids include sleeves that increase the size of knife or fork handles so that they can be gripped more easily by people with bad arthritis of the hands, extensions to brushes so that the patient can brush the hair at the back of their head even if their shoulders are stiff (Figure 8.5b), and dressing sticks that can help people pull clothes up or down when their hands will not reach to the right point. Many people have great difficulty opening bottles and jars and turning faucets on and off because of pain and weakness of the wrist or hand; many simple aids can overcome these problems, such as faucet turners and special bottle and jar openers.

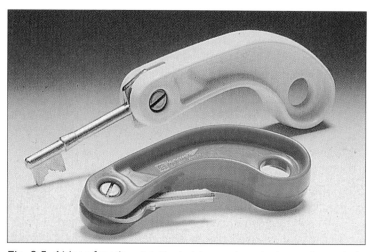
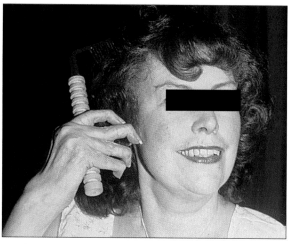

Fig. 8.5 Aids to function. (a) Key holders make gripping easier and give extra leverage for turning.
(b) Extension to a brush helps this patient with rheumatoid arthritis groom her hair. (Courtesy of Homecraft Supplies Ltd, UK.)

faucet turners and special bottle and jar openers.

Some of the many simple ways of compensating for functional limitations are shown in Figure 8.6.

STRATEGIES TO COMPENSATE FOR FUNCTIONAL LIMITATIONS			
Functional limitation	Potential disability	Underlying impairments	Adaptive aids and devices
Tipping head	Drinking	Pain and limited cervical ROM	Use straw or glass with cutout for the nose
Turning head	Driving	Reduced ROM with ankylosis of vertebral joints or hyperostosis, C1–2 arthritis	Larger rear view mirror
Reaching	Eating, cooking, hygiene, washing hair	Shoulder or elbow pain, limited ROM, weakness (Milwaukee shoulder; RA)	Use long-handled or angled utensils (combs and brushes, spoons) and back-scrubbing aids
Grip	Eating, cooking, personal hygiene, dressing, shopping	Arthritis of wrist and finger joints, atrophy of musculi interossei, stiffness, limited ROM, weakness and decreased sensorium	Replace small knobs with big handles Replace buttons, shoelaces, belts, bra hooks with Velcro fasteners Select clothes that are easy to put on: slip-on shoes, clip-on ties, zippers with big ring-pulls Use large and sharp chef's knife or knife with vertical grip; wall-mounted electric opener for cans; and lid lifter to break the suction on vacuum lids
Carrying	Shopping, household activities	Pain, weakness and reduced endurance of upper extremity	Use wheeled carriers or carts for carrying small loads
Balance and stability with standing and moving	Going out, shopping, traveling	Weakness, numbness and balance disturbance, joint dysfunction	Use a cane Use attachments to canes and crutches to improve stability and grip Prevent slipping with suction-cup mat or nonskid tape on the bottom of the bathtub Use single lever faucets and shower caddys Use terry-cloth robe to dry after bathing Shower seat
Rising from sitting	Bathing, sitting	Hip or knee pain and quadriceps weakness	Raised toilet seat and stool; safety rails or bars on the wall; toilet armrest
Walking	Moving around apartment, shopping, traveling	Hip and/or knee pain and muscle weakness	Canes, crutches and walkers Wheelchair for longer distances
Climbing stairs	Moving around the house, shopping, traveling	Hip or knee pain, weakness (RA, OA, degenerative spinal stenosis, spondyloarthropathies)	Consider home elevator and ramps Install rails and split-risers to raise half of each step
Bend or lift (while standing)	Household activities	Pain, reduced ROM of spine or hip	Long-handled reaching aids, dust pans, dusters and mops
Bend knee (while sitting)	Dressing	Pain, muscle weakness, limited ROM of knee or hip	Use long-handled shoehorn, garter snaps or spring clothespins on a piece of tape for helping to put on socks

Fig. 8.6 Some adaptive aids and devices that can be used to compensate for specific functional impairments.

DRUG THERAPY

- Drugs can be given systematically (injections, tablets and suppositories) or locally (rub-ons and injections).
- Systemic drug therapy is symptomatic (analgesics and anti-inflammatory agents) or disease specific (such as hypouricemic agents for gout or antirheumatic drugs for rheumatoid arthritis). See Chapter 9.
- Local therapy is dominated by corticosteroid injections.
- The indication for corticosteroid injections is persistent local inflammation and pain.
- Long-acting crystalline preparations are used for joints and bursae, but less potent preparations should be used for periarticular injections.
- Local anesthetic can be mixed with steroids, and may help confirm the correct site of an injection.
- Injections should never be given if there is suspicion of local infection, and great care must always be taken to avoid sepsis.
- The therapist must be familiar with the procedure. See Section 2.
- The benefit is aided by resting the area for some 48 hours after the injection.

DRUG THERAPY

SYSTEMIC DRUGS

Drug therapy can be symptomatic (relief of pain or stiffness) or disease specific. In metabolic diseases such as hyperuricemia, drugs to lower the serum uric acid (allopurinol or a uricosuric agent) can be combined with a specific anti-inflammatory drug [e.g. colchicine or a nonsteroidal anti-inflammatory drug (NSAID)] to suppress pain and inflammation. In OA, purely analgesic agents such as acetaminophen are often more appropriately used initially, since NSAIDs are associated with significant morbidity. In several recent studies, acetaminophen has been shown to be of benefit in up to 30% of patients who have OA of the knee previously treated with NSAIDs. If inflammatory episodes arise in OA, NSAIDs may be beneficial but therapy should be reviewed frequently and the dose reduced or discontinued as appropriate.

LOCAL DRUGS, INCLUDING CORTICOSTEROID INJECTIONS

Systemic drugs are covered further in Chapter 9. In addition to systemic drug therapy, musculoskeletal problems can be treated locally. Local rubefacients (creams, gels or other applications which the patient rubs onto the painful area) are widely available and very popular with patients. Drugs can also be injected into joints and periarticular tissues. A variety of agents are available, but by far the most important are local corticosteroid injections.

Corticosteroid injections are frequently used to achieve local anti-inflammatory activity. The indications for their use include persistent inflammation at a single site in the absence of a contraindication, such as suspicion of infection (see below). Synovial joints and other cavities are generally injected with a long-acting, crystalline form of corticosteroid such as triamcinolone hexacetonide or acetonide. These agents are taken up by the synovial lining cells, and allow continued local release into the targeted area. Only a relatively small proportion escapes into the general circulation, but during the first 24 hours after injection patients may experience flushing or other evidence of a corticosteroid 'pulse'. For periarticular injections, particularly subcutaneous bursae and de Quervain's tenosynovitis, methylprednisolone acetate is used, as the more potent triamcinolone hexacetonide is likely to induce skin atrophy. Local anesthetic is sometimes mixed with corticosteroids for such injections. In the case of some periarticular lesions, for example rotator cuff lesions around the shoulder, this has the advantage of confirming the correct placement of the injection, as the local anesthetic results in almost immediate relief of the problem if the injection is placed correctly.

Corticosteroid doses vary with the structure injected. For each of the described procedures below a dose range is shown based on the use of methylprednisolone acetate 40mg/ml. If the more potent triamcinolone hexacetonide 20mg/ml is used, the lower figure of the range is applicable.

Corticosteroid injections are used in joints, bursae, tendon sheaths, and entheses. Some of these procedures are easy to perform, while others are technically demanding or have dubious results. Specific information on their use for regional pain syndromes is covered in Section 2. Rest of the injected site for 48 hours following the procedure is generally recommended. Additional rest may lead to better results and should be considered under special circumstances.

SURGERY

In the chronic rheumatic diseases, physicians must work closely with orthopedic surgeons to establish the optimal time for surgical intervention (Fig. 8.7). Modified interventions such as arthroscopic debridement, tendon synovectomy and joint synovectomy need to be reviewed carefully to see if they could reduce the need for arthroplasty in the future. Timing of surgery needs to be assessed carefully and, in particular, the sequence of surgery performed on various joints, particularly in the chronic rheumatoid, needs to be carefully evaluated.

CURRENT SURGICAL PROCEDURES FOR THE TREATMENT OF PATIENTS WITH ARTHRITIS		
Surgical procedure	Common indications	Expected outcome
Joint debridement	Loose bodies and other causes of mechanical joint dysfunction (knee, shoulder, hip, ankle)	Improved mechanical function and decreased pain
Joint debridement and penetration of subchondral bone	Joint pain associated with loss or degeneration of articular cartilage (knee)	Variable
Joint synovectomy	RA, PVNS, synovial chondromatosis, hemophilia (knee, elbow, wrist, shoulder, ankle)	Temporary and, in some cases, long-term decrease in synovitis and possibly reduced rate of articular cartilage destruction
Tenosynovectomy	RA and rarely other causes of tenosynovitis, including PVNS (wrist and hand)	Reduced pain and swelling, improved muscle tendon unit function
Tendon, ligament and joint capsule reconstruction	Joint subluxation due to RA (MCP joints)	Improved joint stability and alignment
	Tendon ruptures due to RA (wrist and hand)	Improved muscle tendon unit function
Osteotomy	OA (hip and knee)	Reduced pain and, in some cases, formation of a new articular surface and regression of osteophytes
Joint replacement	Advanced joint degeneration due to OA, trauma, inflammatory diseases, bone necrosis (shoulder, elbow, hip, knee)	Pain relief, improved function
Joint fusion (including spinal fusion)	Advanced joint degeneration or instability due to OA, trauma, inflammatory diseases, bone necrosis (hand, wrist, shoulder, hip)	Pain relief, restoration of alignment and stability (loss of motion and possible increased risk of degeneration of other joints)
Peripheral nerve decompression or transposition	Localized nerve compression (ulnar and median nerves)	Reduced pain, improved function
Spinal cord and nerve decompression	Existing or impending spinal cord and nerve root compression (cervical spine)	Decreased pain, improved function

Fig. 8.7 Current surgical procedures used for the treatment of patients who have arthritis. (PVNS = pigmented villonodular synovitis.)

DIETARY THERAPY, COMPLEMENTARY AND HOLISTIC MEDICINE

- Many patients are convinced that diet is the cause/cure for their arthritis, but the presence of arthritis in all cultures and throughout history belies a huge role for diet.
- Those with gout or osteoarthritis should lose weight if overweight.
- Diets rich in fish or plant oils, rather than meat oils, may reduce pain and inflammation somewhat in some patients.
- Occasional patients appear to have a genuine, specific dietary issue affecting their arthritis.
- A wide variety of popular complementary techniques are widely available, although there is little or no scientific evidence to support the efficacy of the majority of these treatments.
- Homeopathy is an example of an age-old popular complementary technique used to treat arthritis.
- Holistic medicine is a concept that stresses cooperation between traditional and complementary practitioners, and the involvement of spirit and mind, as well as the body, in the management of disease.

DIETARY THERAPY, COMPLEMENTARY AND HOLISTIC MEDICINE

Dietary, alternative, traditional, and complementary approaches to management are used by an extraordinarily large number of patients who suffer from musculoskeletal conditions. In managing patients affected by musculoskeletal disorders, it is usually desirable to discuss with them the combination of traditional with alternative therapies.

DIET

Many patients who have rheumatic diseases are convinced that diet is either the cause or the potential cure for their arthritis, or both. That rheumatic diseases are worldwide and have been present in all cultures and in people of all different dietary habits for centuries does not dispel these beliefs.

In practice, very little evidence suggests any role of diet for the majority of patients. Exceptions are the treatment of obesity in those who have lower limb OA or gout, and the use of diets high in fish oils, rather than meat oils, to slightly reduce pain and stiffness in those affected by inflammatory disorders. Exclusion diets and specific supplements are of no value to the majority, although it is also apparent that a small number of patients seem to be convinced that a specific dietary factor has a major effect on their arthritis; as the situation is unclear, it is inappropriate to deny these observations.

COMPLEMENTARY TECHNIQUES

A wide variety of complementary techniques are both widely available and popular with patients with musculoskeletal problems. They range from traditional Eastern healing techniques, through physical approaches such as osteopathy and chiropracty, to medicine-based approaches such as herbalism and homeopathy.

HOMEOPATHY

Homeopathy is a system of treatment developed from the natural 'law' (magic) of similia similibus curantur (like is cured by like). Thus, a substance that can cause symptoms in the healthy can cure similar symptoms in the sick. Practitioners consult compendiums called repertories and texts on materia medica to determine the remedy that best matches the total picture of the symptoms. Healing begins by eliminating the immediate symptoms and then progressing to the older, underlying symptoms.

Remedies are prepared from plant and other sources in alcohol, and filtered to give a 'mother tincture' from which dilutions are made – the shaking of each dilution is thought to be important. About 500 remedies are in regular use. Classic homeopaths use a similimum and not a potentiation of an apparent causal agent, while modern homeopaths use combinations of several or many substances and may include low dilutions of herbal products.

HOLISTIC MEDICINE

Holistic medicine is a system of health care that emphasizes personal responsibility, fosters a cooperative relationship among all those involved, and aims for optimal attunement of body, mind, emotions, and spirit. The focus is on prevention, lifestyle, psychotherapeutics, social context of cause of illness, diet, exercise, meditation, family involvement, clinical ecology, assisting nature, and the promotion of good health. The concept of holism differs between alternative practitioners (who apply it to diagnosis and management of individuals) and medical complementary services and practices.

NATUROPATHY

Naturopathy is a system of treatment of ailments that utilizes the 'vital curative force' and employs nature's agencies, forces, processes, and products. Nature-based treatments date back to the dawn of healing.

Naturopathy is a mixture of traditional folk wisdom, empiricism, and selections of biomedical science. The basic principles are:
- healing power of nature is fundamental;
- treat the cause rather than the effect (disease);
- ill health results from lowering of resistance because of diet, spinal displacement, stress, accumulation of toxins, and deficiencies of vitamins, minerals, and other essentials;
- promotion of harmony of body, mind, and emotion (treat the whole person);
- new principles of living (various old and new therapies), with the focus on prevention.

Diagnosis is achieved on the basis of history, observation, iris examination, assessment of 'vital reserve', nutritional assessment, and hair analysis. Naturopaths frequently treat rheumatic symptoms by employing counseling with a selection of modification of lifestyle, diet and nutritional advice, herbal medicine, homeopathy, Bach flower remedies, supplements (vitamins, minerals, biochemical remedies), exercises, massage and manipulation, hydrotherapy, and numerous other therapies, which include acupuncture.

CHIROPRACTIC AND OSTEOPATHY

Chiropractic and osteopathy are among a number of physical, manipulative techniques that are popular, particularly for the treatment of back disorders. Chiropractic is based on the belief that subluxed vertebrae interfere with the proper flow of nervous impulses, and so prevent the 'innate intelligence' (vital force?) from passing through the body. Thus, the affected tissue or organ undergoes dysfunction (disease). Currently, subluxations are believed to be structural or functional and to be caused by physical or psychic stress, and chemical factors.

The diagnostic technique involves history, static palpation of muscles and vertebrae, motion palpation of individual vertebral segments, measurements (especially limb length), posture analysis, skin temperature analysis, and spinal radiography. Treatment includes massage, vertebral and soft-tissue mobilization, vertebral thrusting, stretching, and applied kinesiology.

HERBAL MEDICINE

The medicinal, aromatic, and savory properties of plants (leaf, seed, stem, flowers, root, bark) have been valued by humans for aeons. In traditional and tribal medicine, herbs have had religio-magical uses, often with ceremony, and also empirically-based therapeutic roles. Healers passed on knowledge orally and by text. The usefulness of many herbs (e.g. willow bark) was identified by the application of symbolic magic, and that of others by 'intuitive revelations'. Herbal medicine constitutes a large part of traditional medicine, is relied upon by the majority of the world's population, and is also extensively used in the industrialized nations.

While symbolic, magic, and placebo effects are important, herbalists believe in several therapeutic principles (applied to rheumatism), which including detoxification:
- restoration of balance of the 'vital force';
- nourishment and stimulation;
- antirheumatic actions.

The whole plant should be used in herbal remedies, not an isolated, pure, active drug extract, because the other active substances are necessary for efficacy and safety. In Chinese and other herbal practices, each patient requires a different combination of herbs prepared or administered by different methods. Herbal preparations are available from naturopaths, traditional and nonmedical practitioners, natural product stores, and pharmacies. They may be taken or used as whole herbs, powders, teas (infusions, decoctions), capsules, tablets, extracts, tinctures, oils, salves and ointments, enemas, and baths. Proprietary herbal mixtures are frequently combined with nutritional supplements, fish oils, minerals, and vitamins.

Some popular herbs for rheumatism include aloe vera, alfalfa, celery, comfrey, dandelion, devil's claw, evening primrose oil, feverfew, garlic, ginger, horse-radish, kelp, parsley, Paraguay tea, willow bark, wintergreen, and yucca.

9

PRINCIPLES OF DIAGNOSIS AND MANAGEMENT

DRUGS USED IN THE MANAGEMENT OF RHEUMATIC DISORDERS

This chapter provides a brief summary of the main classes of drugs used in the treatment of the rheumatic diseases, and includes notes on dosages, side-effects, and cautions and contraindications to their usage.

ANALGESICS

Analgesics are commonly used for the immediate relief of pain in rheumatic disorders. They are the primary form of drug management in osteoarthritis and are typically given in combination with nonsteroidal anti-inflammatory drugs (NSAIDs) or antirheumatic drugs for chronic inflammatory syndromes. It is important to avoid analgesics that have addictive potential. In musculoskeletal disorders, analgesics are often best used on an 'on-demand' basis for the prevention or relief of activity-related pain, rather than by regular dosing.

MONITORING

Generally, analgesics are free of side effects when used as prescribed and do not require routine monitoring (Fig. 9.1).

KEY POINTS

- The classes of drugs used in rheumatic diseases include analgesics, nonsteroidal anti-inflammatory drugs, corticosteroids, antirheumatic agents, and drugs used for osteoporosis, fibromyalgia, and gout.
- As with all drugs, it is important to recognize the potential side effects, contraindications, and interactions of these agents.
- Many of the drugs used in the treatment of chronic inflammatory rheumatic disorders must be monitored carefully.

ANALGESICS			
Drug	Dosage	Side effects	Cautions and contraindications
Acetaminophen	1000–4000mg/day in 3–4 doses	Fasting, drinking alcohol, and/or taking excessive amounts of acetaminophen may result in liver or kidney damage	A history of alcohol abuse, kidney disease, hepatitis, or other liver disease
Acetaminophen with codeine	1200–2400mg acetaminophen combined with 60–480mg of codeine per day in 2–4 doses. Take with food	Constipation, dizziness or lightheadedness, drowsiness, nausea, fatigue or weakness, vomiting. Chronic use may cause psychologic and physical dependence	A history of drug or alcohol abuse; asthma; head injury; prostate or gastric problems; liver, kidney or thyroid disease; sensitivities to acetaminophen, codeine or sulfites
Propoxyphene (dextropropoxyphene) hydrochloride	65mg every 3–4h as needed, no more than 390mg/day	Dizziness or lightheadedness, drowsiness, nausea, vomiting	Current or previous serious depression, use of tranquilizers or antidepressants
Tramadol hydrochloride	50–400mg/day in 2–4 doses	Dizziness, nausea, constipation, headache, sleepiness	Liver disease, asthma, kidney disease, history of drug or alcohol abuse

Fig. 9.1 Analgesics. (Adapted with permission from Klippel JH, Weyand CM and Wortmann RL, Primer on the Rheumatic Diseases, 11E, Atlanta, GA: Arthritis Foundation, 1997.)

NONSTEROIDAL ANTI-INFLAMMATORY DRUGS AND SALICYLATES				
	Drug	Dosage	Side effects	Cautions and contraindications
Nonsteroidal anti-inflammatory drugs	Diclofenac potassium Diclofenac sodium Etodolac	75–100mg/day in a single dose 100–150mg/day in 2 doses 400–1200mg/day in 1–4 doses	Abdominal pain, diarrhea, dizziness, drowsiness, fluid retention, gastric ulcers and bleeding, greater susceptibility to bruising or bleeding, heartburn, indigestion, lightheadedness, nausea, nightmares, rash, ringing in ears Side effects may be more pronounced for people with pre-existing heart or kidney disease. May cause confusion in elderly people with kidney impairment.	Sensitivity or allergy to aspirin, nonacetylated salicylates, or similar drugs; kidney or liver disease; heart disease; high blood pressure; asthma; peptic ulcers; use of anticoagulants
	Fenoprofen calcium	900–2400mg/day in 3–4 doses; never more than 3200mg/day		
	Flurbiprofen	200–300mg/day in 2–3 doses		
	Ibuprofen	Adults, 1200–3200mg/day in 3–4 doses; children, 35–45mg/kg/day in divided doses		
	Indomethacin	50–200mg/day in 2–4 doses		
	Ketoprofen	150–300mg/day in 3–4 doses		
	Ketorolac[†]	Oral: up to 40mg/day in 4–6 doses Injected: up to 120mg/day in 4 doses		
	Meclofenamate sodium	200–400mg/day in 3–4 doses		
	Mefecamic acid*	1000mg/day in 4 doses		
	Nabumetone	500–2000mg/day in 1 or 2 doses		
	Naproxen	Adults, 500–1500mg/day in 2–3 doses; children, 15–20mg/kg/day in divided doses		
	Naproxen sodium	550–1650mg/day in 2–3 doses		
	Oxaprozin	1200–1800mg/day in a single dose		
	Piroxicam	20mg/day in a single dose		
	Sulindac	300–400mg/day in 2 doses		
	Tolmetin	Adults, 1200–1800mg/day in 3 doses; children, 25–30mg/kg/day in divided doses		
Salicylates	Aspirin	Adults, 1300–4000mg/day in 4 doses; children, 75–90mg/kg/day in divided doses	Abdominal cramps and pain, deafness, gastric ulcers, heartburn or indigestion, increased bleeding tendency, nausea or vomiting, ringing in ears Use of alcohol may increase the risk of gastric ulcers and bleeding, as well as kidney and liver damage Side effects may be more pronounced for people with pre-existing heart or kidney disease. May cause	Sensitivity or allergy to aspirin or nonacetylated salicylates, kidney or liver disease, heart disease, high blood pressure, asthma, peptic ulcers, use of
	Choline magnesium trisalicylate	3000mg/day in 2–3 doses		
	Choline salicylate	3480–6960mg/day in 3–4 doses		
	Diflunisal	500–1000mg/day in 2 doses		
	Magnesium salicylate	2600–4800mg/day in 3–6 doses		
	Salsalate	1500–3000mg/day in 2–3 doses		
	Sodium salicylate	1950–3900mg/day in 3–4 doses		

* This medication is for short-term pain relief and should not be used for more than 7 days.

[†] This medication is for short-term pain relief and should not be used for more than 3 days. Dosage should be adjusted for people who weigh <50 kg, and it [†] should be used with caution in elderly patients.

Fig. 9.2 Nonsteroidal anti-inflammatory drugs (NSAIDs) and salicylates. (Adapted with permission from Klippel JH, Weyand CM and Wortmann RL, Primer on the Rheumatic Diseases, 11E, Atlanta, GA: Arthritis Foundation, 1997.)

NONSTEROIDAL ANTI-INFLAMMATORY DRUGS

Symptomatic relief of pain and stiffness is provided by NSAIDs for most of the inflammatory articular and periarticular disorders. The response is not immediate, but the vast majority of patients treated with a NSAID respond within 7–10 days, so it is reasonable to wait about 2 weeks to assess the response. To minimize gastrointestinal complaints, NSAIDs should be given with food. Elderly patients and patients who have renal disease should be given NSAIDs with caution, since they may reduce renal blood flow and cause fluid retention. It is important to review the need for NSAIDs periodically and to avoid automatic re-prescribing.

Several different routes of NSAID administration are available, including oral, rectal, by injection, and locally. The all important gastrointestinal side-effects are largely caused by systemic blood levels, so rectal or systemic administration does not remove the risk of this or renal side-effects. In contrast, the amount of systemic absorption from local administration to a joint, in the form of a cream or gel that contains an NSAID, is very small. These creams and gels have the added advantage of helping patients to feel more in control of their drug usage, as they can rub the drug onto the painful joint when they feel the need.

Agents that are used to relieve pain by rubbing things onto the skin over the painful area (rubefacient) have been used for centuries and are widely available over the counter. Most contain substances that produce mild local vasodilatation (and hence heat). There is now good evidence for their efficacy. In some countries a variety of such creams and gels with added NSAIDs are also available, but there is not a great deal of evidence to indicate that they are superior to the cheaper, simple alternatives.

MONITORING

Ulcerations of the gastrointestinal tract, including both gastric and duodenal ulcers, are the most important serious complication of NSAID use, and are particularly likely to occur in older female patients, those who have a history of previous peptic ulceration, those on concomitant corticosteroid therapy, smokers, and those who have multiple organ failure. Patients being given a systemic drug need to be monitored carefully for severe or persistent abdominal pain or evidence of gastrointestinal bleeding. Since NSAIDs have a number of important interactions with other drugs, dosages may need to be altered and specific toxicities monitored (Figs 9.2–9.4).

The general advice given is to avoid the use of NSAIDs in people who are at a high risk of peptic ulceration, however, alternatives do exist. For example, co-prescribing a 'gastroprotective agent' (such as misoprostel) can reduce the risk. In addition, new types of NSAID are being developed (the so-called selective COX-2 inhibitors) which may be less gastrotoxic.

Care also needs to be taken with the potential renal toxicity of NSAIDs, particularly in the elderly, who can develop renal failure as well as fluid retention. In older people renal function should be assessed before initiating NSAID therapy, and regularly thereafter.

DRUGS AFFECTING NSAIDs		
Drug implicated NSAID affected	**Effect**	**Approach to management**
Antacids Indomethacin ? other NSAIDs	Variable effects of different preparations: aluminum-containing antacids reduce rate and extent of absorption of indomethacin; sodium bicarbonate increases rate and extent of absorption of indomethacin.	No action required unless marked reduction in absorption results in poor response to NSAID; dose may need to be increased in this case. Not as important with those NSAIDs that have enteric coating or slow- release profiles.
Probenecid Probably all NSAIDs	Reduction in metabolism and renal clearance of NSAIDs and acyl glucuronide metabolites which are hydrolyzed back to parent drug.	May be used therapeutically to increase the response to a given dose of NSAID.
Cholestyramine Naproxen and probably other NSAIDs	Anion exchange resin binds NSAIDs in gut reducing rate (? and extent) of absorption.	Separate dosing times by 4h; may need bigger than expected dose of NSAID.
Metoclopramide NSAIDs Aspirin	Increased rate and extent of absorption of aspirin in patients with migraine.	May be used therapeutically.

Fig. 9.3 Some of the drugs that can affect nonsteroidal anti-inflammatory drugs (NSAIDs).

NSAIDs AFFECTING OTHER DRUGS		
Drug affected **NSAID implicated**	**Effect**	**Approach to management**

Oral anticoagulants
  Phenylbutazone
  Oxyphenbutazone
  Azapropazone
	Inhibition of metabolism of S-warfarin, increasing anticoagulant effect.	Avoid NSAIDs if possible. Careful monitoring where unavoidable.

Lithium Probably all NSAIDs	Inhibition of renal excretion of lithium, increasing lithium serum concentrations and increasing risk of toxicity.	Use sulindac or aspirin if NSAID unavoidable. Careful monitoring of lithium concentration and appropriate dose reduction.

Oral hypoglycemic agents
  Phenylbutazone
  Oxyphenbutazone
  Azapropazone
	Inhibition of metabolism of sulfonylurea drugs, prolonging half-life and increasing risk of hypoglycemia.	Avoid this group of NSAIDs if possible; if not possible, monitor blood sugar closely.

Phenytoin
  Phenylbutazone
  Oxyphenbutazone
 	
  Other NSAIDs
	Inhibition of metabolism of phenytoin, increasing plasma concentration and risk of toxicity.
	
	Displacement of phenytoin from plasma protein, reducing total concentrations for the same unbound (active) concentration.
		Avoid this group of NSAIDs if possible; if not possible, intensify therapeutic drug monitoring.
		
		Careful interpretation of phenytoin total concentration; measurement of unbound concentration may be helpful.

Methotrexate Probably all NSAIDs	Reduced clearance of methotrexate (mechanism unclear), increasing plasma concentration and risk of severe toxicity.	This is only relevant to high-dose methotrexate used in cancer chemotherapy.
Sodium valproate Aspirin	Inhibition of valproate metabolism increasing plasma concentration.	Avoid aspirin; close monitoring of plasma concentration if other NSAID used.
Digoxin All NSAIDs	Reduction in renal function in susceptible individuals, reducing aminoglycoside clearance and increasing plasma concentration.	Avoid NSAIDs if possible; if not possible, frequent checks of digoxin plasma concentration and plasma creatinine.
Aminoglycosides All NSAIDs	Reduction in hypotensive effect, probably related to inhibition of renal prostaglandin synthesis (producing salt and water retention) and vascular prostaglandin synthesis (producing increased vasoconstriction).	Close plasma concentration monitoring and dose adjustment.

Antihypertensive agents, β-blockers, diuretics, ACE inhibitors, vasodilators
  Indomethacin
  Other NSAIDs
	Reduction in natriuretic and diuretic effects; may exacerbate congestive cardiac failure.	Avoid all NSAIDs in treated hypertensive patients if possible; if not possible, monitor carefully. May need additional antihypertensive therapy.

Diuretics
  Indomethacin
  other NSAIDs
	Gastrointestinal tract mucosal damage, together with inhibition of platelet aggregation, increasing risk of GI bleeding in patients on anticoagulants.	Avoid NSAIDs in patients with cardiac failure; monitor clinical signs of fluid retention.

Anticoagulants All NSAIDs	Potentiation of hypoglycemic effects (mechanism unknown).	Avoid all NSAIDs if possible.

Hypoglycemic agents
  Salicylate
  (high dose)
		Monitor blood sugar level.

Fig. 9.4 Some of the interactions between nonsteroidal anti-inflammatory drugs (NSAIDs) and other drugs.

SYSTEMIC CORTICOSTEROIDS

Corticosteroids have anti-inflammatory and, in high dosages, immunosuppressive properties. They are a valuable class of drugs for the management of select acute and chronic forms of inflammatory rheumatic diseases. Assessment by a rheumatologist is recommended before using corticosteroids for arthritis or diffuse rheumatic syndrome.

Corticosteroids can be administered in many ways; in addition to oral dosing, 'pulses' of intravenous corticosteroid are sometimes used in severe, systemic, inflammatory rheumatic disorders, and local injection therapy is popular for regional problems, as outlined in Chapter 8.

MONITORING

High-dose and/or chronic therapy may be associated with substantial toxicities. Weight gain, change in body habitus (moon facies, buffalo hump, etc.), hypertension, and diabetes are seen early; cataracts, thinning of the skin with easy bruising, osteoporosis, and osteonecrosis are potential late complications (Fig. 9.5).

ANTIRHEUMATIC DRUGS

Antirheumatic drugs are used in the management of chronic inflammatory arthropathies, such as rheumatoid arthritis and related diseases, and systemic rheumatic syndromes, such as lupus. The choice of drugs is largely determined by the severity and extent of disease, and requires assessment by a rheumatologist to help in the development of a plan of management and periodic monitoring of the drug response.

MONITORING

A large number of toxicities are associated with antirheumatic drugs and require careful, drug-specific monitoring (Fig. 9.6).

CORTICOSTEROIDS			
Drug	Dosage	Side effects	Cautions and contraindications
Cortisone Dexamethasone Hydrocortisone Methylprednisolone Prednisolone Prednisolone sodium phosphate (liquid only) Prednisone Triamcinolone	Dosages of corticosteroids are highly variable and determined by the rheumatic disease to be treated. In general, the lowest dose that successfully controls the condition should be used. Corticosteroids should be taken with food or an antacid. A single daily dose should be taken with breakfast. It is very important that corticosteroids, when used long-term, not be stopped abruptly; dosage must be tapered gradually	Cushing's syndrome (weight gain, moon-face, thin skin, muscle weakness), osteoporosis, cataract, hypertension, increased appetite, elevated blood sugar, indigestion, insomnia, mood changes, nervousness or restlessness, cramps, immune suppression/infection	Active infection (or inactive tuberculosis), hypothyroidism, herpes simplex of the eye, hypertension, osteoporosis, gastric ulcer, diabetes

Fig. 9.5 Corticosteroids. (Adapted with permission from Klippel JH, Weyand CM and Wortmann RL, Primer on the Rheumatic Diseases, 11E, Atlanta, GA: Arthritis Foundation, 1997.)

DISEASE-MODIFYING ANTIRHEUMATIC DRUGS					
Drug	Dosage	Side effects	Cautions and contraindications	Monitoring	
				System review	Laboratory
Auranofin (oral gold)	3–9mg/day in single dose or in 2–3 doses	Abdominal or stomach cramps or pain, bloated feeling, decrease in or loss of appetite, diarrhea or loose stools, gas or indigestion, mouth sores, nausea or vomiting, skin rash or itching, photosensitivity	Adverse reaction to gold-containing drugs, inflammatory bowel disease, kidney or liver disease	Symptoms of myelosuppression*, edema, rash, diarrhea	CBC, platelet count, urine dipstick for protein every 4–12 weeks
Azathioprine	50–150mg/day in 1–3 doses, based on body weight. Take with food.	Loss of appetite, nausea or vomiting, skin rash, bone marrow suppression, infection, malignancy, pancreatitis	Kidney or liver disease, concomitant use of allopurinol, pregnancy	Symptoms of myelosuppression*	CBC and platelet count every 1–2 weeks with changes in dosage, and every 1–3 months thereafter
Cyclophosphamide	50–150mg/day orally in a single morning dose. Fluid intake (2–3L/day) and emptying bladder before bedtime is important.	Infertility in men and women, loss of appetite, bone marrow suppression, infection, hemorrhagic cystitis, malignancy	Kidney or liver disease, any active infection, pregnancy	Symptoms of myelosuppression*, hematuria	CBC and platelet count every 1–2 weeks with changes in dosage, and every 1–3 months thereafter
Cyclosporin	2.5–5mg/kg/day in 1–2 doses	Bleeding, tender, or enlarged gums; fluid retention, hypertension; increase in hair growth; loss of renal function; loss of appetite; trembling or shaking of hands; tremors	Sensitivity to castor oil (if receiving drug by injection), liver or kidney disease, active infection, hypertension	Edema, blood pressure every 2 weeks until dosage stable, then monthly	Creatinine every 2 weeks until dose is stable, then monthly; periodic CBC, potassium, and liver function tests
Hydroxychloroquine sulfate	200–600mg/day in 1–2 doses. Take with food.	Diarrhea, loss of appetite, nausea, stomach cramps or pain, skin rash, retinopathy, neuromyopathy	Allergy to any antimalarial drug, retinal abnormality, G6PD deficiency, pregnancy	Visual changes, funduscopic and visual fields every 6–12 months	
Methotrexate	7.5–25mg orally or intramuscularly per week in a single dose	Cough, diarrhea, hair loss, loss of appetite, unusual bleeding or bruising, fever, pneumonitis, infection, stomatitis	Bone marrow suppression, liver and lung disease, alcoholism, immune-system deficiency, active infection, pregnancy	Symptoms of myelosuppressiona, shortness of breath, nausea/vomiting, lymph node swelling	CBC, platelet count, aspartate aminotransferase, albumin, creatinine every 4–8 weeks
D-Penicillamine	125–250mg/day in a single dose to start, increased to not more than 1500mg/day in 3 doses. Take on an empty stomach.	Diarrhea, joint pain, lessening or loss of sense of taste, loss of appetite, fever, hives or itching, mouth sores, nausea or vomiting, skin rash, stomach pain, lymphadenopathy, bone marrow suppression, unusual bleeding or bruising, weakness	Penicillin allergy, blood disease, kidney disease	Symptoms of myelosuppression*, edema, rash	CBC, urine dipstick for protein every 2 weeks until dosage stable, then every 1–3 months
Sulfasalazine	2–3g/day in 2–4 doses	Stomach pain, achiness, diarrhea, dizziness, headache, light sensitivity, itching, appetite loss, liver abnormalities, lowered blood count, nausea or vomiting, rash	Allergy to sulfa drugs or aspirin, kidney or liver disease, blood disease, bronchial asthma	Symptoms of myelosuppression*, photosensitivity, rash	CBC every 2–4 weeks for first 3 months, then every 3 months
Gold sodium thiomalate (injectable) Aurothioglucose (injectable)	10mg in a single dose the first week, 25mg the following week, 25–50mg/week thereafter. Frequency may be reduced after 1g total dose.	Photosensitivity; irritation or soreness of tongue; metallic taste; skin rash or itching; soreness, swelling, or bleeding of gums; unusual bleeding or bruising; white spots on lips or in mouth or throat; oral ulcers; proteinuria; bone marrow suppression	Kidney disease, bone marrow suppression, colitis	Symptoms of myelosuppression*, edema, rash, oral ulcers, diarrhea	CBC, platelet count, urine dipstick every 1–2 weeks for first 20 weeks, then at the time of each (or every other) injection

*Symptoms of myelosuppression include fever, symptoms of infection, easily bruisability and bleeding.

Fig. 9.6 Disease-modifying antirheumatic drugs (DMARDS). (Adapted with permission from Klippel JH, Weyand CM and Wortmann RL, Primer on the Rheumatic Diseases, 11E, Atlanta, GA: Arthritis Foundation, 1997, and from the American College of Rheumatology Ad Hoc Committee on Clinical Guidelines. Guidelines for monitoring drug therapy in rheumatoid arthritis. Arthritis Rheum. 1996;39:723–31.)

DRUGS USED IN OSTEOPOROSIS

Calcium and vitamin D are generally recommended as baseline therapy for the prevention and/or treatment of osteoporosis. The use of other bone-modifying drugs is typically based on abnormalities evident on measurements of bone mineral density, as well as clinical considerations. Rapid developments are occurring in this field, with the introduction of several new agents.

MONITORING

Generally, drugs used for osteoporosis are free of side effects when used as prescribed and do not require routine monitoring (Fig. 9.7).

DRUGS USED IN FIBROMYALGIA

Both antidepressants and muscle relaxants are used in the management of fibromyalgia.

OSTEOPOROSIS MEDICATIONS			
Drug	Dosage	Side effects	Cautions and contraindications
Alendronate	10mg/day in a single dose. Take with a full glass of water first thing in the morning. Do not eat or drink anything else, take any other medications or lie down for at least 30 minutes after taking the drug.	Irritation and ulcers of the throat and esophagus, bone pain or tenderness, diarrhea, difficulty swallowing, nausea, taste changes	Swallowing or gastric-emptying difficulties, hypercalcemia, pregnancy, kidney disease, intestinal or bowel disease
Calcitonin (injection)	100IU/day in a single dose	Diarrhea, flushing of skin, local inflammation at injection site, loss of appetite, nausea, stomach pain, vomiting, allergic reaction	
Calcitonin (nasal spray)	200IU/day in a single dose. Use alternate nostrils daily. It is necessary to activate the pump prior to each dose.	Nasal irritation, diarrhea, flushing of the skin, loss of appetite, nausea, stomach pain, vomiting, allergic reaction	
Calcium	Females: children: 800mg/day adolescents: 1500mg/day adults: 1200mg/day pregnancy: 1500mg/day Males: children: 800mg/day adolescents: 1000mg/day adults: 500–1000mg/day	Rare constipation, intestinal colic, or kidney stones	Kidney stones
Conjugated estrogens	Taken daily or in 4-week cycles of 0.625mg/day for 3 weeks followed by 1 week of rest from drug. Women who have not had a hysterectomy should take this drug in conjunction with progestin.	Abdominal cramps, breast swelling and tenderness, loss of appetite, nausea, rapid weight gain, stomach bloating, edema	Undiagnosed vaginal bleeding; breast cancer or other estrogen-dependent cancer; a family history of breast cancer; problems related to blood circulation or blood clotting
Vitamin D	400–800IU/day		

Fig. 9.7 Osteoporosis medications. (Adapted with permission from Klippel JH, Weyand CM and Wortmann RL, Primer on the Rheumatic Diseases, 11E, Atlanta, GA: Arthritis Foundation, 1997.)

MONITORING

Generally, drugs used for fibromyalgia are free of side effects when used as prescribed and do not require routine monitoring (Fig. 9.8).

DRUGS USED IN GOUT

Drug therapy of gout is directed toward the treatment of the acute attack with NSAIDs (or occasionally colchicine or corticosteroids) and secondarily toward the correction of the hyperuricemia, that causes the attacks. Gout drugs are generally given with food to minimize gastrointestinal complaints.

MONITORING

Periodic monitoring of uric acid and renal function after beginning treatment to lower uric acid is recommended. Allopurinol is rarely associated with liver or bone marrow toxicity, or vasculitis (Fig. 9.9).

FIBROMYALGIA MEDICATIONS				
	Drug	Dosage	Side effects	Cautions and contraindications
Antidepressants: tricyclics	Amitriptyline hydrochloride	10–100mg/day in a single dose at bedtime	Difficulty concentrating, dizziness, drowsiness, dry mouth, headache, increased appetite (including craving for sweets), nausea, sleep disturbances, unpleasant taste, urinary retention, weakness or tiredness, weight gain	A history of seizures, urinary retention, heart problems, glaucoma or other chronic eye conditions; use of thyroid medication or another antidepressant
	Doxepin hydrochloride	10–100mg/day in a single dose at bedtime		
	Nortriptyline	10–100mg/day in a single dose at bedtime		
Muscle relaxants	Cyclobenzaprine	10–30mg/day in 1–3 doses	Dizziness or lightheadedness, drowsiness, dry mouth. Alcohol, other antidepressants, or monoamine oxidase inhibitors may increase risk of side effects.	Glaucoma, urinary retention, cardiac or peripheral vascular disease, hyperthyroidism

Fig 9.8 Fibromyalgia medications. (Adapted with permission from Klippel JH, Weyand CM and Wortmann RL, Primer on the Rheumatic Diseases, 11E, Atlanta, GA: Arthritis Foundation, 1997.)

GOUT MEDICATIONS			
Drug	Dosage	Side effects	Cautions and contraindications
Allopurinol	100–400mg/day in a single dose with food	Hives, itching, liver-function abnormalities, bone marrow suppression, nausea, skin rash or sores. Acute attacks of gout are a common initial reaction, but can be minimized if taken along with colchicine.	Kidney disease: concomitant, use of azathioprine or mercaptopurine. Discontinue medication at the first sign of a rash, which may indicate an allergic reaction.
Colchicine	0.6–1.2mg/day in 1–3 doses for prevention. 0.5–0.6mg every 1–2h (no more than 8 doses per day) to stop acute attacks. Take with food and encourage fluid intake.	Diarrhea, nausea, and vomiting, stomach pain	History of alcohol abuse; intestinal disease; kidney or liver disease; low white blood cell count or low platelet count
Probenecid and colchicine	1 tablet (500mg probenecid and 0.5mg colchicine) 2–3 times per day. Take with food and encourage fluid intake.	Diarrhea, nausea and vomiting, stomach pain, headache, joint pain and swelling, loss of appetite, nausea, skin rash, vomiting. Drug may interfere with urine glucose tests.	History of alcohol abuse; intestinal disease; kidney or liver disease; low white blood count; blood disease; use of antinoplastics, heparin, NSAIDs, nitrofurantoin, or zidovudine
Probenecid	500–3000mg/day in 2–3 doses. Take with food.	Headache, joint pain and swelling, loss of appetite, nausea, skin rash, vomiting. Drug may interfere with urine glucose tests.	Blood disease; kidney disease; kidney stones; use of antineoplastics, heparin, NSAIDs, nitrofurantoin or zidovudine
Sulfinpyrazone	200–800mg/day in 2–4 doses. Take with food.	Bone marrow suppression, rash, abdominal pain	Ulcers; anemia; low white blood cell count; use of other sulfa drugs, insulin or anticoagulants

Fig. 9.9 Gout medications. (Adapted with permission from Klippel JH, Weyand CM and Wortmann RL, Primer on the Rheumatic Diseases, 11E, Atlanta, GA: Arthritis Foundation, 1997.)

REGIONAL PAIN AND MONOARTICULAR DISORDERS

AN INTRODUCTION TO MONOARTICULAR JOINT PAIN

Pain in a single joint area is one of the most common forms of presentation of a musculoskeletal disorder in primary care.

One of the most important issues in diagnosis is to find out which structures are giving rise to the pain. Unfortunately, pain localization provides very little help with this, as pain that arises from the commonly affected articular or periarticular tissues is of a visceral type, and difficult to define anatomically, in contrast to the well-localized, somatic pain that arises from the skin. Furthermore, the pain may radiate, either proximally or distally, from the site of the pathology. The precise site of any local tenderness and other examination tests are a better guide to anatomic localization.

In general, regional pain originates from one of three anatomic sites:

- pain referred from another structure;
- pain that arises from periarticular tissues ('soft-tissue rheumatism');
- pain that emanates from the joints themselves, because of acute or chronic forms of arthritis.

In Section 2 of *Primary Care Rheumatology*, the common causes of pain in a single joint area are presented in two formats:

- First, the problems are considered region by region, concentrating on common disorders of the periarticular tissues.
- Second, some of the important causes of an acute monoarticular arthritis, such as gout and septic arthritis, are described.

Forms of acute or chronic monoarticular joint disease that occur principally in children or older people are dealt with in Sections 7 and 8, respectively, and other forms of chronic arthritis that can present as a monoarticular disease are covered in Sections 3 and 4.

DIAGNOSIS

Diagnosis of regional musculoskeletal pain requires two steps:

1. Rule out any dangerous or urgent 'not-to-be-missed' condition. In practice, this means either an acute, inflammatory arthritis that might be sepsis, or a severe traumatic condition in which there might be major bony or soft tissue injury.
2. Establish the anatomic structures that give rise to the pain.

This requires three areas of knowledge and/or skill:

- knowledge of what is common in different patient groups (age, sex, etc.);
- skills to examine the region adequately to define the cause of pain (the authors recommend the 'look, feel, move' approach to examination of each region);
- knowledge of what investigations are available and when they might help (in practice, investigations are rarely necessary, unless there is a risk of a serious, 'not-to-be-missed' disorder, such as acute inflammation or a fracture).

MANAGEMENT

Management of regional musculoskeletal disorders is usually straightforward, with two major principles to the management of disorders in each region:

1. Deal with the cause. Many of the common periarticular disorders are related to overuse or to some form of minor or repetitive trauma, and removal of the cause is the first step to consider.
2. Treat local inflammation if it is present – and treat it locally not systemically. Local inflammation is the pathologic cause of many periarticular disorders, in which case local rubrifacients or local injections may help, and in most instances systemic treatment is not indicated.

LAYOUT OF CHAPTERS DEALING WITH REGIONAL PAIN

The background described above explains the layout of each of the chapters dealing with regional pain. It is also appropriate to consider the diagnosis of regional pain disorders using an algorithm to remember the practical steps that need to be taken, as set out below.

There are two key diagnostic questions:

1. Is there any chance that a serious, 'not-to-be-missed' disorder is causing this patient's regional pain?
2. Where is the pain coming from – is it articular, periarticular, or referred in origin, and which structural component in or around the joint is causing the problem?

Once the diagnosis is made, a further management question that should be asked is:

- Is there an obvious, remedial cause of this patient's regional problem, such as repetitive use, overuse, injury, or some other mechanical abnormality?

DIAGNOSTIC ALGORITHM FOR MONOARTICULAR JOINT PAIN

Many patients present with pain localized to one joint site.
The first step is to rule out dangerous 'not-to-be missed' disorders.
This can be facilitated through asking two questions:

1. Is there any history of significant trauma that might have resulted in fracture or major soft-tissue injury?

2. Is there evidence of severe local inflammation (heat, redness, or marked soft-tissue swelling)?

YES | NO | NO | YES

In most cases there is no evidence of severe local inflammation, and no significant local trauma.

In such cases, the main challenge is to define the anatomic site of the lesion that is causing the monoarticular pain; this can usually be defined from the history and a careful examination of the joint.

3. Is the disorder articular or periarticular?

A radiograph should be obtained to exclude a fracture, and other specialized investigations such as arthroscopy may be necessary.

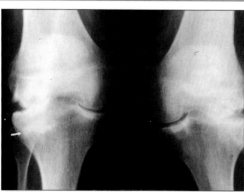

Fig. 1 Radiograph obtained to detect fracture.

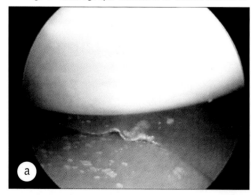

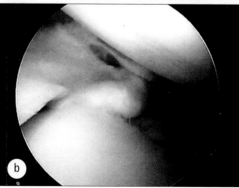

Figs 2a and b Arthroscopy if internal derangement of joint is suspected.

Results of acute joint trauma may include:

Intra-articular or periarticular fractures

Intra-articular or periarticular soft-tissue injuries, e.g. ligament rupture, capsular tear, meniscal

Synovial or bursal fluid needs to be examined from any large accumulation that can be aspirated, and examined for evidence of blood, crystals, or infectious organisms. Other specialized investigations may be needed, and synovial biospy is occasionally required to make a definitive diagnosis.

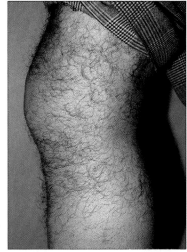

Fig. 3 Heat swelling or redness.

Causes of monoarticular joint pain with severe local inflammation include:

- Gout, pseudogout (other forms of crystal arthritis) •
Acute or chronic septic arthritis
- Traumatic arthritis
- Bleeding disorder, e.g. hemophilia
- Rare synovial disorders, e.g. foreign bodies, tumors
- Monoarticular presentations of polyarthritis

Articular disorders

Characterized by:
Tenderness over the joint line
Pain during or at the end range of movement in any direction

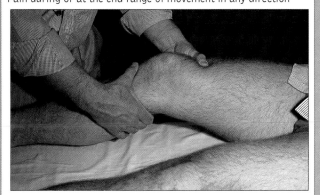

Fig. 4 The Lachman test for tears of the cruciate ligaments.

Typical disorders:
- Monoarticular osteoarthritis
- Internal mechanical derangement of the joint
- Uncommon soft-tissue or bone disorders within the joint

Periarticular disorders

Characterized by:
Point tenderness at the site of the lesion
Pain exacerbation on a particular movement

They include:
- Bursitis
- Tendinitis (and tendon-sheath inflammation)
- Ligament or capsular damage
- Enthesopathies (inflammation at tendon or ligament insertions)
- Nerve entrapment

REGIONAL PAIN AND MONOARTICULAR DISORDERS

10

PAIN IN THE SHOULDER

Pain in the shoulder region is extremely common. It may arise from the glenohumeral or acromioclavicular (AC) joints, or from periarticular structures, or it may be referred from the neck, thorax, or abdomen.

COMMON CAUSES OF SHOULDER PAIN

In practice, the most common disorders seen are periarticular conditions, especially rotator cuff lesions (tendinitis, cuff tears, or subacromial bursitis), and capsulitis (sometimes known as 'frozen shoulder'). Figure 10.1 provides a rough guide to the most common causes by age group and anatomic origin of the pain, but considerable overlap is found in the conditions between age groups. In addition, different periarticular disorders frequently coexist (capsulitis with some form of rotator cuff disease, for example). Pain can be referred to the shoulder from the neck, thorax, or abdomen.

KEY POINTS

- The most frequent causes of shoulder pain are periarticular lesions (rotator cuff tendinitis and adhesive capsulitis).
- In addition to these periarticular conditions, pain in the shoulder is often referred from the neck or other structures and can be caused by the many forms of arthritis that affect both the acromioclavicular and the glenohumeral joint.
- Most shoulder disorders can be diagnosed clinically, without the need for any investigations.
- A conservative approach to management is appropriate for most cases.
- Physical therapy, injections, and surgery are all widely used, but their value and indications for shoulder disease are controversial.

COMMON CAUSES OF SHOULDER PAIN BY AGE, AND ORIGIN AND TYPE OF PAIN			
Age (years)	Type of pain		
	Periarticular	Articular	Referred
<30	Rotator cuff (tendinitis)	Glenohumeral instability	
30–50	Capsulitis	Inflammatory arthritis	Cervical spondylosis
	Rotator cuff (tendinitis, calcific, periarthritis)	Acromioclavicular arthritis	Biliary disease
>50	Capsulitis	Glenohumeral osteoarthritis	Cervical disease
	Rotator cuff (tears)	Acromioclavicular arthritis	Lung tumors
			Subphrenic abscess

Fig. 10.1 Common causes of shoulder pain defined by age, and origin and type of pain.

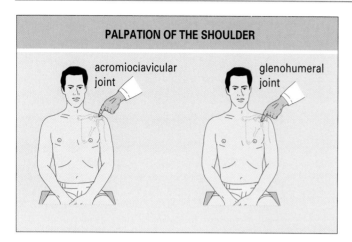

PALPATION OF THE SHOULDER

acromioclavicular joint

glenohumeral joint

Fig. 10.2 The acromioclavicular (left) and glenohumeral (right) joints can be palpated to elicit tenderness of the local joint line. One finger is pressed on the groove between the clavicle and acromion (left) or the groove between the coracoid process and humeral head (right).

EXAMINATION OF THE SHOULDER

- *Look.* Observing the patient undressing may indicate the extent of shoulder disease. The shoulder should be inspected from the anterior, posterior, and lateral aspects, particularly for swelling, deformity, and muscle wasting. Also, note the position in which the neck is held.
- *Feel.* Palpation is used to define any areas of local tenderness, and specifically the AC joint and glenohumeral joint should be palpated (Fig. 10.2).
- *Move.* Shoulder movement should be assessed as shown in Figure 10.3. True glenohumeral joint disease and capsulitis are characterized by limitation of all movements, but preferentially internal rotation is limited. Rotator cuff lesions are characterized by pain on active abduction of the shoulder, particularly in mid range (the so-called painful arc), and by pain on tests of impingement of the shoulder onto the cuff apparatus (Fig. 10.4).

Specific tendon lesions can be further defined by tests that stress individual tendons (Fig. 10.5). The neck (and in some cases the abdomen) is examined to exclude pain referred to the shoulder.

INVESTIGATIONS

Investigations are not indicated in most shoulder disorders. Only if the condition is very severe, when surgical intervention may be considered, or if there is concern about the possible diagnosis of a serious disorder, such as sepsis or tumor, should investigations be undertaken.

- The first investigation to consider is the plain radiograph. This may show evidence of arthritis of the glenohumeral or acromioclavicular joint, but can also visualize calcific tendinitis (Fig. 10.6) and provide indirect evidence of damage to the rotator cuff through upward subluxation of the humeral head.
- If surgery is being contemplated further imaging may be required to elucidate the exact anatomical abnormalities related to shoulder pain. Arthrography, arthroscopy, and magnetic resonance imaging (MRI) are available and all can show evidence of damage to soft tissues in the rotator cuff and other peri-articular structures as well as cartilage and bone lesions (Figs 10.7 & 10.8). MRI is usually the investigation of choice for patients with severe persistent shoulder pain of unknown origin.
- *If a large effusion is present* it may need aspirating so that the synovial fluid can be examined.
- *Blood tests* have no place in the investigation of shoulder pain, with the exception of bilateral shoulder pain and stiffness due to polymyalgia rheumatica, which may be confirmed by finding a very high ESR.

ASSESSMENT OF SHOULDER MOVEMENT

Active elevation	Abduction/lateral rotation	Extension/internal rotation

Maneuver	Arms in air
Assessment	Degree of elevation
Normal angle	–
Active/passive	Active

The patient is asked to place each arm together or in turn in the air as high as he/she can. Failure to achieve total elevation (in the absence of muscle paralysis) indicates limitation of glenohumeral joint motion. Where the failure appears to be the result of pain (such as a painful arc), a tendinitis may be present.

Maneuver	Hands behind head
Assessment	–
Normal angle	–
Active/passive	Active

The patient is asked to place both hands on the back of his/her neck. If they cannot reach it, then there is limitation of glenohumeral abduction and/or lateral rotation. If failure appears to result from pain, consider a painful arc caused by a supraspinatus/infraspinatus tendinitis.

Maneuver	Hands behind back
Assessment	–
Normal angle	–
Active/passive	Active

The patient is asked to place both hands behind his/her lower back region. If they cannot reach it, then there is limitation of glenohumeral extension and/or medial rotation. If failure appears to result from pain, consider a painful arc caused by a subscapularis tendinitis.

If any of these three shoulder maneuvers appears restricted, a more detailed shoulder examination is required

Glenohumeral external rotation	Glenohumeral abduction	Glenohumeral flexion

The examiner gently steadies the patient's right scapula with his left hand, while he passively rotates the patient's right shoulder laterally with his right hand, again using the humerus held vertically as the axis of rotation. The angle of lateral rotation achieved is estimated by eye. A range less than 70° indicates restricted shoulder motion.
The test is repeated on the opposite side.

The examiner gently steadies the patient's right scapula with his left hand, while he passively flexes the patient's right shoulder with his right hand, again measuring by eye the angle of flexion achieved.
The test is repeated on the opposite side.

The examiner gently steadies the patient's right scapula with his left hand, while he passively abducts the patient's right shoulder with his right hand, again measuring by eye the angle of abduction achieved.
The test is repeated on the opposite side.

Fig. 10.3 Assessment of shoulder movement.

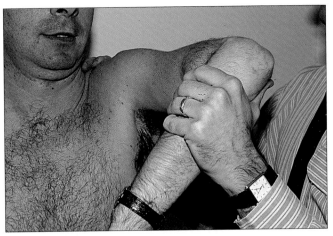

Fig. 10.4 **Rotator cuff lesions are often accompanied by painful impingement of the upwardly subluxating humerus onto the acromion.** Evidence for this as a cause of pain is elicited by impingement tests, for example by forced, passive, internal rotation and abduction of the shoulder, as shown here.

TESTS TO DETECT LESIONS OF SPECIFIC TENDONS IN AND AROUND THE ROTATOR CUFF

Tendon	Test
Supraspinatus	Resisted abduction with the arm abducted to 90°
Subscapularis	Resisted internal rotation
Infraspinatus/teres minor	Resisted external rotation
Biceps	Resisted supination with the elbow flexed to 90°

Fig. 10.5 Tests to detect lesions of specific tendons in and around the rotator cuff.

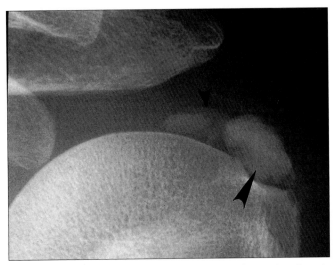

Fig. 10.6 Calcific tendinitis: formative phase (arrowhead) and resorptive phase.

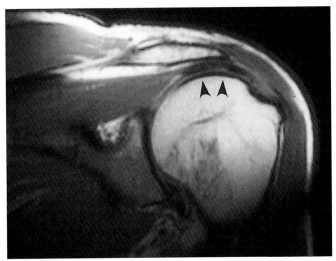

Fig. 10.7 **Rotator cuff tears can be confirmed by magnetic resonance imaging.** The image here shows a focal defect in the undersurface (arrowheads) of the supraspinatus tendon, consistent with a partial tear.

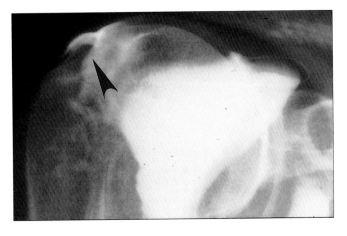

Fig. 10.8 The arthrogram illustrates leakage of the dye into the supraspinatus tendon, indicative of a partial tendon tear (arrowhead).

TYPICAL CASE: ROTATOR CUFF TENDINITIS

Jane is a 43-year-old housewife who presents with a history of gradual onset of aching pain in her right shoulder; she thinks the condition may have started to develop when she was decorating her new house, while painting ceilings. Recently, the pain has become worse, even though she has finished the decorating.

The pain is felt on the outside of her shoulder, and spreads down the lateral side of the arm to the elbow. It often wakes her at night, particularly when she rolls onto her right side. She has difficulty dressing (particularly fastening her bra) and doing anything with the arm raised.

On examination she has a painful arc, and stress tests indicate that the supraspinatus tendon is involved.

You infiltrate the area with corticosteroid and local anesthetic, and the presence of anesthetic produces immediate relief of all symptoms, which confirms that you have injected the appropriate anatomic site. You advise a period of a few days rest after the injection, and Jane's problem is solved.

OTHER ROTATOR CUFF LESIONS

TEARS

Partial rotator cuff tendon tears can occur with trauma at any age, but full-thickness tears and spontaneous tears mostly occur in older people. The symptoms are similar to those of people who have tendinitis, but, in addition, the history may be one of sudden onset associated with a specific movement or activity, and restriction of certain shoulder movements or activities. Muscle wasting may be seen.

The pathology can be confirmed using MRI, arthrography, or arthroscopy.

Partial tears can be managed conservatively with rest, and corticosteroid injections should be avoided. Complete tears can be surgically repaired, but which patients benefit from this procedure is unclear, as is when it should be carried out. Impingement is a common consequence of cuff tears.

ACUTE CALCIFIC PERIARTHRITIS

Some calcification of the rotator cuff tendons, particularly the supraspinatus, is common and often asymptomatic. Acute calcific periarthritis is an uncommon disorder caused by crystals being shed from these deposits, which results in acute severe inflammation in the rotator cuff region (Fig. 10.9).

Symptoms begin suddenly, often with no history of trauma. The shoulder quickly becomes extremely painful and tender, and redness and swelling may be present. The pain may be excruciating. The symptoms subside spontaneously within a few days, and nonsteroidal anti-inflammatory drugs (NSAIDs) or colchicine can be used to help resolution. Aspiration of the toothpaste-like material responsible is sometimes indicated, but corticosteroid injections should be avoided, as they can make the calcification worse.

Some patients suffer recurrent attacks, and sites other than the shoulder are occasionally involved.

IMPINGEMENT SYNDROME

Impingement describes a situation in which the head of the humerus comes into contact with the acromium or acromioclavicular joint. It results from loss of the supraspinatus tendon which usually separates these structures, resulting in superior migration of the humeral head on elevation and abduction with attendant pain (see Fig. 10.4), or from the presence of osteophytes on the inferior part of the acromioclavicular joint. It can cause persistent severe pain on shoulder use.

FEATURES OF ROTATOR CUFF TENDINITIS

- A spectrum of disorders affecting the rotator cuff tendons and subacromial bursa.
- The condition may present acutely in young people with glenohumeral instability (see Section 7), or with a sudden rupture in the elderly, but more commonly presents as an aching pain around the shoulder, sometimes triggered by a period of unusual activity.
- The pain is felt on the outer side of the shoulder, and may radiate down the lateral side of the arm to the elbow. It is often marked at night, is made worse by activities that involve elevation of the arm, and can restrict activities considerably.
- Rotator cuff tendinitis is often complicated by capsulitis, which is likely to develop if patients rest the arm for long periods.
- Damage to the rotator cuff may lead to upward subluxation of the humerus and impingement of this bone on the acromion (impingement syndrome).
- Careful clinical examination is usually sufficient to make an accurate diagnosis of the anatomic site involved.
- Nonsteroidal anti-inflammatory drugs and rest may help, injections of corticosteroid often improve the situation, and physical therapy can be beneficial, but treatment is difficult, and many cases persist for many months in spite of these measures.
- Persistence with an aggravating activity is likely to make treatment impossible.
- Surgery is occasionally necessary in severe cases.

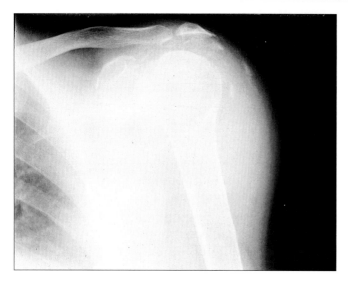

Fig. 10.9 Anteroposterior radiograph of the shoulder during an attack of severe calcific periarthritis. The deposit becomes indistinct and ill-defined as the crystals are shed into the surrounding tissues. In this elderly patient, the communication between the shoulder joint and the subacromial bursa led to a large effusion of the glenohumeral joint and a huge extension of the bursa into the upper arm, as shown by the soft-tissue swelling seen in the radiograph.

FEATURES OF ADHESIVE CAPSULITIS

- An ill-understood, ill-defined disorder.
- Rare in those under 40 years of age, and most common in women in the sixth decade of life.
- Characteristically passes through three stages – a painful phase of 3–8 months, an adhesive phase of 4–6 months, and a resolution phase of 1–3 years.
- The adhesive and resolution phases are characterized by global restriction of shoulder movements, which is the basis for diagnosis.
- Investigations are unnecessary and unhelpful.
- Treatment is difficult – corticosteroid injections, physical therapy, manipulation, and a variety of other techniques are used, with varying results.
- The majority of cases eventually resolve, and recurrence is unusual.

2 TYPICAL CASE: CAPSULITIS OF THE SHOULDER

Sally is a 62-year-old bank clerk who first noticed some shoulder discomfort 5 months ago. Although the pain was often quite severe, her activities were not restricted, and Sally took no action.

However, a few weeks before presentation she noticed that, although the pain was improving, it was becoming increasingly difficult to move the shoulder, and some work and home activities were becoming very difficult.

Examination shows severe global restriction of movements, justifying the term 'frozen shoulder'.

You explain to Sally that many treatment options are available, but the effects are limited and the condition nearly always resolves completely and spontaneously within a few months. As the pain is not too bad now, Sally decides against any treatment. You advise her about some exercises to maintain and improve movement (see Shoulder Self-Help Leaflet, page 339).

One year later, she is back to normal.

SHOULDER JOINT DISORDERS

THE ACROMIOCLAVICULAR JOINT

The acromioclavicular (AC) joint is a frequent cause of 'shoulder' pain, a condition which is often missed. In younger people, AC disease may be the result of subluxation and trauma, and in older people it is usually caused by osteoarthritis (OA), but other forms of arthritis can also affect this joint, including septic arthritis. Diagnosis is confirmed by point tenderness over the joint, and resolution of symptoms is effected by infiltration of local anesthetic. Osteolysis of the clavicle occasionally occurs.

THE GLENOHUMERAL JOINT

The shoulder joint is frequently affected by inflammatory arthropathies such as rheumatoid arthritis (RA), and effusions and painful restriction of movement (preferentially internal rotation) occur. Although OA can occur in the elderly, it is relatively uncommon. A rare, special disorder of the shoulder that occurs in elderly women is characterized by large, blood-stained effusions in the shoulder and severe bony destruction; it is sometimes known as Milwaukee shoulder. In addition, the shoulder can develop septic arthritis, particularly in drug addicts.

MANAGEMENT OF SHOULDER JOINT LESIONS

The management of common periarticular disorders of the shoulder is difficult, but fortunately most cases are self-limiting.

- *Education and self-help* are important. Being able to reassure patients that the condition is not serious, and helping to educate them on how to maintain shoulder mobility are particularly important.
- *Physical therapy* can be helpful, particularly in the mobilization of the shoulder with adhesive capsulitis, but there is a paucity of good evidence on the precise indications for physical therapy and little guidance can be given as to which patients should be referred.
- *Drugs* have some role to play. Analgesics and NSAIDs can help reduce pain from any form of shoulder disorder, particularly in the acute phase or if there is a flare of symptoms, but they should not be given over the long term.
- *Local injection therapy* is widely used (see below), although the benefits of this procedure are disputed, and, as with physical therapy, it is not clear exactly which patients are most likely to benefit. However, many practitioners believe that injections are much more likely to be of value in the early phases of a rotator cuff disorder or capsulitis, rather than in established cases.
- *Surgery* can be used for the repair of some rotator cuff lesions or severe cases of impingement or arthritis. Operations available include tendon repairs, debridement or removal of part of the acromium to relieve impingement syndrome (both of which may be done arthroscopically), or shoulder replacement.

ASPIRATION AND INJECTION TECHNIQUES FOR DISORDERS OF THE SHOULDER REGION

Injections of corticosteroids are frequently used in the treatment of rotator cuff disorders, capsulitis of the shoulder, and arthritis of both the glenohumeral and the acromioclavicular joint.

 COMPLICATIONS OF CORTICOSTEROID INJECTIONS

Any injection of corticosteroid can result in facial flushing a few hours later. This occurs in some 40% of cases and is transient and inconsequential, but it can cause concern if the patient has not been warned. A flare-up of the condition which is being treated occasionally occurs (in about 5% of cases): this develops within a few hours of the injection and lasts for up to 1–2 days.

Rarely, a corticosteroid injection results in a more serious complication such as infection, tendon rupture, skin atrophy, or joint damage. Each of these uncommon but severe complications is more likely if the technique used is poor. The following measures are recommended:

- Use a good aseptic technique to reduce the risk of infection.
- Avoid repeated injections around tendons and never inject corticosteroids into the body of a tendon, to reduce the risk of subsequent rupture.
- Do not use strong, long-acting crystalline preparations when injecting periarticular structures close to the skin, as these can cause unsightly skin atrophy.
- Avoid repeated intra-articular injections to reduce the risk of accelerated joint damage or osteonecrosis.

SUBACROMIAL BURSA AND ROTATOR CUFF REGION
Indications. Injection may be indicated in subacromial impingement and some cases of rotator cuff tendinitis and calcific periarthritis.

RECOMMENDATIONS FOR REFERRAL

Subspecialty
Referral to a rheumatologist is rarely indicated, unless an inflammatory arthritis is suspected or it is felt that an aspiration or local injection may be needed, and if you do not have sufficient familiarity or confidence with the procedure to do it yourself.

Physical therapy/rehabilitation
Patients with capsulitis should be referred to physical therapy for mobilization of the shoulder and to be taught exercises to continue with at home to maintain shoulder movement. Physiotherapists may also wish to use techniques such as interferential therapy to aid recovery. Physical therapists can also help patients with rotator cuff lesions by teaching them to use the shoulder without stressing the cuff apparatus unduly, and avoiding those mechanical stresses that may precipitate the condition.

Orthopedic surgery
Surgery is only indicated in those patients with persistent pain and/or disability caused by a structural problem around the shoulder, who have not responded to conservative therapy, including physical therapy.

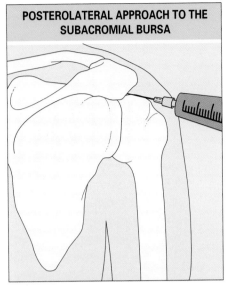

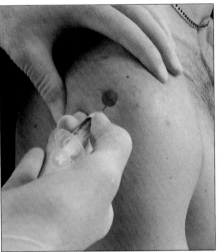

Corticosteroid dose. Methylprednisolone 30–40mg (No. 22 or No. 25 needle).
Approach. Several possible entries are available. Two are described here, the posterolateral approach and the anterior approach. Adequate muscle relaxation is important, as it allows a better palpation of the gap between the acromion and humeral head.

- Posterolateral approach. The needle is aimed anteromedially, ensuring that it passes under the acromion (Fig. 10.10). Easy flow indicates bursal injection.
- Anterior approach. A front of lidocaine (lignocaine) is required in this approach. The needle is aimed anteroposteriorly, flush with the inferior surface of the acromion, 1cm lateral to the AC joint (Fig. 10.11). Once the tough coracoacromial ligament is passed, tissue resistance to the lidocaine ceases. Easy flow indicates a bursal location of the needle.

Precautions. Use a chair with armrests, have an assistant present, and watch for fainting.

Note: Subacromial bursa injection is technically difficult, with only about 50% of injections on target. However, even if the bursal sac is not entered, the results may be excellent.

ACROMIOCLAVICULAR JOINT

Indications. Aspiration in acute arthritis; injection in OA, RA, and spondylo-arthropathy.
Corticosteroid dose. Methylprednisolone 10–20mg (No. 23 butterfly or No. 22 needle). Aspiration should be attempted before injection (for aspiration alone use a No. 20 needle).
Approach. Aim the needle perpendicular to the articular cleft, advance it by 0.5cm, and aspirate or inject to distend joint.
Precautions. The procedure is difficult because the AC joint is very narrow and has a partial meniscus. Septic AC arthritis should be suspected in drug addicts and in patients who have, or have recently had, an indwelling subclavian catheter. If sepsis is suspected, corticosteroids should not be injected.

Fig. 10.10 Posterolateral approach to the subacromial bursa.

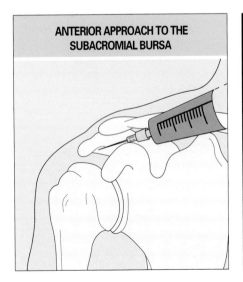

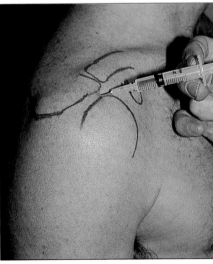

Fig. 10.11 Anterior approach to the subacromial bursa.

GLENOHUMERAL JOINT

Indications. Aspiration in acute arthritis; injection in RA, spondyloarthropathy, the initial stages of frozen shoulder, and OA.

Corticosteroid dose. Methylprednisolone 40–60mg (No. 22 needle). Aspiration should be attempted before injection. In the frozen shoulder, injection into the joint may be difficult on account of the capsular restriction. For aspiration alone use a No. 20 or larger needle.

Approach. Two entry methods are described, the posterior approach, which is often preferred because it causes less apprehension and pain, and the needle is farther away from neurovascular structures, and the anterior approach.

- Posterior approach. The patient should be sitting. The posterior margin of the acromion is palpated. The needle is then inserted posteroanteriorly 1cm below and 1cm medial to the posterior corner of the acromion, aiming toward the coracoid process until bone is touched at the articular space (Fig. 10.12).

- Anterior approach. Again, the patient should be sitting (landmarks are lost in the recumbent position), with the arm hanging at the side of the body, elbow flexed 90°, and forearm in the sagittal plane. The needle is entered antero-posteriorly 1cm distal and 1cm lateral to the coracoid process (Fig. 10.13). Prior to each advancement of the needle some lidocaine is injected, so the needle is moved through an anesthetized front. Once the bone is touched (which happens soon after the capsular toughness is felt), the forearm is very gently and passively brought into internal rotation as the needle is pushed into the articular space.

Precautions. Use a chair with armrests, have an assistant present, and watch for fainting.

Special complications. Vasovagal attacks can occur. Prior to the procedure patients should be asked about previous fainting upon venipuncture or other minor procedures – any such experience dictates a posterior approach. Misplaced anterior injections may encounter neurovascular structures, increasing the likelihood of a vasovagal attack.

Note: Glenohumeral joint aspiration may be difficult. In cases of acute arthritis in which a 'dry tap' results, the procedure should be repeated under fluoroscopic or echo control.

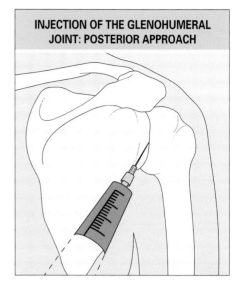

INJECTION OF THE GLENOHUMERAL JOINT: POSTERIOR APPROACH

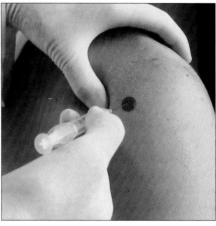

Fig. 10.12 Injection of the glenohumeral joint – posterior approach.

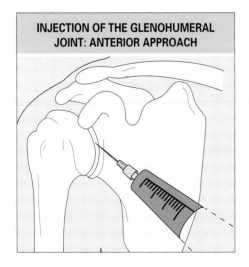

INJECTION OF THE GLENOHUMERAL JOINT: ANTERIOR APPROACH

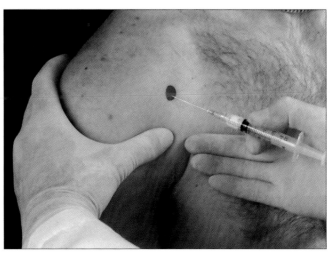

Fig. 10.13 Injection of the glenohumeral joint – anterior approach.

REGIONAL PAIN AND MONOARTICULAR DISORDERS

11

PAIN IN THE ELBOW

Pain in the elbow is common in adults, but the number of causes is limited. Diagnosis is generally simple, and is based on the pain characteristics and localization of any point tenderness or swelling. Management is largely based on physical measures (to reduce stress on the affected part) and local injection techniques. Lateral epicondylitis ('tennis elbow') is the most common condition. The main causes of elbow pain are outlined in Figure 11.1.

EXAMINATION OF THE ELBOW JOINT

Look. The elbow should be inspected anteriorly, laterally, and posteriorly, and in comparison with the contralateral elbow, for evidence of local swelling or deformity, such as an abnormal carrying angle (which can occur in syndromes such as Turner's), or a fixed-flexion deformity (an early feature of elbow arthritis).
Feel. Tenderness over the epicondyles or olecranon may indicate the presence of the common periarticular conditions. Joint tenderness can be sought by first locating the radial head, and then palpating the joint space around it during rotation of the elbow.
Move. Active and passive movements should be examined to detect abnormalities of flexion or extension, which can occur in arthritis and hypermobility (Fig. 11.2).

Evidence for pain on restricted wrist movement should be sought to diagnose lateral (resisted wrist extension) or medial (resisted wrist flexion) epicondylitis (Fig. 11.3).

NEUROLOGIC EXAMINATION AND OTHER JOINTS

The radial nerve passes just anterior to the lateral epicondyle, the ulnar nerve just behind the lateral epicondyle, and the medial nerve anterior to the joint line. All can be involved in severe elbow disease.

The neck and shoulder need examination to rule out referred pain.

KEY POINTS

- Elbow pain is common, and usually is caused by lateral or medical epicondylitis (tennis or golfer's elbow) or olecranon bursitis.
- Less commonly, elbow pain is referred from the neck or shoulder, or is caused by arthritis of the elbow joint.
- Diagnosis is easy on clinical grounds, and is based mainly on the localization of any tenderness or swelling, and the presence of pain exacerbated by movements that stress the medial or lateral epicondyle.
- Investigations are unnecessary.
- Management is relatively simple and is based on the use of splints to reduce stress on the epicondyles, or local injection therapy.

MAIN CAUSES OF ELBOW PAIN	
Periarticular disorders:	Lateral epicondylitis Medial epicondylitis Olecranon bursitis
Articular:	Inflammatory arthritis Osteoarthritis (relatively uncommon)
Referred:	From the shoulder or neck

Fig. 11.1 The main causes of elbow pain.

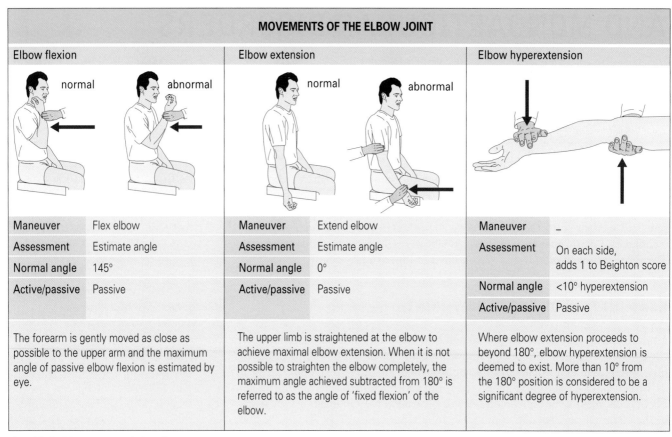

MOVEMENTS OF THE ELBOW JOINT		
Elbow flexion	**Elbow extension**	**Elbow hyperextension**
normal abnormal	normal abnormal	
Maneuver — Flex elbow	Maneuver — Extend elbow	Maneuver — –
Assessment — Estimate angle	Assessment — Estimate angle	Assessment — On each side, adds 1 to Beighton score
Normal angle — 145°	Normal angle — 0°	Normal angle — <10° hyperextension
Active/passive — Passive	Active/passive — Passive	Active/passive — Passive
The forearm is gently moved as close as possible to the upper arm and the maximum angle of passive elbow flexion is estimated by eye.	The upper limb is straightened at the elbow to achieve maximal elbow extension. When it is not possible to straighten the elbow completely, the maximum angle achieved subtracted from 180° is referred to as the angle of 'fixed flexion' of the elbow.	Where elbow extension proceeds to beyond 180°, elbow hyperextension is deemed to exist. More than 10° from the 180° position is considered to be a significant degree of hyperextension.

Fig. 11.2 Movements of the elbow joint.

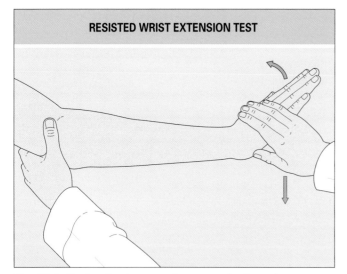

RESISTED WRIST EXTENSION TEST

Fig. 11.3 Resisted wrist extension to test for lateral epicondylitis. The examiner asks the patient to try to extend the wrist, but prevents movement by fixing the wrist; this puts tension on the lateral epicondyle without moving the elbow and reproduces the pain of lateral epicondylitis.

INVESTIGATIONS

Investigation is not generally necessary. If there is a major mechanical problem with the elbow, such as locking or severe restriction of movement, there may be arthritis, osteochondritis, loose bodies or a fracture – each of which can be visualized by a plain radiograph. If there is a large, warm effusion in the olecranon bursa, there may be a risk of sepsis or crystal synovitis, and these can only be diagnosed by aspirating the fluid for *synovial fluid examination* including staining for bacteria, culture and polarized light microscopy.

1 ## TYPICAL CASE: LATERAL EPICONDYLITIS OF THE ELBOW

Sue is a 41-year-old accountant who is generally fit and well, but is currently off work and at home looking after her 6-month-old first-born son, Pete.

She first noticed the gradual onset of discomfort around her right elbow 6 weeks ago. This gradually worsened, the pain spreading into her forearm, and for the past 4 weeks it has been extremely uncomfortable to carry anything in her right hand. This is causing increasing difficulty in looking after Pete. She wants help, quickly.

Careful questioning reveals that the pain is more on the outside than the inside of the elbow, that there has been no swelling, and that she is otherwise fine, with no further musculoskeletal or other type of problems, and no shoulder or neck pain.

On examination, you find severe local tenderness over the lateral epicondyle, and you can exacerbate the pain with resisted wrist extension (see Fig. 11.3).

You diagnose 'tennis elbow' (lateral epicondylitis) in spite of the fact that Sue has never played tennis in her life.

As Sue needs quick relief you inject the area (see below) as well as providing a forearm splint. Within a few days the problem has resolved.

OTHER COMMON CAUSES OF ELBOW PAIN

Referred pain from the shoulder or neck can cause elbow symptoms – look for restriction of movement of the neck or shoulder, and movement of these areas causing the elbow pain.

Other periarticular disorders frequently cause elbow pain, particularly medial epicondylitis and olecranon bursitis (Fig. 11.4). Medial epicondylitis (or golfer's elbow) is very similar to tennis elbow, but less common, and localized to the medial epicondyle. Olecranon bursitis is a common inflammatory bursitis that can result from trauma, or from part of an inflammatory arthropathy such as rheumatoid arthritis (Fig. 11.5) or gout; occasionally, it is septic. Localized tenderness and swelling over the olecranon bursa are the characteristic features.

FEATURES OF LATERAL EPICONDYLITIS

- Lateral epicondylitis ('tennis elbow') is the commonest cause of elbow pain, affecting 1–3% of the population, both sexes, and being seen most frequently in patients between 40 and 60 years of age (it is rare in those younger than 30 years of age).
- Onset is usually insidious and unconnected with any trauma or activity, although those who play a lot of racket sports are frequently affected.
- Pain is maximal around the lateral epicondyle, but can spread up and down the arm.
- Grip is impaired because of pain, which results in various degrees of disability.
- Resisted wrist extension exacerbates the pain (see Fig. 11.3).

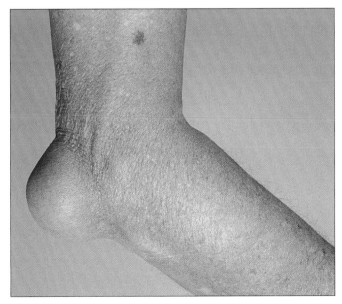

Fig. 11.4 Olecranon bursitis. A soft, sometimes tender swelling over the tip of the elbow.

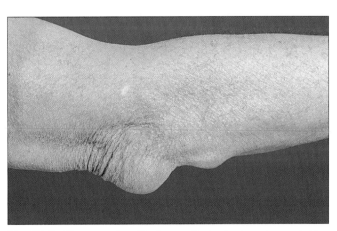

Fig. 11.5 Olecranon bursitis in a patient who has rheumatoid arthritis. A rheumatoid nodule is also shown.

Inflammatory arthritis of the elbow can occur in any of the inflammatory poly-arthritides, and may result in severe joint damage.

Osteoarthritis of the elbow is relatively uncommon, and largely affects men.

In children, trauma or overuse (especially in teenagers involved in throwing sports) can cause osteochondritis of the radial head, and traumatic partial sub-luxation of the radial head can occur in those who have joint hypermobility.

 MANAGEMENT

Medial and lateral epicondylitis can be treated by using forearm splints that reduce the pressure on the relevant muscle origins, by ultrasound, or by local injections of corticosteroids (see below).

INJECTIONS AROUND THE ELBOW REGION

Injection of corticosteroids is frequently used to treat medial or lateral epi-condylitis, olecranon bursitis or elbow joint lesions.

! COMPLICATIONS OF CORTICOSTEROID INJECTIONS

Any injection of corticosteroid can result in facial flushing a few hours later. This occurs in some 40% of cases and is transient and inconsequential, but it can cause concern if the patient has not been warned. A flare-up of the condition which is being treated occasionally occurs (in about 5% of cases): this occurs within a few hours of the injection and lasts for up to 1–2 days.

Rarely, a corticosteroid injection results in a more serious complication such as infection, tendon rupture, skin atrophy or joint damage. Each of these uncommon but severe complications is more likely if the technique used is poor:

- Use a good aseptic technique to reduce the risk of infection.
- Avoid repeated injections around tendons and never inject corticosteroids into the body of a tendon to reduce the risk of subsequent rupture.
- Do not use strong, long-acting crystalline preparations when injecting periarticular structures close to the skin, as these can cause unsightly skin atrophy.
- Avoid repeated intra-articular injections to reduce the risk of accelerated joint damage or osteonecrosis.

TENNIS ELBOW

Indications. Failure of conservative treatment.

Corticosteroid dose. Methylprednisolone 10–20mg (No. 22 needle).

Approach. At the most tender point (Fig. 11.6). Pass the needle to periosteal contact and infiltrate with 2–3ml lido-caine (lignocaine). Failure to eradicate pain on resisted wrist dorsiflexion indicates the wrong injection site – reposition the needle and reinfiltrate with lidocaine. The corticosteroid should be infiltrated deeply, at the tenoperiosteal junction.

Precautions. Avoid injecting too superficially.

Special complications. Transient increase in pain in 40% of patients. Repeated corticosteroid infiltrations may result in

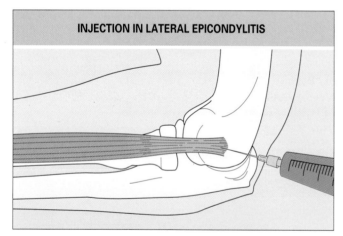
INJECTION IN LATERAL EPICONDYLITIS

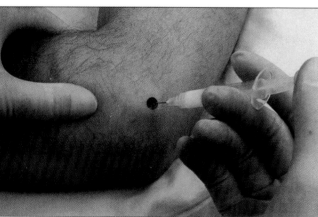

Fig. 11.6 Injection of corticosteroid and local anesthetic into the common extensor tendon origin at the lateral humeral epicondyle.

chronic pain, and skin atrophy is common if the injection is place too superficially.

Note: The current trend is to be conservative, and avoid infiltrations.

Lack of improvement with lidocaine infiltration suggests an alternative diagnosis, such as compressive neuropathy of the deep branch of the radial nerve or cervical radiculopathy.

ELBOW JOINT

Indications. Aspiration in acute arthritis, injection in rheumatoid arthritis and psoriatic arthritis.

Corticosteroid dose. Methylprednisolone 30–40mg (No. 22 needle). Aspiration should be attempted before injection. For aspiration alone use a No. 20 or No. 18 needle, depending on the suspected diagnosis.

Approach. Three entries are commonly used. For all entries the elbow is held flexed at 90°.

- Posterior approach. The depression in the midline between the two halves of the triceps tendon is palpated at the back of the elbow. The needle is passed perpendicular to the skin into the olecranon fossa (Fig. 11.7).
- Inferolateral approach. The midpoint cleft between the olecranon tip and the lateral epicondyle is palpated. The needle is inserted perpendicularly, aiming at the center of the joint.
- Lateral approach. The radiocapitular joint may be entered from the side, just proximal to the radial head. The needle is passed tangentially between the two bones, rather than directly (Fig. 11.8).

Precautions. No neurovascular structures are in the vicinity.

Complications. None.

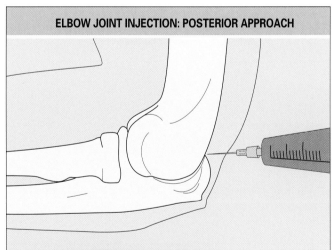

ELBOW JOINT INJECTION: POSTERIOR APPROACH

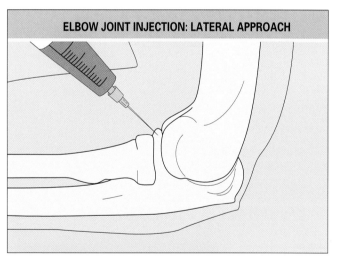

ELBOW JOINT INJECTION: LATERAL APPROACH

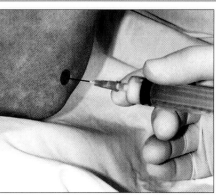

Fig. 11.7 Elbow joint injection: posterior approach.

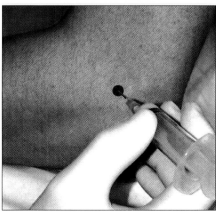

Fig. 11.8 Elbow joint injection: lateral approach.

Referral is rarely necessary.

Physical therapy/rehabilitation

Physiotherapists may help with the provision of splints for tennis elbow, and education about avoidance of activities that might be exacerbating elbow problems.

Subspecialty

Referral to rheumatology or orthopedic surgery may be considered in severe intractable cases, when conservative therapy has failed.

OLECRANON BURSA

Indications. For the diagnosis of effusion and for treatment of aseptic bursitis (traumatic or idiopathic) in cases that are refractory to conservative treatment. A negative bursal fluid culture is required for the procedure to be performed.

Corticosteroid dose. Methylprednisolone acetate 20mg (No. 22 needle). Aspiration should be attempted before injection. For aspiration alone use a No. 20 needle.

Approach. Lateral through normal skin, aiming at the center of the bursa.

Precautions. Taps at the tip of the bursa may create a chronic leak. Medial entries may damage the ulnar nerve.

Note: In traumatic or idiopathic olecranon bursitis, conservative treatment is recommended, namely to avoid leaning on the elbow, for 3 months. Intrabursal corticosteroids may be tried in cases that fail to resolve.

REGIONAL PAIN AND MONOARTICULAR DISORDERS

12

PAIN IN THE WRIST AND HAND

The hand has been called the 'patient's calling card' by rheumatologists, because examination of the patterns of skin, joint, and other changes in the hand provides so much information as to the diagnosis, activity and severity of rheumatic diseases. Most forms of arthritis affect the hand; some of the specific patterns of involvement are outlined in Chapter 3 (Pattern recognition).

Pain in the wrist and hand can be caused by arthritis of the wrist or small joints of the hand or by periarticular disorders, and it can be referred from the neck. The focus of this chapter is the common periarticular disorders.

Common causes of wrist and hand pain are summarized in Figure 12.1.

EXAMINATION

Look. The patient is asked to hold their hands out in front of them, backs up; examine carefully for joint or periarticular swellings, and for any skin disorder. After asking them to turn the hands over (noting any trouble with supination), examine the palmar aspect. Next ask the patient to make a fist, noting any pain, difficulty, or restriction of movement.
Feel. Palpate the joints for signs of tenderness and swelling, and also palpate any other swellings, for example in the palmar fascia. Squeeze across the metacarpophalangeal joints (Fig. 12.2), as this is the most sensitive way to detect

KEY POINTS

- Common periarticular causes of pain in the wrist and hand, include de Quervain's tenosynovitis, trigger finger, carpal tunnel syndrome, and Dupuytren's contracture.
- These conditions can be diagnosed clinically, and investigations are unnecessary.
- They need to be differentiated from arthritis of the wrist of hand, and from referred causes of wrist and hand pain.
- These disorders are often related to overuse, and one treatment option is to change behavior to prevent the activities that cause the problem.
- Other treatment options include temporary splinting to rest overused structures, other forms of physical therapy, local injections, and surgery.
- Referral is reserved for patients with suspected inflammatory arthritis or patients who are being considered for surgery (i.e. those who have severe intractable pain or functional problems), or if an injection is indicated but the general physician is not able to carry this out.

COMMON CAUSES OF WRIST AND HAND PAIN	
Pain type	Cause
Arthritis	See Chapter 3 (Pattern recognition) and chapters on specific diseases
Periarthritis:	
Tendinitis	De Quervain's tendinitis Trigger finger
Fasciitis	Dupuytren's contracture
Nerve entrapment	Carpal tunnel syndrome
Referred pain	Cervical spine disorders Cardiac Shoulder–hand syndrome Bone and vascular lesions

Fig. 12.1 Common causes of wrist and hand pain.

COMPOSITE COMPRESSION TEST

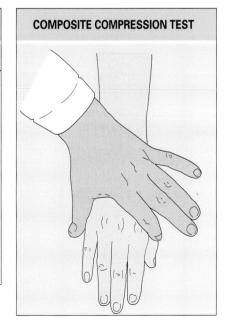

Fig. 12.2 The 'composite compression' test to elicit tenderness in a group of small joints. A gentle squeeze is applied across the knuckles. If pain is elicited, this indicates that one or more of the joints encompassed is inflamed. Each one can be palpated individually to determine the culprit.

MOVEMENTS OF THE WRISTS AND FINGERS

Finger flexion (MCPs, PIPs, DIPs)

Maneuver	Make a fist
Assessment	Ability/inability to embed finger tips into palm
Normal angle	–
Active/passive	Active

The patient is asked to make a fist and to try to bury the fingers in the palm. With the volar aspect uppermost the observer can immediately see if one or more fingers fail to reach the palm, indicating that a reduced range of flexion exists in one or more small finger joints (MCPs, PIPs, or DIPs) of the respective digit(s). There is simultaneous assessment of joint swelling, redness, tenderness on palpation and whether movement elicits pain.

Finger extension (MCPs, PIPs, DIPs)

Maneuver	Prayer sign
Assessment	Contact of digits
Normal angle	–
Active/passive	Active

The patient is asked to place the palms of both hands together in the position of prayer. Full small finger joint extension is denoted by complete contact of all digits along their whole length. When a gap remains between the fingers, this indicates the presence of fixed flexion, affecting one or more small finger joints in the affected finger(s).

Finger hyperextension, fifth MCP >90°

Maneuver	–
Assessment	On each side, adds 1 to Beighton score
Normal angle	<90°
Active/passive	Passive

With the hand placed flat on a table, the little finger is gently extended as far as it will go, short of causing pain. If an angle of 90° of extension or more is achieved, the fifth MCP is deemed to be hypermobile.

Wrist flexion

Maneuver	Bend wrist palmarly
Assessment	Estimate angle
Normal angle	60–90
Active/passive	Passive

With the forearm outstretched, the hand is gently coaxed downward until the maximal range of wrist flexion is achieved, short of causing pain. The angle achieved is estimated by eye.
There is simultaneous assessment of joint swelling, redness, tenderness on palpation and whether the movement elicits pain.

Wrist extension

Maneuver	Bend wrist dorsally
Assessment	Estimate angle
Normal angle	60–90°
Active/passive	Passive

With the forearm outstretched, the hand is gently coaxed upward until the maximal range of wrist extension is achieved, short of causing pain. The angle achieved is estimated by eye.

Thumb apposition to volar aspect of wrist

Maneuver	–
Assessment	On each side, adds 1 to Beighton score
Normal angle	–
Active/passive	Passive

The thumb is passively moved toward the volar aspect of the forearm. Where contact is made the thumb–wrist complex is deemed to demonstrate hypermobility.

Fig. 12.3 Movements of the wrist and fingers. (MCP, metacarpophalangeal; PIP, proximal interphalangeal; DIP, distal interphalangeal.)

inflammation of these joints, which occurs as an early feature of diseases such as rheumatoid arthritis.

Move. Examine the range of movement of the wrist and fingers, as shown in Figure 12.3.

INVESTIGATIONS

Special investigations are rarely needed. If arthritis is suspected a plain radiograph may be indicated – however, it is important to note that the definitive features of arthritis do not appear on the radiograph until the disease has been present for many months – so an X-ray is no help in early diagnosis. If difficulty is encountered in the diagnosis of a possible nerve entrapment syndrome, nerve conduction studies may be indicated.

 TYPICAL CASE: DE QUERVAIN'S TENOSYNOVITIS

Richard is a 41-year-old bank clerk who does a lot of bowling. He has had months of discomfort around his right wrist, worsening on activity, and now comes to see you because the pain is becoming increasingly problematic and interfering with his bowling scores.

On examination, you notice a visible swelling of the affected tendon sheaths (Fig. 12.4), and on palpation the area is tender.

Your initial treatment with a splint and course of non-steroidal anti-inflammatory drugs proves unhelpful. You then inject the area with local corticosteroid (see below), which cures the problem.

FEATURES OF DE QUERVAIN'S TENOSYNOVITIS

- Tendinitis of the abductor pollicis longus and extensor pollicis brevis.
- Common, particularly in women in the age range 30–50 years.
- Usually related to overuse or repetitive trauma (previously known as 'nappy wrist').
- Presents with pain, on activity, over the radial side of the wrist.
- Tenderness, and sometimes swelling, of the affected tendon sheaths.
- May respond to alterations of activity, splinting, and local treatment.
- Responds well to local infiltration of corticosteroids.

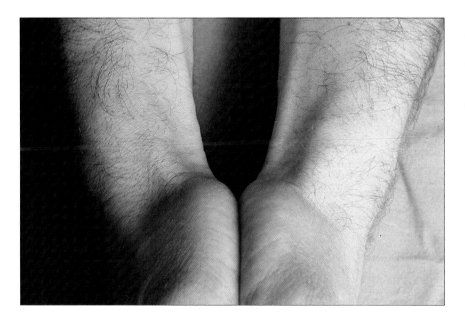

Fig. 12.4 De Quervain's tenosynovitis. Note the swelling caused by the tenosynovitis of abductor pollicis longus and extensor pollicis brevis of the left wrist.

FEATURES OF TRIGGER FINGER (OR THUMB)

- Stenosing tendinitis of the flexor tendons of the finger or thumb.
- Common condition, usually associated with overuse, particularly with activities that involve gripping.
- Presents with discomfort in the palm on usage.
- As the condition develops, the affected finger or thumb starts to catch, and becomes stuck in the flexed position.
- As the digit is straightened out, the patient may feel a painful pop or catching sensation.
- Palpation may reveal thickening of the tendon sheath, nodule formation, or crepitus.
- Can be treated with alteration of activities and splintage.
- Often responds well to local injection of corticosteroid.

FEATURES OF CARPAL TUNNEL SYNDROME

- Most common entrapment neuropathy in the body.
- Caused by pressure on the median nerve in front of the wrist.
- Most common in women of middle age, and most commonly affects the dominant hand.
- Can be caused by a large number of possible lesions around the wrist joint, including any form of arthritis; also associated with some metabolic disorders and other conditions, including pregnancy.
- Often related to overuse, as in musicians and keyboard workers.
- Causes an aching discomfort in the wrist and hand, which may spread up the forearm.
- Patients may develop paresthesia and numbness in the distribution of the median nerve, although these symptoms do not always fit the expected nerve distribution.
- Characteristic, distressing symptom is pain and paresthesia at night, which disturbs sleep.
- Signs may include sensory loss in the nerve distribution and, in advanced cases, wasting and weakness of the thenar eminence, as well as positive Tinel's sign and Phalen's maneuver.
- Wrist splinting, especially at night, is helpful.
- Often responds well to local corticosteroid injection.
- Surgical decompression is needed for severe or intractable cases, and should be considered if any motor signs (wasting and weakness) are present.

2 TYPICAL CASE: TRIGGER FINGER

Tony is a 48-year-old plumber who complains that the second finger of his right hand often becomes stuck down, and that he has to force it straight, which causes him pain. The problem began some weeks ago, soon after he took on a special job that involved much more lifting and carrying than usual for him.

On examination you note the characteristic flexion deformity of the finger (Fig. 12.5), and on palpation a tender nodule on the flexor tendon sheath is obvious, just proximal to the metacarpophalangeal joint.

You inject the area with corticosteroid (see below), with good results.

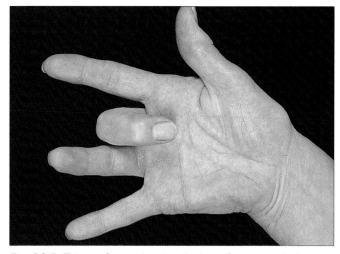

Fig. 12.5 Trigger finger showing the long finger caught in flexion. The patient was able to straighten the finger with force and an audible click could be felt and heard.

3 TYPICAL CASE: CARPAL TUNNEL SYNDROME

Erica is a 38-year-old secretary who does a lot of keyboard work. During her first pregnancy, 3 years ago, she first developed carpal tunnel syndrome (CTS) in her right hand. The same symptoms have recurred. The most troublesome symptom is the pain at night which wakes her – she has to hang her arm out of the bed or shake it to relieve the discomfort. She also has discomfort and tingling in her index finger and thumb during the day when working on the keyboard, and the aching sometimes spreads up her forearm.

Examination shows some reduced sensation in the distribution of the median nerve (Fig. 12.6), and both Tinel's sign and Phalen's maneuver are positive (Figs 12.7 and 12.8). No other abnormal signs or symptoms are found.

You diagnose CTS related to work, but not associated with any other disorder. You provide her with a wrist splint to use at night, which helps for a while, but the symptoms worsen, so you inject the carpal tunnel area with corticosteroid (see below), which relieves Erica's problem.

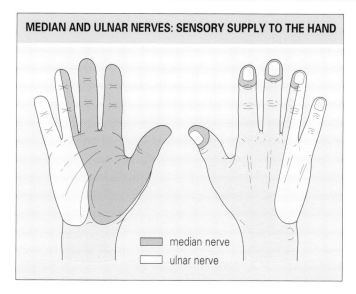

MEDIAN AND ULNAR NERVES: SENSORY SUPPLY TO THE HAND

median nerve
ulnar nerve

Fig. 12.6 Median and ulnar nerve innervation of the hand. The radial three digits and half of the ring finger are supplied by sensory branches of the median nerve. The fifth finger and half of the ring finger are supplied by sensory branches of the ulnar nerve.

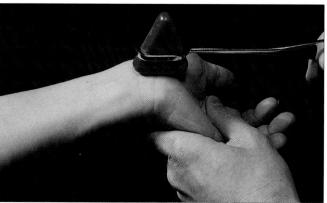

Fig. 12.7 Tinel's sign. The wrist is held in extension while gentle percussion is performed over and just proximal to the transverse carpal ligament.

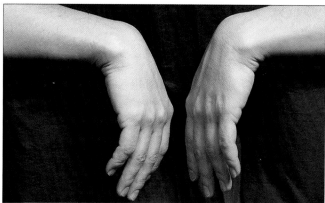

Fig. 12.8 Phalen's (wrist flexion) maneuver. With the wrists held in unforced flexion for 30–60s, a positive test reproduces or worsens the patient's symptoms.

TYPICAL CASE: DUPUYTREN'S CONTRACTURE

Andrew is a fit 47-year-old banker who has noticed that the little finger of his hand seems to be becoming bent. On examination you notice the flexion deformity (Fig. 12.9), and obvious thickening of the fascia is found on palpation. On direct questioning, Andrew remembers that his father had a similar problem.

You explain the nature of the condition to Andrew; it needs no treatment, but Andrew should keep stretching his finger to prevent the condition from becoming worse.

℞ MANAGEMENT OF PERIARTICULAR WRIST AND HAND PROBLEMS

Most of the common periarticular disorders of the hand and wrist are related to overuse. The types of recurrent activity that are causing the problem may be obvious, in which case education and advice to help patients alter their behavior appropriately may cure the problem.

FEATURES OF DUPUYTREN'S CONTRACTURE

- Nodular thickening of the palmar fascia, which draws one or more fingers into flexion contracture.
- Most common in men and on the ulnar side of the hand, often bilateral.
- Fibrous nodules can be felt in the fascia.
- Has a genetic component, is more common in men than women, and incidence rises with increasing age.
- The cause is unknown – various associations have been suggested, but the vast majority of cases are idiopathic.
- Runs a variable course.
- Often needs no treatment (other than stretching the fingers to reduce the rate of progressive flexion), but this depends on severity and rate of progression.
- Advanced or severe disease can be treated surgically, but there is a risk of recurrence, particularly in younger people and those who have bilateral disease.

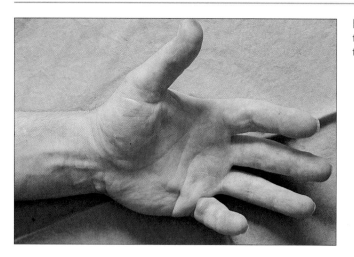

Fig. 12.9 Dupuytren's contracture of the palmar fascia. Note the thickening of the fascia in the palm and the contracture of the little finger.

Overuse problems of this sort can be treated by resting the affected structures, and splinting can be particularly valuable for de Quervain's tenosynovitis, trigger finger, and CTS (when a wrist splint worn at night is often an effective intervention). In contrast, Dupuytren's contracture may benefit from stretching exercises to help prevent progression of the contracture. Other physical techniques such as ultrasound can be of value in some difficult cases of tendinitis.

Drugs have little or no place in the treatment of these disorders, with the exception of the local injection techniques described below.

Surgery can be considered for any of these conditions if they are particularly troublesome. It is rarely necessary to operate on de Quervain's tenosynovitis or trigger finger, but in occasional cases the disorders cause such functional difficulty as to warrant this intervention. In CTS, surgery should be considered if motor signs are present, or in anybody who has severe pain and paresthesia unresponsive to other treatments (splints or injection). Dupuytren's contracture can also be treated surgically, although recurrence is common after the procedure.

INJECTION THERAPY FOR THESE COMMON WRIST AND HAND DISORDERS

Injections are commonly used for these disorders.

 COMPLICATIONS OF CORTICOSTEROID INJECTIONS

Any injection of corticosteroid can result in facial flushing a few hours later. This occurs in some 40% of cases and is transient and inconsequential, but it can cause concern if the patient has not been warned. A flare-up of the condition which is being treated occasionally occurs (in about 5% of cases): this occurs within a few hours of the injection and lasts for up to 1–2 days.

Rarely, a corticosteroid injection results in a more serious complication such as infection, tendon rupture, skin atrophy or joint damage. Each of these uncommon but severe complications is more likely if the technique used is poor:
- Use a good aseptic technique to reduce the risk of infection.
- Avoid repeated injections around tendons and never inject corticosteroids into the body of a tendon to reduce the risk of subsequent rupture.
- Do not use strong, long-acting crystalline preparations when injecting periarticular structures close to the skin, as these can cause unsightly skin atrophy.
- Avoid repeated intra-articular injections to reduce the risk of accelerated joint damage or osteonecrosis.

DE QUERVAIN'S TENOSYNOVITIS

Indications. Most instances of inflammation of the common sheath of the abductor pollicis longus and extensor pollicis brevis result from hand overuse. Corticosteroid injections are highly successful in these cases if there is failure of symptom improvement with alterations of activity and splinting.

Corticosteroid dose. Methylprednisolone acetate 20–30mg (No. 25 needle).

Approach. The needle is aimed toward the radial styloid, which underlies the sheath. The needle is then pulled back in millimeter stages and injection attempted. Successful injection distends the sheath distally to the metacarpal base.

Precautions. Make sure that the corticosteroid remains within the sheath. Do not infiltrate grossly thickened sheaths, as mycobacterial infection may be present.

Special complications. Skin hypopigmentation frequently complicates this procedure. Skin atrophy, leading to recurring ecchymosis, is particularly prevalent in elderly patients.

FLEXOR TENDON SHEATHS

Indications. Injection in trigger finger; flexor tenosynovitis in rheumatoid arthritis and psoriatic arthritis.

Corticosteroid dose. Methylprednisolone 15–20mg mixed with lidocaine (lignocaine) 1–2ml; (No. 25 or No. 27 needle, or No. 23 butterfly).

Approach. Just distal to palmar crease (thumb), proximal palmar crease (index finger), distal palmar crease (long, ring, and little fingers) with needle held at a 45° distal inclination (Fig. 12.10).

Precautions. Avoid intratendinous injection. Reciprocal needle movements upon gentle finger motion indicate tendon engagement; withdraw needle in millimeter stages, free the needle and inject. Up to three injections given 3 weeks apart are allowed.

Special complications. Superficial extravasation may produce asymptomatic, focal, palmar fat atrophy. Large published series comment on a lack of tendon rupture and iatrogenic infection.

CARPAL TUNNEL SYNDROME

Indications. Injection treatment can be helpful in all etiologies of CTS, except acute cases caused by fracture, hemorrhage, infection, and CTS of late pregnancy. However, conservative therapy (splints and avoidance of precipitating activities) should be attempted first.

Corticosteroid dose. Methylprednisolone 30–40mg, mixed with lidocaine (lignocaine) 2–3ml (No. 22 or No. 25 needle, or No. 23 butterfly).

Approach. Just distal to the distal wrist crease and just medial to palmaris longus (PL) tendon (Fig. 12.11). If the PL tendon is absent (25% of people lack the PL tendon), use the midline. The needle is inserted to a depth of 1cm with a 45° distal inclination and a 45° lateral inclination.

Precautions. Paresthesias indicate median nerve engagement; if they are severe, reposition the needle or abort the procedure. Reciprocal needle motion upon gentle finger motion (which should be rehearsed beforehand) indicates tendon engagement; again, reposition the needle.

Special complications: Temporary increases in parasthesiae may occur even when the injection is correctly positioned.

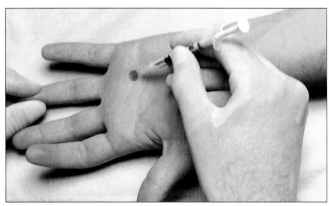

INJECTION OF THE FLEXOR DIGITAL TENDON SHEATH IN TRIGGER FINGER

flexor tendon sheath

proximal pulley

Fig. 12.10 Injection of the flexor digital tendon sheath in trigger finger.

INJECTION OF THE CARPAL TUNNEL

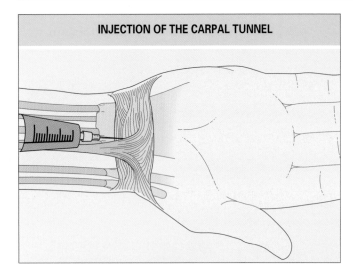

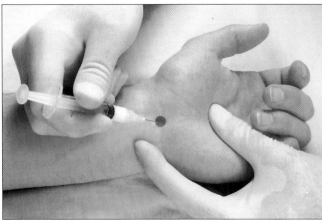

Fig. 12.11 Injection of the carpal tunnel.

RECOMMENDATIONS FOR REFERRAL

Subspecialty

If you are suspicious of early inflammatory arthritis (such as early rheumatoid arthritis), referral to a rheumatologist for definitive diagnosis and the establishment of a treatment plan is indicated. If there is a joint or periarticular problem that you feel may benefit from an injection, but you are not familiar or confident with the procedure, you may refer for treatment.

Physical therapy/rehabilitation

Physical modalities can be of great help in the treatment of tendinitis – ultrasound and splintage can be useful in acute stages, and mobilizing exercises may help those who have developed contractures. Splints can be of value if there are functional problems.

Orthopedic surgery

Surgical treatment is indicated in cases of tendinitis or carpal tunnel syndrome with severe longstanding pain and/or functional problems that have not responded to conservative therapy. In addition, some cases of carpal tunnel syndrome with very severe pain (in pregnancy for example) warrant urgent decompression, and patients with motor signs should be referred for surgical decompression.

REGIONAL PAIN AND MONOARTICULAR DISORDERS

13

PAIN IN THE HIP

Hip problems are common at all ages. Although a large number of causes are possible, only a small number are common – in young and middle-aged adults, trochanteric bursitis and osteoarthritis (OA) predominate, and in the elderly femoral neck fractures are common.

COMMON CAUSES OF HIP PAIN

Pain in the hip region may be referred from the spine or abdomen, originate from osseous lesions, such as fractures or osteonecrosis, arise from periarticular tissues (principally bursae), or derive from the hip joint itself (principally OA; Fig. 13.1).

PAIN LOCALIZATION AND PATTERNS

'Hip pain' covers a number of different locations and patterns of pain. Resolution of the different pain patterns, including the factors that exacerbate or relieve hip pain (exacerbation of OA hip pain by exercise, for example), is a major step to diagnosis (Fig. 13.2).

KEY POINTS

- Hip pain is common in all age groups.
- Pain may be referred from the spine or intra-abdominal structures, arise from periarticular tendons or bursae, or result from hip pathology. These causes can generally be differentiated on clinical examination, although a plane radiograph may be necessary to help define hip joint pathology.
- The most common causes in adults are trochanteric bursitis and osteoarthritis of the hip.
- Periarticular problems can be treated simply by rest and removal of any mechanical cause, or by local injection therapy.
- Treatment of osteoarthritis of the hip is similar to that described for the knee joint, but anyone who has severe pain or disability ('cannot sleep, cannot walk, or cannot work') caused by hip disease should be considered for joint replacement surgery.

COMMON CAUSES OF HIP PAIN		
Intra-articular	Periarticular	Referred
Osteoarthritis	Trochanteric bursitis	Thoracolumbar spine
Osteonecrosis	Adductor tendinitis	Intra-abdominal
	Nerve entrapment (meralgia paresthetica)	
	Fractured neck of femur	
	Paget's and other bone diseases	

Fig. 13.1 Common causes of hip pain.

PAIN LOCALIZING TO DIFFERENT AREAS AROUND THE HIP	
Region of pain	Cause of pain – main (less common)
Lateral pain	Trochanteric bursitis (hip pathology, thoracolumbar disease)
Groin pain	Hip pathology – pain often radiates anteriorly to the knee (bursitis, tendinitis, hernias)
Buttock pain	Thoracolumbar disease, ischiogluteal bursitis, sacroiliac joint (hip pathology)

Fig. 13.2 Pain localizing to different areas around the hip. Main and less common causes.

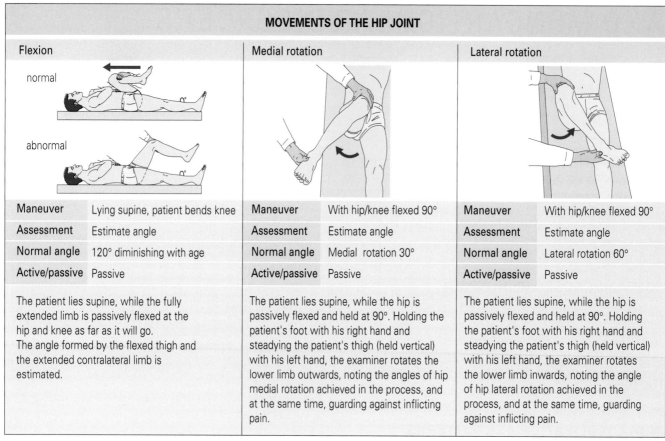

MOVEMENTS OF THE HIP JOINT		
Flexion	**Medial rotation**	**Lateral rotation**
normal / abnormal		
Maneuver — Lying supine, patient bends knee	**Maneuver** — With hip/knee flexed 90°	**Maneuver** — With hip/knee flexed 90°
Assessment — Estimate angle	**Assessment** — Estimate angle	**Assessment** — Estimate angle
Normal angle — 120° diminishing with age	**Normal angle** — Medial rotation 30°	**Normal angle** — Lateral rotation 60°
Active/passive — Passive	**Active/passive** — Passive	**Active/passive** — Passive
The patient lies supine, while the fully extended limb is passively flexed at the hip and knee as far as it will go. The angle formed by the flexed thigh and the extended contralateral limb is estimated.	The patient lies supine, while the hip is passively flexed and held at 90°. Holding the patient's foot with his right hand and steadying the patient's thigh (held vertical) with his left hand, the examiner rotates the lower limb outwards, noting the angles of hip medial rotation achieved in the process, and at the same time, guarding against inflicting pain.	The patient lies supine, while the hip is passively flexed and held at 90°. Holding the patient's foot with his right hand and steadying the patient's thigh (held vertical) with his left hand, the examiner rotates the lower limb inwards, noting the angle of hip lateral rotation achieved in the process, and at the same time, guarding against inflicting pain.

Fig. 13.3 Movements of the hip joint.

EXAMINATION

Look. Inspect the patient standing and walking to assess gait, and note any obvious pelvic tilt, leg length inequality, or other abnormality.

Feel. Palpate the hip with the patient lying supine, paying particular attention to the inguinal area (to detect tenderness of the hip joint, or other abnormalities such as inguinal hernias) and the greater trochanter (for trochanteric bursitis).

Move. The range of movement of the hip joint can be assessed with the maneuvers shown in Figure 13.3. Hip pathology tends to cause preferential, painful limitation of medial (internal) rotation.

In addition, it may be necessary to examine the spine and the abdomen for possible causes of referred pain, and to measure leg length – discrepancies of leg length being both an important cause of back and hip pain, and a possible result of hip pathology.

INVESTIGATIONS

Not everyone who has hip pain (even if there is hip joint pathology) needs to be investigated. If the examination suggests a primary periarticular cause, no further investigation is necessary. If the examination suggests hip joint pathology (i.e. painful limitation of movements, particularly internal rotation of the hip), a plain radiograph may be indicated to define the type of pathology. The radiograph aids differentiation of different types of arthritis from other intra-articular or bony pathologies such as osteonecrosis or fractures. Any other form of investigation is rarely necessary. In cases of severe or intractable pain and/or functional limitation, but where the plain radiograph is normal, other investigations that might be considered include scintigraphy or magnetic resonance imaging (to show, for example, early osteonecrosis) as well as blood tests to help detect the presence of an inflammatory arthropathy, and occasionally aspiration of the joint.

1 TYPICAL CASE: TROCHANTERIC BURSITIS

Joan is an obese, 53-year-old woman with a history of gradual onset of a deep, aching sensation lateral to the right hip that is made worse by activity, and bothers her at night. Recently, she developed a slight limp. A family history of arthritis has helped to convince Joan that her hip joint is 'falling to pieces'.

On examination, hip movements are normal, and no pain occurs on full internal rotation of the hip, which makes hip disease extremely unlikely. However, severe point tenderness is found over the greater trochanter.

You diagnose trochanteric bursitis, reassure Joan that nothing is wrong with her hip, inject local corticosteroids into the tender area, advise a few days' rest, and Joan's problems resolve.

2 TYPICAL CASE: OSTEOARTHRITIS OF THE HIP JOINT

Jim is a 57-year-old car mechanic who, some 10 years ago, first developed an aching pain in his groin when walking. This became troublesome, with some pain that radiated down the front of his thigh, and his wife has noticed that he seems to be limping a little at times, particularly first thing in the morning.

He first consulted you 7 years ago. On examination, you found less internal rotation of the right hip than of the left, and this maneuver caused pain. No other abnormal signs were present.

You arranged a radiograph, which showed early osteoarthritis of the hip (Fig. 13.4). You advised him about the condition, and advised him about footwear and the use of acetaminophen as needed for pain.

Jim managed perfectly well with this regime until quite recently. However, over the past 3 months he has had increasing pain and disability – he is now being woken at night by pain, is unable to put his socks on, and cannot walk far without developing severe pain. A new radiograph shows advanced hip OA (Fig. 13.5). You refer him to an orthopedic surgeon, who successfully replaces the hip, which relieves all of Jim's pain (Fig. 13.6).

FEATURES OF TROCHANTERIC BURSITIS

- A common condition of adults, more frequent in women than in men.
- Causes a deep aching and sometimes burning pain on the lateral aspect of the hip, made worse by exercise, often severe at night, and relieved by rest.
- Some patients develop a limp.
- Tenderness over the greater trochanter is present.
- Predisposing factors include obesity, mechanical back pain, hip disease (note – trochanteric bursitis and hip osteoarthritis often coexist), leg-length abnormalities, trauma, and some athletic activities, which include jogging.
- Rest, nonsteroidal anti-inflammatory drugs, local ultrasound, and physical therapy can all help, but local infiltration with corticosteroids and local anesthetic, combined with a few days' rest, is probably the preferred treatment in uncomplicated cases.

FEATURES OF OSTEOARTHRITIS OF THE HIP

- Common condition that is slightly more frequent in men than in women, and occasionally presents as early as in the 20–30 age group, but peaking in incidence in the fifth and sixth decades.
- More common in Caucasians than in Asians or Africans.
- Predisposing factors include childhood hip disorders (slipped epiphysis, congenital dislocation, Legg–Perthes disease), acetabular dysplasias and leg-length anomalies, farming, and other work that involves heavy lifting and carrying.
- Usually presents with use-related groin pain, which often radiates to the knee, but can present with lateral or posterior hip pain.
- Inactivity stiffness is usually present, and on examination movements are limited and painful – the earliest sign is restricted internal (medial) rotation of the hip.
- Painful and restricted hip movement causes difficulty with walking, dressing (particularly putting shoes and socks on), and sexual intercourse.
- Shortening of the affected leg may develop.
- The natural history is very variable – most cases stay relatively mild for many years, but many do at some stage progress to severe joint damage.
- Conservative management is appropriate in the early phases; late disease can cause very severe pain and disability, the only satisfactory treatment for which is hip replacement.

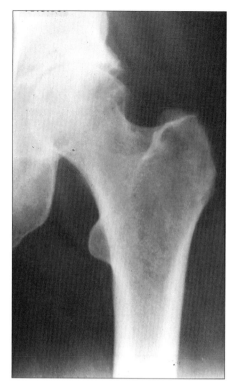

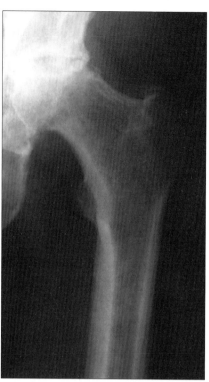

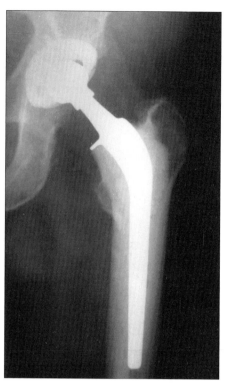

Fig. 13.4 Radiograph of the hip showing relatively early osteoarthritis of the superior pole of the hip. Note the narrowing of the joint space, sclerosis of bone of the acetabulum, and osteophyte formation at the superior pole of the acetabulum.

Fig. 13.5 Radiograph of the hip showing advanced osteoarthritis of the superior pole of the hip. Osteonecrosis and collapse of the head of the femur superiorly are complicating features.

Fig. 13.6 The same hip joint as in Figure 13.5 after resection and successful replacement. The metal femoral component was fixed with cement and an uncemented acetabular component containing polyethylene liner.

OTHER CAUSES OF HIP PAIN

Inflammatory arthropathies can cause pain and restricted movement in a similar pattern to that associated with OA. Ischiogluteal bursitis is associated with activities that cause friction over the ischial tuberosity (previously known as 'Weaver's bottom') and buttock pain with local tenderness over the ischial tuberosity. Adductor tendinitis is common in athletes (the common cause of 'groin strain') and causes groin pain with tenderness over the adductor origins. Meralgia paresthetica is a nerve entrapment syndrome of the lateral cutaneous nerve of the thigh, and causes anterior groin and thigh pain and paresthesias. The hip is also one of the joints most prone to osteonecrosis, which should be suspected in any high-risk patient (i.e. in particular those on long-term cortico-steroid therapy, alcoholics, and people who have sickle cell disease).

In the elderly, special consideration must be given to the possibility of other bone diseases, which include fractured neck of femur, Paget's disease, and bony metastases.

 MANAGEMENT

PERIARTICULAR PROBLEMS, INCLUDING TROCHANTERIC BURSITIS
Periarticular problems around the hip may be related to overuse or some specific mechanical factor, in which case rest and some behavioral change to reduce the risk factor may be all that is needed. In more persistent cases, a course of non-steroidal anti-inflammatory drugs (NSAIDs) and local physical therapy

techniques (such as local ultrasound therapy) may help. However, local injection therapy is often the most effective intervention. Referral is not recommended.

 COMPLICATIONS OF CORTICOSTEROID INJECTIONS

Any injection of corticosteroid can result in facial flushing a few hours later. This occurs in some 40% of cases and is transient and inconsequential, but it can cause concern if the patient has not been warned. A flare-up of the condition which is being treated occasionally occurs (in about 5% of cases): this occurs within a few hours of the injection and lasts for up to 1–2 days.

Rarely, a corticosteroid injection results in a more serious complication such as infection, tendon rupture, skin atrophy or joint damage. Each of these uncommon but severe complications is more likely if the technique used is poor:

- Use a good aseptic technique to reduce the risk of infection.
- Avoid repeated injections around tendons and never inject corticosteroids into the body of a tendon to reduce the risk of subsequent rupture.
- Do not use strong, long-acting crystalline preparations when injecting peri-articular structures close to the skin, as these can cause unsightly skin atrophy.
- Avoid repeated intra-articular injections to reduce the risk of accelerated joint damage or osteonecrosis.

INJECTION OF THE TROCHANTERIC 'BURSA'

Indications. Trochanteric 'bursitis' syndrome.

Corticosteroid dose. Methylprednisolone 30–40mg mixed with 3ml of lidocaine (lignocaine) 1%. [No. 22 3.8cm needle; a spinal needle may be required in obese patients.]

Approach. With the patient lying on his or her opposite side, the greater trochanter is identified by distal-to-proximal palpation along the femur. The point of maximal tenderness is usually located at the posterior corner of the greater trochanter. The needle is inserted vertically to make periosteal contact (Fig. 13.7).

- Step 1. Lidocaine should be infiltrated radially to cover the base of a cone 3cm in diameter, half on bone and half in the proximal soft tissues.
- Step 2. If pain is relieved, the mixture of corticosteroid and lidocaine is infiltrated in the same area. Experienced physicians may skip Step 1.

Precautions. The needle should be of sufficient length to reach the bone.

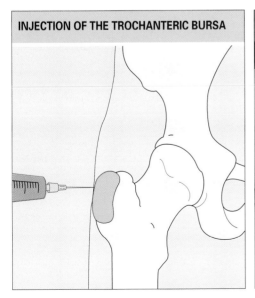
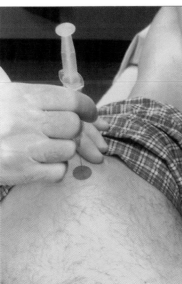

Fig. 13.7 Injection of the trochanteric bursa.

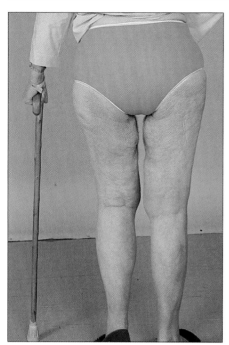

Fig. 13.8 Use of a cane, stick, or other walking aid. This patient, who has hip osteoarthritis, found that she could reduce the pain in her damaged right hip by leaning on the stick in the left hand as she walked. The reduction in loading can be huge, and the effect on symptoms and confidence with walking very beneficial.

OSTEOARTHRITIS OF THE HIP

The treatment objectives and principles of the management of OA of the hip are the same as those described in more detail in Chapter 14.

Particularly valuable help can come from:

- shock-absorbing shoes and a cane in the contralateral hand to help painful loading of the hip when walking (Fig. 13.8);
- education, empowerment for self-help, general exercises and weight loss for the obese (it is important to advise patients to continue or increase activity and not to rest the joint – increased exercise can relieve pain and disability and no evidence shows that it causes further damage to the joint);
- physical therapy, including hydrotherapy, is particularly useful in more advanced cases and in those whose limitations of hip movement have become significant;
- simple analgesics or courses of NSAIDs may help, but indomethacin should be avoided as some evidence indicates that that this drug can accelerate progression of hip OA.

Consideration for arthroplasty is appropriate for anyone who has severe pain or disability from hip OA. Although no clear indications as to who should or should not have a joint replacement are established, the old adage that 'anyone who cannot sleep, cannot walk, or cannot work' because of hip disease should have a prosthesis provides some help: severe rest or night pain, and severe disability that interferes materially with everyday activities are indications for referral to consider surgery. Older people and obese people can do well with operations, but severe intercurrent disease may be a contraindication.

RECOMMENDATIONS FOR REFERRAL

Subspecialty

Indications for possible referral to a rheumatology service include those cases in which isolated hip disease appears to be due to an inflammatory arthropathy, cases with generalized arthritis and a particular problem with the hip, those in whom you suspect osteonecrosis, and cases of severe hip osteoarthritis in whom surgery is contraindicated.

Physical therapy/rehabilitation

Physiotherapy can be of great value to patients with mild or early osteoarthritis – mobilizing exercises, muscle-strengthening exercises, and advice about activities and the use of appropriate footwear and walking aids can all be facilitated by therapists. In addition, people with severe arthritis in whom surgery is contraindicated may benefit greatly from a rehabilitation program.

Orthopedic surgery

As outlined above, any patient with severe OA, osteonecrosis or hip arthritis should be considered for surgery if there are no major contraindications.

REGIONAL PAIN AND MONOARTICULAR DISORDERS

14

PAIN IN THE KNEE

COMMON CAUSES OF KNEE PAIN

The major causes of knee pain can be classified according to the age of the patient, as well as into referred, periarticular, or articular causes, as shown in Figure 14.1.

EXAMINATION OF THE KNEE JOINT

Look. The knee is inspected with the patient standing, so that any malalignment or posterior swelling (such as Baker's cyst) can be seen, and so that the gait can be examined. The knees are also examined with the patient on an examination table, where any quadriceps wasting or anterior swelling can be seen, as well as any scars or other obvious abnormalities.

COMMON CAUSES OF KNEE PAIN IN DIFFERENT AGE GROUPS			
	Cause		
Age group	Intra-articular	Periarticular	Referred
Adolescence (10–18 years)	Osteochondritis dissecans Torn meniscus Anterior knee pain syndrome Patellar malalignment	Osgood–Schlatter's disease Sinding-Larsen–Johansson syndrome Osteomyelitis Tumors	Slipped upper femoral epiphysis
Early adulthood (18–30 years)	Torn meniscus Instability Anterior knee pain syndrome Inflammatory conditions	Overuse syndromes Bursitis	Rare
Adulthood (30–50 years)	Meniscal tears Early degeneration following injury or meniscectomy Inflammatory arthropathies	Bursitis Tendinitis	Osteoarthritis of the hip (may be secondary to hip dysplasia or injury)
Older age (>50 years)	Osteoarthritis Inflammatory arthropathies	Bursitis Tendinitis	Osteoarthritis of the hip

Fig. 14.1 Common causes of knee pain in different age groups.

Feel. Feel for any heat over the joint and palpate any swellings. Look for point tenderness, particularly over the joint line and at ligament and tendon insertion points around the knee. Small effusions can be detected by the 'bulge sign' (Fig. 14.2).

Move. Flexion and extension are examined with the patient on an examination table (Fig. 14.3).

You should also feel for crepitus on movement and examine for ligamentous instability (Figs 14.4–14.6). In addition, the hip and spine may need examination to exclude referred pain (hip disease is often mistaken for knee disease because of pain referral).

INVESTIGATIONS

Most knee disorders can be diagnosed from the history and examination, and investigations are unnecessary in the majority of cases. If examination suggests a periarticular cause, no investigation is necessary; similarly, radiographs add nothing to the clinical diagnosis of osteoarthritis (OA) unless surgery is being considered.

THE BULGE SIGN IN THE KNEE

Fig. 14.2 The bulge sign in the knee. The back of the hand gently wafts the fluid from one side of the knee to the other. This is most helpful in detecting small knee effusions.

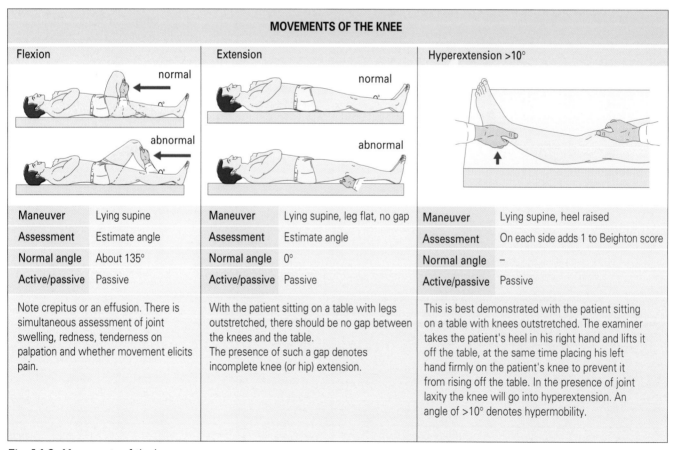

MOVEMENTS OF THE KNEE

Flexion		Extension		Hyperextension >10°	
normal		normal			
abnormal		abnormal			
Maneuver	Lying supine	Maneuver	Lying supine, leg flat, no gap	Maneuver	Lying supine, heel raised
Assessment	Estimate angle	Assessment	Estimate angle	Assessment	On each side adds 1 to Beighton score
Normal angle	About 135°	Normal angle	0°	Normal angle	–
Active/passive	Passive	Active/passive	Passive	Active/passive	Passive
Note crepitus or an effusion. There is simultaneous assessment of joint swelling, redness, tenderness on palpation and whether movement elicits pain.		With the patient sitting on a table with legs outstretched, there should be no gap between the knees and the table. The presence of such a gap denotes incomplete knee (or hip) extension.		This is best demonstrated with the patient sitting on a table with knees outstretched. The examiner takes the patient's heel in his right hand and lifts it off the table, at the same time placing his left hand firmly on the patient's knee to prevent it from rising off the table. In the presence of joint laxity the knee will go into hyperextension. An angle of >10° denotes hypermobility.	

Fig. 14.3 Movements of the knee.

If the history and examination suggest an articular problem with significant mechanical problems (for example, locking, instability or major restriction of movement) then *imaging studies* are indicated to make the diagnosis. A plain radiograph should be performed first, and will aid the diagnosis of some of the less common bony disorders, as well as confirming the presence of osteoarthritis. Soft tissue lesions such as meniscal (cartilage) injuries and ligament damage can only be diagnosed by other imaging procedures, specifically arthroscopy or magnetic resonance imaging (MRI). These investigations are indicated if surgical intervention is being considered; which one is preferred varies in different centers, depending on experience and availability.

If there is a large, warm or tense effusion in the joint or a bursa it should be aspirated for *examination of the synovial fluid* to exclude infection or crystal-induced synovitis.

KNEE PAIN IN CHILDREN

Knee pain in children below 10 years of age is uncommon, but always significant. Knee pain, particularly anterior knee pain, is common in adolescence and some young adults (see Chapter 38).

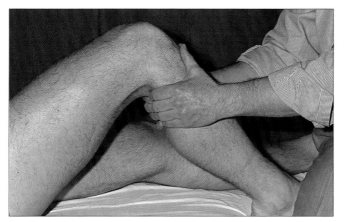

Fig. 14.4 The anterior drawer test for the detection of instability of the anterior cruciate ligament. The examiner is testing whether the tibia can be pulled forward on the femur.

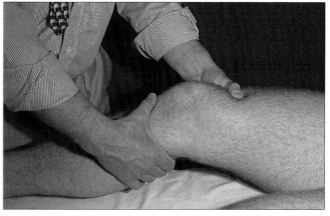

Fig. 14.5 The Lachman test for cruciate ligament instability. The examiner is testing whether the tibia can be rocked backward and forward on the femur.

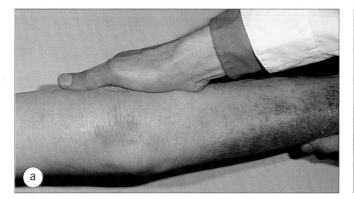

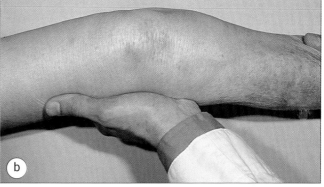

Fig. 14.6 Testing the stability of the collateral ligaments of the knee joint. (a, b) With the knee slightly flexed to avoid normal 'locking', lateral pressure is applied to establish whether the knee will rock from side to side.

KNEE PAIN IN EARLY ADULTHOOD

Knee pain in early adulthood is rarely referred from the hip and is most commonly related to trauma or overuse. Ligamentous and meniscal injuries predominate, and periarticular disorders, such as bursitis, are common.

1 TYPICAL CASE: ATHLETIC INJURY TO THE KNEE JOINT

Jack is a 31-year-old builder who plays a lot of soccer on the weekends and in the evenings. Last night, while he was playing, he twisted his knee during a tackle, heard it 'pop', and felt immediate, severe pain. He was carried off the field. On examination you find an effusion in the knee, and he is obviously very anxious about moving the knee. Tests for instability caused by rupture of the anterior cruciate ligament are positive (see Figs 14.4 & 14.5). You diagnose ligament rupture and refer Jack to the local orthopedic surgeon.

A subsequent MRI scan shows that Jack has also torn his medial meniscus (Fig. 14.7). He is operated on to repair the anterior cruciate ligament rupture and the meniscal tear.

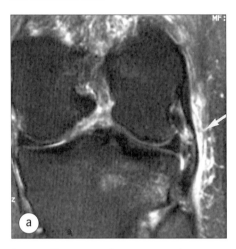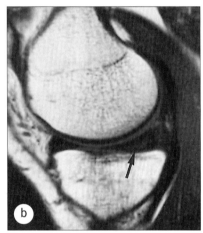

Fig. 14.7 Imaging ligaments and menisci with magnetic resonance imaging (MRI). (a) Coronal fat-suppressed T2-weighted image of the knee shows an intact fibular collateral ligament (white arrow). Surrounding high-signal intensity fluid is indicative of sprain. (b) Meniscal tear appears as a linear band of increased signal (black arrow) within the otherwise low-signal intensity meniscus on sagittal T1-weighted MRI.

2 TYPICAL CASE: PREPATELLAR BURSITIS OF THE KNEE

Pete is a 39-year-old carpet layer who has had a period of particularly hard work since a rush of business resulting from a local carpet factory's closing-down sale. He complains of a painful swelling over the front of his knee, which prevents him from kneeling to carry on his work.

On examination he has an obvious, well-circumscribed, hot, fluctuant swelling over the front of the knee (Fig. 14.8), and you also notice thickening of the skin caused by recurrent trauma to that area of his knee at work. Nothing suggests gout or sepsis, but you aspirate the bursa and send the fluid for microscopy and microbiologic examination, to be on the safe side. The tests come back negative, and after a short period of rest and avoidance of kneeling, the condition settles completely.

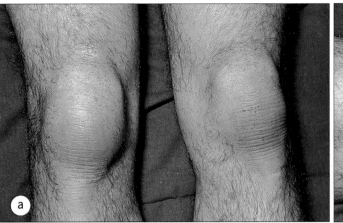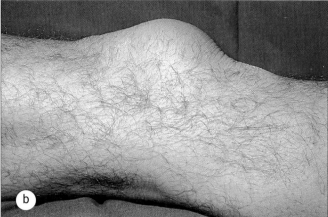

Fig. 14.8 Prepatellar bursitis. (a) Anterior and (b) lateral views of a red, swollen, painful prepatellar bursa.

KNEE PAIN IN OLDER ADULTS

Knee pain in older people may be referred from the hip (which is usually an OA hip) or more rarely from the spine. Periarticular disorders may occur, particularly anserine bursitis or medial ligament syndrome. However, by far the most common and most important cause of knee pain in this group is OA of the knee.

3 TYPICAL CASE: OSTEOARTHRITIS OF THE KNEE JOINT

Candida is an obese, 56-year-old woman who works for a very demanding boss. Over the past few years she has noticed the insidious development of some discomfort and stiffness in her right knee; she has come to see you now because this has deteriorated over recent months, and made it difficult for her to run up and down stairs to respond to the constant demands of her boss. She also describes some limitation of walking any distance as a result of the pain, difficulty climbing in and out of the bath, and stiffness of the knee after periods of inactivity and first thing in the morning.

On examination you find quadriceps wasting and modest swelling around the knee, which feels bony on palpation. On movement there is pain and some restriction of full flexion, as well as marked crepitus.

OTHER CAUSES OF KNEE PAIN IN OLDER ADULTS

Inflammatory arthritis of any sort can affect the knee joint, and the elderly may suffer from bursal or ligament injuries.

THE MEDIAL KNEE PAIN SYNDROME (ANSERINE BURSITIS)

In addition, a number of elderly people develop knee pain with tenderness that is largely confined to the medial side of the knee joint, just below the joint line (Fig. 14.10). This pain may derive from either of two local structures, the anserine bursa or the insertion of the medial collateral ligament or pes anserinus. It is difficult to differentiate these causes, and medial pain and tenderness of this sort may complicate OA of the knee joint. Rest may help, but in resistant cases, injection of a small amount of corticosteroid into the lesion may be needed.

FEATURES OF OSTEOARTHRITIS OF THE KNEE JOINT

- An extremely common disorder, particularly in middle-aged and elderly women.
- Risk factors include age, obesity, and previous injury to the knee, as well as a familial predisposition to osteoarthritis.
- Characterized by the gradual onset of use-related pain and inactivity stiffness in one knee. Usually becomes bilateral with time.
- Usually affects either the medial compartment of the tibiofemoral joint, which results in a varus deformity, or the lateral facet of the patellofemoral joint, or both.
- Some cases slowly progress to develop severe pain and disability.
- Diagnosis can be made from the clinical picture, which includes the characteristic examination findings of crepitus and some bony lipping or swelling without marked inflammation of the joint or any other obvious cause of knee pain (such as referred pain from the hip). Radiographs confirm the diagnosis and can be used to help assess the severity of joint damage (Fig. 14.9).
- Treatment depends on the amount of pain, the degree of disability, and the extent of the joint damage (see Management of Osteoarthritis of the Knee Joint, below).

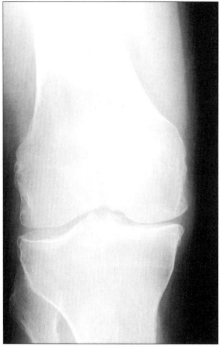

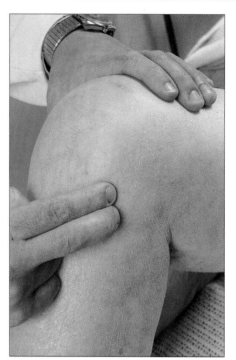

Fig. 14.10 **Identifying the cause of pain in osteoarthritis.** One of the prerequisites to good therapy is to establish the cause of symptoms in a joint with 'osteoarthritis'. Symptoms arise from periarticular problems that result in severe local tenderness, rather than from the joint. In the case illustrated, the symptoms are caused by anserine bursitis and stretching of the capsule at its insertion on the medial aspect of the knee. However, local pathology must be carefully distinguished from referred tender spots, which are commonly identifiable around damaged joints. True periarticular pathology results in severe point tenderness with other signs, such as reproduction of the pain on certain movements that stress the structures involved.

Fig. 14.9 **Anteroposterior radiograph of the knee joint.** Established osteoarthritis of the medial tibiofemoral compartment of the joint is shown. Note the narrowing of the joint space on the medial side, and the osteophytes.

MANAGEMENT OF KNEE OSTEOARTHRITIS

- Education of patients and carers, self-help, and empowerment are important in the management of knee osteoarthritis – many people who have early-to-mild disease need no other help.
- A wide range of physical approaches help patients to reduce impact loading on the knee while maintaining a full range of movement and good muscle strength, as well as general fitness and activity.
- Simple analgesics and rubefacients are appropriate for pain control; some patients may be helped more by nonsteroidal anti-inflammatory drugs, but these agents should be used with care.
- Surgery is indicated for most people who have severe knee osteoarthritis.
- Dietary considerations are important – obese patients should lose weight, and some vitamin and other dietary supplements may be of some value

 ## MANAGEMENT OF OSTEOARTHRITIS OF THE KNEE JOINT

OBJECTIVES OF THERAPY

The main objectives in the treatment of knee OA are:

- To reduce pain and other symptoms, such as anxiety or stiffness, with minimum risk.
- To minimize the impact of the condition on the patient's life, reducing disability and handicap where possible.
- To limit the risk of progression by reducing those insults to the knee thought to contribute to further joint damage.

EDUCATION AND SUPPORT

Education of patients and carers is very important. Many people fear severe disability and a wheelchair-bound life, although this is an extremely rare outcome of knee OA. Other patients are concerned that any further usage of the knee will cause more damage, whereas movement and continuing activity are, in actuality, good for both knee and patient – patients should be advised to keep active and keep movement up, but to avoid high-impact loading to the joint as much as possible. It has been shown that education and continuing contact and support of patients who have knee OA is a cost-effective way of reducing pain and disability.

Also, the patients can take a number of measures to help themselves (see Self-Help Leaflet, page 340).

PHYSICAL AND OTHER NONPHARMACOLOGIC FORMS OF THERAPY

Abnormal mechanical loading of the joint, in part causes OA of the knee. Obesity, as well as major injuries to the joint, are major risk factors for the progression as well as initiation of the disease. Reduction of weight in the obese is therefore important, as are measures that reduce abnormal loading on the joint. These measures can include:

- Shock-absorbing insoles to shoes.
- Other shoe alterations, such as lateral heel wedges.
- Exercises to keep the quadriceps muscle strong, and thus help stabilize the joint.
- Braces, strapping, and orthoses, which can reduce the common sensation of 'giving way' by increasing proprioception, as well as protect the unstable or deformed knee.
- Use of a cane in the hand on the opposite side to the worst knee, to reduce loading on it.
- Generally keeping fit, and maintaining as full a range of motion of the joint as possible is also important.

In more severe cases other walking aids or orthoses may help, as can changes to the home/work environment, such as bathroom aids or stair rails.

DRUG THERAPY

Current guidelines for the treatment of knee OA recommend the use of simple analgesics, such as acetaminophen, as the first-line drug therapy. If symptoms persist despite this and other conservative measures, a course of a nonsteroidal anti-inflammatory drugs (NSAIDs) may be indicated, but it must be remembered that those patients most likely to suffer knee OA (elderly women) are also the group most susceptible to the damaging side effects of these drugs .

Rubefacients (agents to rub on the painful joint) can provide useful symptomatic relief with the advantages that they do not lead to significant absorption of drugs, they avoid systemic side-effects, and they give the patient a modicum of control over the condition (they can be rubbed into the knee joint when required). Many such agents are available over the counter, some of which contain small amounts of an active ingredient that produces local vasodilation and warmth. In addition, prescription agents containing either capsaicin or a non-steroidal anti-inflammatory agent are becoming available in many countries, but there is no evidence to suggest that they are more efficacious than the simpler, cheaper agents available over the counter.

Agents injected into OA knee joints include corticosteroids and hyaluronan products. Corticosteroids may be useful for symptomatic flares associated with an effusion and for providing short-term relief prior to a major life event or to the use of physical therapy for rehabilitation, but should not be used regularly. The place of hyaluronan injections has yet to be established.

Periarticular injections sometimes help (see anserine bursitis injection, below), and other drugs to help symptoms, such as antidepressants, are occasionally indicated.

SURGERY

A number of surgical procedures are available for knee OA, including:

- Lavage with or without debridement – producing temporary symptomatic relief.
- Osteotomy – preferred for those patients under 60 years of age who place major physical demands on the joint, and who have predominant involvement of one part of the tibiofemoral joint.
- Knee replacements, which can be unicompartmental or total.

Surgery is indicated for those who have severe pain or disability, who are unresponsive to other measures, and who also have significant joint damage. Some evidence indicates that knee replacement surgery is currently under-utilized, despite the outcome generally being excellent.

DIETARY AND COMPLEMENTARY TECHNIQUES

Obese patients are advised to lose weight. A large number of vitamin and dietary supplements are on sale with the recommendation that they are good for OA. The evidence for the efficacy of most of these products is either poor or non-existent, but there is some support for the use of some dietary supplements, such as glucosamine, and it may be of value to maintain good dietary levels of vitamins C and D.

A number of other complementary techniques, such as relaxation, may help with the pain and stiffness of knee OA, particularly in mild cases.

MONITORING PROGRESSION AND OUTCOME

Knee OA is not always inexorably progressive – it frequently stabilizes, and patients may adapt to the problems and lower their expectations with time. However, some patients do experience severe pain or disability, which can develop gradually without the patient complaining or realizing how disabled they are becoming.

It is important to keep an eye on patients who have knee OA for these reasons, and because of the risk of side effects to therapy, particularly those of NSAIDs if they are being used, and to monitor the degree of pain, amount of disability, and severity of joint damage. This can be done clinically, with no need for regular radiographs or other investigations.

ASPIRATION AND LOCAL INJECTION THERAPY IN AND AROUND THE KNEE JOINT

Aspiration and injection of the knee joint or anserine bursa is often indicated.

 ## COMPLICATIONS OF CORTICOSTEROID INJECTIONS

Any injection of corticosteroid can result in facial flushing a few hours later. This occurs in some 40% of cases and is transient and inconsequential, but it can cause concern if the patient has not been warned. A flare-up of the condition which is being treated occasionally occurs (in about 5% of cases): this occurs within a few hours of the injection and lasts for up to 1–2 days.

Rarely, a corticosteroid injection results in a more serious complication such as infection, tendon rupture, skin atrophy or joint damage. Each of these uncommon but severe complications is more likely if the technique used is poor:
- Use a good aseptic technique to reduce the risk of infection.
- Avoid repeated injections around tendons and never inject corticosteroids into the body of a tendon to reduce the risk of subsequent rupture.
- Do not use strong, long-acting crystalline preparations when injecting peri-articular structures close to the skin, as these can cause unsightly skin atrophy.
- Avoid repeated intra-articular injections to reduce the risk of accelerated joint damage or osteonecrosis.

KNEE JOINT

Indications. For diagnosis in any joint effusion. For corticosteroid injection in rheumatoid arthritis (RA), spondyloarthropathies, OA and occasionally in crystal-induced synovitis.

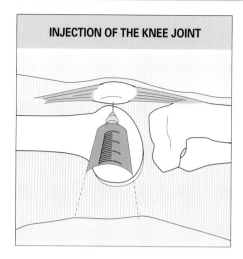

INJECTION OF THE KNEE JOINT

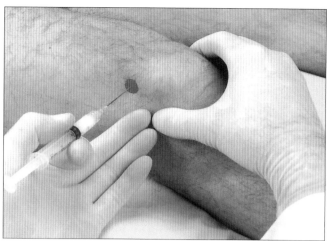

Fig. 14.11
Injection of the
knee joint.

Corticosteroid dose. Methylprednisolone 40–60mg (No. 22 needle). Aspiration should be attempted before injection. For aspiration alone use a No. 20 or No. 18 needle, depending on the clinical suspicion.

Approach. Medial, with the needle aimed at the patellar undersurface, mid-distance between the upper and lower poles of the patella. A medial approach is preferred because the lateral patellofemoral cleft is narrower than the medial, and the joint capsule is tougher laterally than medially. However, many entries to the knee are possible (Fig. 14.11) and the choice is very dependent on personal preference.

Precautions. Beware of superimposed septic arthritis in RA patients. Postpone the injection of an acutely inflamed joint until a negative synovial fluid culture result is available.

INJECTION OF ANSERINE BURSITIS

Indications. The medial knee pain/anserine bursitis syndrome that has not responded to conservative measures.

Corticosteroid dose. Methylprednisolone 20–30mg mixed with lidocaine (lignocaine) 2–3ml, No. 22 needle.

Approach. The injection site is best determined by following the medial tendinous border of the thigh, with the knee in semiflexion, to the tibia where a mark is placed. The knee is then brought to extension and the needle is entered perpendicularly to tibial contact. An area 3cm in diameter is infiltrated adjacent to the periosteum.

Precautions. Paresthesias that extend along the medial leg indicate engagement of the saphenous nerve; reposition the needle.

Note: Since anserine bursitis is almost always secondary (in addition to genu valgum, patellofemoral OA, etc), the condition is expected to recur unless the primary process has also been addressed. A vigorous program of isometric quadriceps exercises should be initiated.

RECOMMENDATIONS FOR REFERRAL

Subspecialty

Referral to a rheumatologist might be considered for cases in which there is diagnostic uncertainty, when the degree of pain or disability seems to be disproportionate to the degree of joint damage evident on examination or on a radiograph, or in milder cases where further advice about conservative management needs to be sought. Patients with severe disease in whom surgery is contraindicated should be referred to a rheumatology service, as well as for rehabilitation.

Physiotherapy/rehabilitation

Physical and occupational therapy can be of great benefit in all stages of the condition, particularly to teach joint protection and exercises to strengthen muscles in the early phase, and to provide advice about walking aids and other rehabilitative measures in more advanced disease. Everyone with knee OA should be taught quadriceps-strengthening exercises and encouraged to continue with them.

Orthopedic surgery

Rapidly progressive disease, severe pain and/or disability unresponsive to conservative measures, as well as severe deformity or instability of the knee joint are indications to consider surgery. There are no clear indications as to the degree of severity that warrants surgical intervention, although, as with the hip, the adage that anyone who cannot walk, work or sleep because of OA should have surgery provides some guidance.

REGIONAL PAIN AND MONOARTICULAR DISORDERS

15

THE ANKLE AND FOOT

The ankle and foot includes three functional units – the hindfoot (ankle and subtalar joints), midfoot (midtarsal joints), and forefoot [metatarsophalangeal (MTP) and interphalangeal (IP) joints] (Fig. 15.1). Disorders of the foot are common in both children and adults, most being static disorders caused by foot deformities or inappropriate footwear, including disorders such as corns and calluses, or injuries such as sprained ankle. In addition, as in other regions of the body, a number or articular, periarticular, and referred causes of pain occur in the ankle and foot.

KEY POINTS

- Ankle and foot problems are common. Most are related to mechanical abnormalities or inappropriate footwear.
- Common causes of pain around the heel are plantar fasciitis, Achilles' tendinitis, and sprained ankle.
- Common causes of forefoot pain are hallux valgus, bunions, and metatarsalgia.
- Management principally involves correction of any mechanical abnormality, with particular attention to footwear. Podiatrists and chiropodists can provide valuable help in the management of foot disorders.

Fig. 15.1 The bones and functional units of the foot.

COMMON CAUSES OF PAIN IN THE ANKLE AND FOOT	
Region	Cause
Heel	Achilles' tendinitis and bursitis Other enthesopathies Tarsal tunnel syndrome Plantar fasciitis Ankle sprains
Arch	Clubfoot and other congenital or ostoechondral lesions Flat feet – pes planus High arched feet – pes cavus
Forefoot	Gout, bunions, hallux valgus, and hallux rigidus (first metatarsophalangeal area) Metatarsalgia Sausage toes in psoriatic arthritis Stress fractures Toe deformities Morton's neuroma

Fig. 15.2 Common causes of pain in the ankle and foot.

109

MOVEMENTS OF FOOT AND ANKLE

Ankle extension

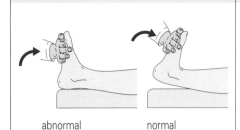

abnormal   normal

Maneuver	Pressure on ball of foot
Assessment	Estimate angle
Normal angle	15°
Active/passive	Passive

The patient points his/her foot toward his/her head as far as it will go, gently encouraged by the examiner's hand. The angle subtended with the right angle to the shin is estimated, and recorded as the angle of ankle flexion. There is simultaneous assessment of joint swelling, redness, tenderness on palpation and whether movement elicits pain.

Ankle flexion

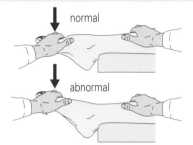

normal

abnormal

Maneuver	Pressure on dorsum of foot
Assessment	Estimate angle
Normal angle	55°
Active/passive	Passive

The patient points his/her foot away from his/her head as far as it will go, gently encouraged by the examiner's hand. The angle subtended with the right angle to the shin is estimated and recorded as the angle of ankle extension. There is simultaneous assessment of joint swelling, redness, tenderness on palpation and whether movement elicits pain.

Subtalar inversion

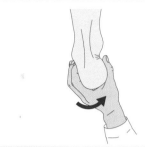

Maneuver	Deviate heel medially
Assessment	Estimate angle
Normal angle	35°
Active/passive	Passive

The patient's heel is grasped between the examiner's thumb and index finger while the examiner's other hand firmly anchors the patient's shin. The heel is then inverted as far as it will go. The angle of inversion is estimated and recorded. There is simultaneous assessment of joint swelling, redness, tenderness on palpation and whether movement elicits pain.

Subtalar eversion

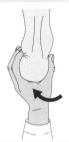

Maneuver	Deviate heel laterally
Assessment	Estimate angle
Normal angle	20°
Active/passive	Passive

The patient's heel is grasped between the examiner's thumb and index finger while the examiner's other hand firmly anchors the patient's shin. The heel is then everted as far as it will go. The angle of eversion is estimated and recorded. There is simultaneous assessment of joint swelling, redness, tenderness on palpation and whether movement elicits pain.

Midtarsal rotation

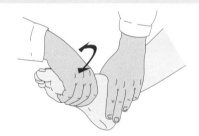

Maneuver	Rotation of forefoot on hindfoot
Assessment	Estimate angle
Normal angle	35°
Active/passive	Passive

The patient's forefoot is grasped between the examiner's right thumb and fingers while the examiner's left hand firmly anchors the patient's heel. The forefoot is then rotated on the hindfoot as far as it will go. The angle of midtarsal rotation is estimated and recorded. There is simultaneous assessment of joint swelling, redness, tenderness on palpation and whether movement elicits pain.

MTPs, IPs

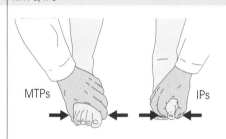

MTPs   IPs

Maneuver	Individual joints moved passively
Assessment	Pain on movement of joints
Normal angle	–
Active/passive	Passive

The metatarsus is gently grasped by the examiner's hand. If this maneuver causes pain, inflammation in one or more MTP joints can be deduced. The MTP joints should then be palpated individually to establish which one (or more) is inflamed. The individual interphalangeal joints (PIPs, DIPs and IP hallux) are individually palpated by the examiner using his index finger and thumb to detect any signs of inflammation.

The examination of the feet cannot be considered complete without observing them in the standard (weight-bearing) position. The following deformities may thereby be recognized:

- Flat feet (pes planus) – flattening of the longitudinal arch of the foot.
- Pronation of the foot (often associated with pes planus).
- Valgus deformity of the hindfoot (eversion of subtalar joint).
- Pes cavus – an exceptionally high longitudinal arch.
- Talipes equinovarus – the heel is raised to produce an 'equine' posture.
- Hallux valgus – great toe pointing away from the midline.
- Subluxation of MTPs – toes deviated upward proximally and curled distally.

Fig. 15.3 Movements of the foot and ankle.

COMMON CAUSES OF PAIN IN THE ANKLE AND FOOT

Instead of using the conventional categories of causes of regional musculo-skeletal pain (articular, periarticular, or referred), the most convenient way to classify disorders of the ankle and foot is to divide them into the main anatomic area involved – heel region, the foot arches, or the forefoot (Fig. 15.2). In addition to the conditions listed, pain can be referred to the foot from the lumbar spine or knee, or be caused by vascular disease.

EXAMINATION

Look. The foot and ankle should be inspected with the patient weight bearing, which brings out deformities such as flat feet, and lying, when it may be easier to see deformities such as cock-up toes. The heel and other parts of the foot need to be inspected for swellings, and the sole of the foot for evidence of abnormal weight bearing such as atypical callus formation.
Feel. The areas of the ankle and foot most likely to cause pain are palpated – in heel and forefoot pain, a careful search for the point of maximum tenderness is particularly important to define the anatomic site of the lesion.
Move. The movements of two of the three main components of the foot are each examined – the ankle and subtalar components of the hindfoot, and midfoot rotation, as shown in Figure 15.3. Movement is less important in the forefoot, palpation being the crucial examination maneuver, but big-toe movements need to be assessed to exclude hallux rigidus (lack of extension of the toe that prevents the 'push-off' needed for normal walking).

INVESTIGATIONS

Special investigations are hardly ever necessary. Ankle and foot disorders can and should be diagnosable from the history and examination alone.

Only if specific bone disorders, such as a stress fracture, are suspected, should *plain radiography* be necessary (although stress fractures take some time to appear as radiographic changes), and very occasionally other special investigations are warranted, such as *nerve conduction studies* for nerve entrapment syndromes.

PAIN AROUND THE HEEL

Pain around the heel is usually caused by inflammation of the Achilles' tendon or plantar fascia where they insert into the calcaneum, or of the associated bursae (Fig. 15.4). It can also arise from ankle arthritis, entrapment of the posterior tibial nerve at the medial side of the ankle (tarsal tunnel syndrome), and a number of other disorders.

In addition, a 'sprained ankle' is a common problem in all age groups.

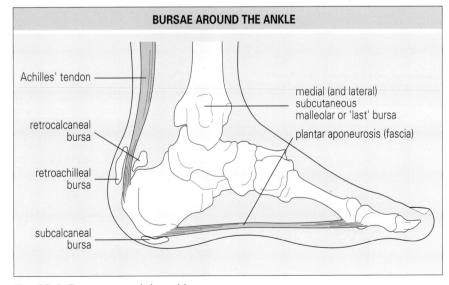

Fig. 15.4 Bursae around the ankle.

FEATURES OF PLANTAR FASCIITIS

- A very common disorder of middle aged or older people.
- A painful, inflammatory lesion at the insertion of the plantar fascia into the calcaneum (or caused by inflammation of the associated bursa).
- Associated with obesity, flat feet, and occupations that lead to repetitive trauma, such as excessive walking (occasionally known as policeman's heel).
- Occasionally part of an enthesopathy (inflammatory disorder of tendon and ligament insertions into bone) caused by inflammatory arthritis.
- Presents with pain under the heel, made worse by standing and walking.
- Point tenderness occurs at the site of insertion of the plantar fascia into the calcaneum.
- Relieved by rest, arch supports, and shoe orthoses that take weight off the area.
- Sometimes treated by local corticosteroid injection into the tender area.

1 TYPICAL CASE: PLANTAR FASCIITIS

Jim is an overweight 54-year-old policeman who has recently had to go back to the 'beat'. A few months ago, he received a shiny new pair of police-issue boots and was told that he had to walk the streets more to help keep crime figures down. Jim did as he was told, until his foot pain made it impossible.

He first noticed the discomfort under his right heel on standing and walking a few weeks ago. It has gradually worsened, and is now bad at night and excruciating when he first puts weight on his foot in the morning.

On examination you find point tenderness over the anteromedial aspect of the plantar surface of the calcaneus. You notice that he has rather flat arches, but find no other abnormalities.

You help Jim to obtain arch supports for his boots, and heel pads to reduce the weight bearing on the affected area. These measures, with a period of rest from having to walk the beat, and some weight loss, lead to resolution of his problems.

2 TYPICAL CASE: ACHILLES' TENDINITIS

Gloria is a 26-year-old ballet dancer who complains of pain and swelling around her heel; it is interfering with her promising dancing career.

On examination you find some swelling and tenderness of the Achilles' tendon, above the insertion into the calcaneum (Fig. 15.5). You advise her to rest from dancing for a short while, to use heel raises when walking to reduce stress on her Achilles' tendon, and you prescribe a course of nonsteroidal anti-inflammatory drugs (NSAIDs). In addition you refer her to physical therapy, where she is treated with local heat and ultrasound, and with stretching exercises. She is also taught the importance of careful stretching of the tendon before any dancing. She is soon able to take up dancing again.

FEATURES OF ACHILLES' TENDINITIS

- A common inflammatory disorder of the Achilles' tendon near to its insertion.
- Often associated with overuse, particularly in dancers and athletes.
- Faulty footwear and rigid shoe heels also contribute to the condition.
- Treated by rest, heel raises to reduce stress on the tendon, stretching exercises and local physical therapy. Nonsteroidal anti-inflammatory drugs can be used. Injections are contraindicated as there is a risk of tendon rupture.

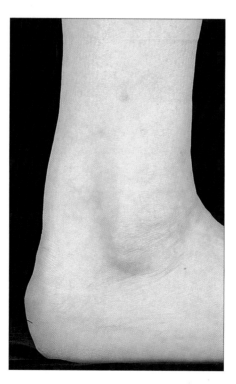

Fig. 15.5 Swelling of the Achilles' tendon.

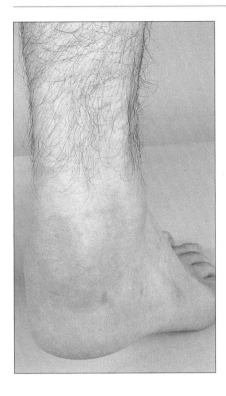

Fig. 15.6 Inflammatory swelling at the insertion of the Achilles' tendon. The patient has Reiter's syndrome and an inflammatory enthesopathy.

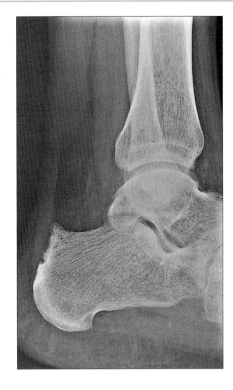

Fig. 15.7 Radiograph of the calcaneum showing irregular bony erosion at the insertion of the Achilles' tendon. This was caused by inflammatory enthesopathy in Reiter's syndrome.

ASSOCIATED DISORDERS AROUND THE ACHILLES' TENDON

The bursae around the tendon insertion can become inflamed, as part of an inflammatory joint disease (including gout) or because of repetitive trauma.

The tendon insertion may become inflamed (an enthesopathy) as a result of trauma or as part of one of the seronegative spondyloarthritides (mainly ankylosing spondylitis and Reiter's disease), when radiographic erosions are seen (Figs 15.6 & 15.7).

Tendon rupture can occur –because of either trauma or a sudden burst of activity in the young patient (e.g. squash playing), or spontaneously in the elderly. A sudden sharp pain is often followed by swelling and bruising. The 'Thompson calf-squeeze test' is positive (when you squeeze the calf muscles with the patient sitting or kneeling on a chair, the foot normally plantar flexes – this does not occur if the tendon is ruptured).

3 TYPICAL CASE: SPRAINED ANKLE

Marion is a 64-year-old, fit woman who ran to catch a bus, caught her foot on the edge of the sidewalk, and 'twisted' her right ankle. Immediate, sharp pain occurred on the lateral side of the ankle, followed by some swelling, and much pain and insecurity on standing.

Careful questioning suggested an inversion injury, and examination showed plenty of swelling and marked tenderness over the lateral malleolus. A radiograph was taken and was normal. Marion was initially treated with ice and ankle elevation for 24 hours, followed by NSAIDs for 5 days and then gentle mobilization and exercises.

FEATURES OF SPRAINED ANKLE

- An extremely common injury that affects all ages, including young people involved in athletic activities, and older people doing normal everyday activities.
- Most often affects the lateral ligaments around the ankle, because of inversion injury (Fig. 15.8).
- Can be complicated by instability and fractures of the malleoli.
- Is graded into three levels of severity – I, local tenderness only; II, some swelling and restriction of movements, with pain on weight bearing; III, severe pain, swelling, tenderness, and bruising, and impossible to weight bear.
- In grade III injuries, or in anyone who shows clinical signs that suggest possible instability (Fig. 15.9) or fracture (bony tenderness), a radiograph should be taken.
- Grade III sprains should be referred to orthopedic surgery.
- Most mild cases recover easily.
- An approach to treatment is shown in Figure 15.10.

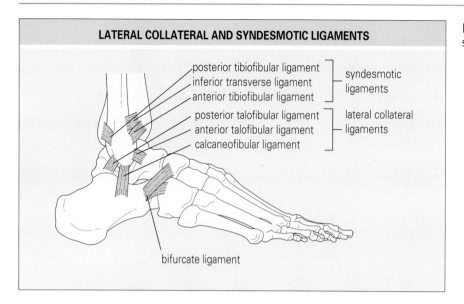

LATERAL COLLATERAL AND SYNDESMOTIC LIGAMENTS

posterior tibiofibular ligament
inferior transverse ligament ⎤ syndesmotic
anterior tibiofibular ligament ⎦ ligaments

posterior talofibular ligament ⎤ lateral collateral
anterior talofibular ligament ⎦ ligaments
calcaneofibular ligament

bifurcate ligament

Fig. 15.8 Lateral collateral ligaments and syndesmotic ligaments of the ankle.

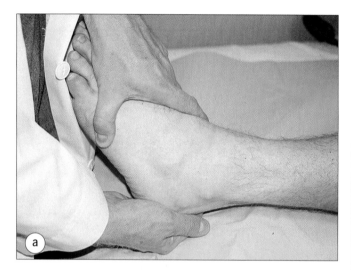

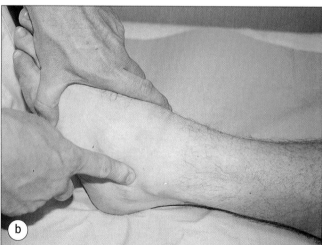

Fig. 15.9 **Passive ankle inversion.** Gentle inversion of the foot (a) with observation and (b) palpations of the talofibular joint. Motion or laxity suggests ligamentous instability.

AN APPROACH TO THE MANAGEMENT OF ACUTE ANKLE SPRAIN (GRADES 1 AND 2)

Immediate

- Rule out instability by examination
- Radiography when indicated

Initial 24–48 hours

- Rest
- Elevation
- Ice
- Compression
- NSAIDs

2–7 days

- NSAIDs
- Modified weight-bearing with ankle support (adhesive taping or air-stirrup support)
- Range of motion, proprioceptive exercise as tolerated

7–28 days

- Progressive mobilization with ankle support
- Additional strengthening exercises

Chronic

- Ankle support if insecurity or mild stability
- Resume athletic training when pain is minimal

Fig. 15.10 An approach to the management of acute ankle sprain.

FOREFOOT DISORDERS

The most vulnerable structure in the forefoot is the first MTP joint, which takes most of the stresses in walking and pushing-off with the foot. It suffers from common deformities (e.g. hallux valgus) and a number of forms of arthritis (especially gout). Pain is also common in the other MTP joints (metatarsalgia), and is usually caused by mechanical disorders and inappropriate footwear, although inflammatory joint diseases, particularly rheumatoid arthritis, frequently affect these joints.

4 TYPICAL CASE: HALLUX VALGUS WITH A BUNION

Marjorie is a 51-year-old charity worker, fond of fashionable shoes. She has noted that her big toes have tended to point outward for as long as she can remember, and her mother suffered from the same problem. Recently, increasing pain has occurred over the outside of the big toe of her right foot, and she is finding it very painful to put her best shoes on.

You notice hallux valgus of both feet, worse on the right than the left. In addition, there is a painful, red, swollen area over the lateral aspect of the base of the right first metatarsal bone (a bunion).

You advise Marjorie about the use of wider shoes and a pad to protect the bunion. This has little effect, and the pain worsens. In addition, Marjorie is becoming increasingly anxious and upset about the 'ugly deformities' of her foot. You refer her to an orthopedic surgeon who carries out a corrective osteotomy with removal of the metatarsal head. Marjorie's problem is solved and she is much happier with the shape of her foot.

FEATURES OF HALLUX VALGUS

- An extremely common deformity of the foot, much more frequent in women than men, in which there is a varus of the first metatarsal and valgus of the toe (Fig. 15.11).
- Has a congenital element, and also is associated with the wearing of tight shoes.
- Often asymptomatic, but frequently leads to pain because of inflammation of the bursa and subcutaneous tissues that overlie the head of the first metatarsal (a bunion), which is subjected to repeated trauma in shoes.
- Shoe alterations and bunion pads may help, but severe symptomatic cases need surgical correction.

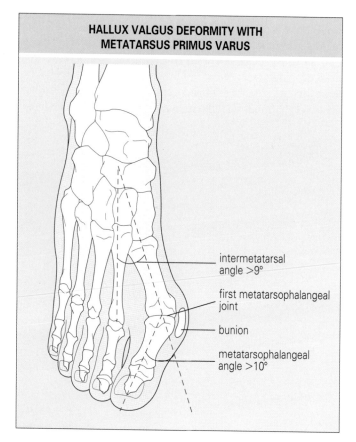

HALLUX VALGUS DEFORMITY WITH METATARSUS PRIMUS VARUS

intermetatarsal angle >9°

first metatarsophalangeal joint

bunion

metatarsophalangeal angle >10°

Fig. 15.11 Hallux valgus deformity.

ASSOCIATED DISORDER: HALLUX RIGIDUS

Hallux rigidus is a less common disorder, mainly seen in the elderly, in which there is marked restriction of movement of the first MTP joint. This can result in a lot of pain and difficulty with walking. Shoe correction may help, but surgery is sometimes needed.

FEATURES OF METATARSALGIA AND MORTON'S INTERDIGITAL NEUROMAS

- Metatarsalgia is common, and Morton's neuromas are not.
- Metatarsalgia is characterized by pain in the ball of the foot on standing and walking.
- Tenderness is found on palpation of the metatarsophalangeal joints.
- Metatarsalgia is usually caused by mechanical abnormalities of foot shape and/or inappropriate footwear.
- Occasionally, metatarsalgia is a presentation of an arthritis, such as rheumatoid disease.
- Occasionally, patients develop severe neurologic pain in one web space of the foot because of nerve entrapment and the development of a neuroma on one of the interdigital nerves (Morton's metatarsalgia).
- The best way to treat common metatarsalgia is with alterations to footwear and activities as appropriate.

5 TYPICAL CASE: METATARSALGIA WITH AN INTERDIGITAL (MORTON'S) NEUROMA

Julia is a 64-year-old woman who has always complained of aching feet. She lives a fairly sedentary life, but will not go out without her smart shoes on.

A few months back, her right foot became much worse, with a lot of aching pain in the ball of the foot, particularly on standing and walking. You advised her to wear wider, better-fitting shoes, but she took no notice. She now complains of a new symptom, that of a burning pain between her third and fourth toes, with tingling and numbness. She finds that massaging the feet helps a bit. You find exquisite tenderness on palpation of the web space between the two affected toes.

You talk further to Julia about shoes, but realize you are wasting your time. She goes to a surgeon who successfully removes the neuroma that has developed on the affected digital nerve, which relieves the problem, but leaves a small area of numbness.

Rx MANAGEMENT OF ANKLE AND FOOT DISORDERS

The basic principles of management of each of the specific disorders have been mentioned under the relevant section. In general, common ankle and foot disorders are largely caused by mechanical problems, and the mainstay of management is correction of any abnormal mechanical stresses, mainly through footwear adjustments. Good management of disorders of the foot requires help from orthotists and podiatrists, who are able to give specialist advice about footwear and also manage local lesions, such as calluses, effectively. This is particularly important in older patients, who often suffer extensively and unnecessarily from foot disorders.

Local injection therapy to any structures in and around the foot should only be undertaken by specialists very familiar with the relevant anatomy and procedures.

RECOMMENDATIONS FOR REFERRAL

Subspecialty
Referral to a rheumatologist is rarely indicated, although patients in whom you suspect an inflammatory arthropathy such as Reiter's disease or rheumatoid arthritis, as well as those who might need injection therapy (which should not generally be attempted in primary care) should be considered for referral.

Physical therapy/podiatry and chiropody
Podiatrists and chiropodists have much to offer people with foot problems, particularly those with mechanical problems leading to callus formation, and those in need of footwear advice and alterations.

Orthopedic surgery
Any patient with a major soft tissue injury (e.g. grade III ankle sprain) or severe progressive disease, should be considered for surgical referral. Severe hallux valgus or rigidus, resulting in persistent pain and/or disability in spite of conservative management, should be considered for operative correction.

REGIONAL PAIN AND MONOARTICULAR DISORDERS

16

GOUT

Gout has been recognized since antiquity, and remains a relatively common condition with a prevalence of around 1% in the adult population. Men are affected more than women (about 5:1), and the peak age is 40–50 in males and over 60 in females. The acute form of gouty attack is the most common manifestation – this is an excruciatingly painful condition, which classically affects the base of the big toe (podagra). Other presentations and chronic tophaceous gout are less common, but can present challenging diagnostic and therapeutic problems.

ACUTE GOUT

TYPICAL CASE: THE PRESENTATION OF GOUT

John is a 47-year-old company director who has mild hypertension, enjoys socializing with his friends, and is slightly overweight. He is otherwise well and on no treatment.

He wakes up in the middle of the night with a painful, pricking sensation at the base of his right big toe. An hour later he is in severe pain. The toe progressively worsens over the next few hours, becoming swollen, bright red (Fig. 16.1), and exceedingly painful, and he calls his doctor out at 5.00 in the morning. He is prescribed a nonsteroidal anti-inflammatory agent.

> **KEY POINTS**
>
> - Gout is a clinical syndrome caused by an inflammatory response to monosodium urate monohydrate crystals, which may form in people who have hyperuricemia.
> - Hyperuricemia may be caused by environmental and/or genetic factors.
> - Gout most commonly affects middle-aged men.
> - Acute gout is a relapsing, self-limiting, severe inflammatory form of arthritis; hyperuricemia is not always present at the time of an acute attack.
> - The chronic form of gout is associated with tophus formation and bone and joint destruction.
> - Gout is commonly associated with obesity, heavy alcohol intake, hypertension, hyperlipidemia, renal impairment, and diuretic use.
> - The main joints affected are the first metatarsophalangeal joints; other sites include the instep, heel, ankle, and knee.

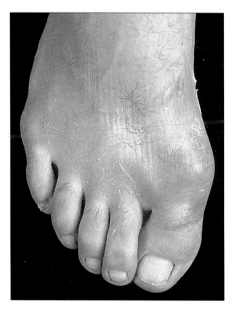

Fig. 16.1 The toe in early acute gout. The first metatarsophalangeal joint is the most commonly affected joint – the intense inflammation of the joint results in severe pain, swelling, and local heat, which develops so quickly that the overlying skin becomes red and shiny.

FEATURES OF ACUTE ATTACK OF GOUT

- Acute gout peaks in men aged 40–50 years.
- Over 50% of acute attacks occur in the first tarsometatarsal joint; other common sites include the instep, heel, ankle, and knee.
- The attack may be heralded by a feeling of tickling or pricking in the affected joint.
- Attacks often begin at night, and some are triggered by trauma.
- The joint becomes red, hot, swollen, and extremely painful within a few hours of onset.
- Systemic signs of inflammation, such as fever and malaise, may occur.
- Attacks nearly always subside spontaneously over a few days, although subsequent desquamation of the skin is common.

The pain is so bad that John cannot walk, and he is furious because he has had to cancel an important company meeting. However, over the next 48 hours the pain and swelling gradually subside, but the skin over the joint starts to desquamate (Fig. 16.2). After 5 days, John is back to normal, and within a month he has forgotten all about the incident.

NATURAL HISTORY AND OTHER CLINICAL FEATURES

Most acute attacks resolve spontaneously within a few days of onset, with or without treatment, although the very severe pain is much relieved by prompt treatment. Between attacks, no symptoms or signs occur. Some people experience only one attack in their whole life. Many develop a pattern in which they suffer one attack every few months. Some go on to have more frequent, recurrent acute attacks of gout, some of which may be polyarticular. A minority develop chronic tophaceous gout, which is characterized by tophi, and described below.

The risk of repeated attacks and of chronic gout depends on the degree and duration of hyperuricemia.

OTHER FORMS OF PRESENTATION OF GOUT

The classic attack of gout is relatively easy to recognize clinically. However, other presentations (polyarticular acute and periarticular gout, and gout in elderly females with renal disease) can cause major problems.

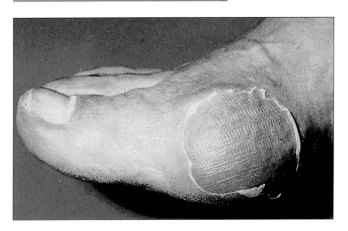

Fig. 16.2 The toe at a later stage in the evolution of an acute attack of gout. As the pain, redness, heat, and swelling subside, often desquamation of the overlying skin occurs.

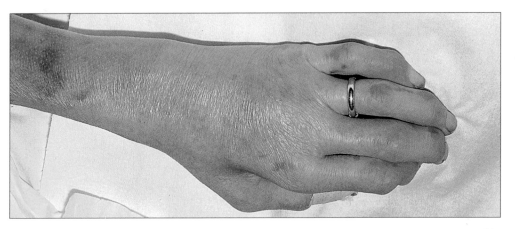

Fig. 16.3 A polyarticular attack of gout results in swelling and redness of the wrist and of several of the interphalangeal joints.

POLYARTICULAR ACUTE GOUT

Some 5% of acute attacks are polyarticular, which causes confusion with other inflammatory arthropathies (Fig. 16.3).

PERIARTICULAR ('SOFT TISSUE') GOUT

Periarticular gout can cause inflammation that is primarily in the subcutaneous tissues, and which simulates a cellulitis (Fig. 16.4).

GOUT IN ELDERLY FEMALES WHO HAVE RENAL DISEASE OR USE DIURETICS

This is a special form of gout, only seen in older people (usually women) who have renal disease and/or use diuretics that contribute to the hyperuricemia. The patients present with tophi – most commonly on the hands around Heberden's nodes, which may ulcerate (Fig. 16.5) – and may not experience any classic acute attacks of gout.

QUESTIONS TO ASK AND THINGS TO LOOK OUT FOR

WHAT IS THE CAUSE OF THE HYPERURICEMIA?

Hyperuricemia is necessary for uric acid crystals to form, but it is not a sufficient cause for gout. Most people with hyperuricemia do not develop gout – furthermore, the hyperuricemia may not be evident at the time of a gout attack. Most typical gout in middle-aged men is associated with mild hyperuricemia caused by a relative deficiency of uric acid excretion by the kidney. A family history of gout is common in such men. However, other risk factors for hyperuricemia need to be considered. Obesity causes hyperuricemia, as does excess alcohol intake. Renal disease and diuretics are both potent causes of hyperuricemia, and diuretic use is one of the main causes of gout in older people. Hyperuricemia and gout can also result from neoplastic disorders and their treatment, and from drugs such as cyclosporine given to prevent transplant rejection – the presentation and clinical features may be atypical in such cases. Other drugs, including low doses of aspirin, can raise uric acid levels. A number of other rare genetic or environmental causes occur, which need only be considered in very young patients or in atypical or severe cases. Gout in premenopausal woman is extremely rare, and anyone with this condition is likely to have a significant metabolic abnormality as the cause.

ARE THERE ANY ASSOCIATED CARDIOVASCULAR RISK FACTORS?

Gout is strongly associated with a number of cardiovascular risk factors (obesity, hypertension, and hyperlipidemia) so the attack of gout may act as a useful pointer to the need for prophylactic measures to be taken to prevent a subsequent cardiovascular crisis, such as a myocardial infarction.

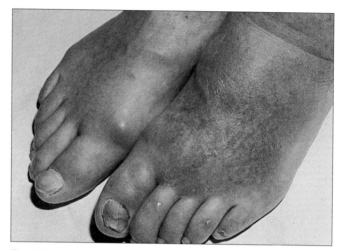

Fig. 16.4 Gouty cellulitis. Inflammation induced by urate crystals occasionally occurs, primarily in the soft tissue of periarticular areas, and causes an appearance similar to that of streptococcal cellulitis.

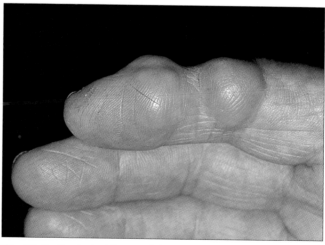

Fig. 16.5 Gouty tophi around the osteoarthritic joints of the hand of an elderly female patient. Her presentation of gout was with these relatively painless tophi.

THE MOST IMPORTANT DIFFERENTIAL DIAGNOSES

- Trauma – including fractures of the small bones of the foot.
- Bursitis or cellulitis of structures around the joint ('poor man's gout').
- Septic arthritis (the most important differential diagnosis – not to be overlooked).
- Other crystal-related arthropathies, such as pseudogout.

! POINTS TO LOOK OUT FOR

- Gout sufferers are often obese – obesity contributes to hyperuricemia, and is also a cardiovascular risk factor.
- Check blood pressure – hypertension is common in middle-aged, male gout patients.
- Check serum lipids – hypertriglyceridemia (type IV lipoproteinemia) is common.
- Inquire about any family history of cardiovascular disease, and about any other potential synergistic risk factors, such as smoking.

ASSOCIATIONS, DIFFERENTIAL DIAGNOSIS, AND INVESTIGATIONS

The acute attack of gout is often easy to diagnose from the history and examination. However, difficulty can arise, particularly with the first attack, with milder attacks, or with atypical or polyarticular attacks.

'Nongout' – a condition characterized by nongouty joint symptoms and hyperuricemia – is often seen in rheumatology clinics; such patients have often been mistreated with allopurinol, sometimes with disastrous results.

Investigations need not be carried out for typical attacks in a patient who is known to have gout. However, when possible, it is valuable to confirm the diagnosis in a first attack, to avoid the trap of 'nongout'. The difficulty is that the diagnosis of gout can only be confirmed by the identification of urate crystals in the synovial fluid - high uric acid levels are not diagnostic of gout. The three relevant investigations are:

- Uric acid levels – these are generally above normal most of the time in most gout patients. However, levels are often normal range, or even low around the time of the acute attack, and most patients who have mild elevations of uric acid do not suffer gout – so this is a very unreliable test for gout in the acute phase. An extremely low level makes gout unlikely, and a very high level makes gout a little more likely – uric acid levels indicate no more than this.
- Radiographs – these are generally normal during acute attacks, and are therefore noncontributory to diagnosis unless used to rule out a differential diagnosis, such as a fracture.
- Synovial fluid crystal identification – this is the definitive test, but requires aspiration of fluid from the acutely painful joint (which may be difficult) and examination by a trained specialist using a polarized light microscope (Fig. 16.6). The primary care physician may not have access to a laboratory where there is someone with special training and interest in synovial fluid crystal identification, which is ideally what is needed.

Other investigations that may be of value include renal function tests and measurement of serum lipid levels, for reasons outlined above.

A PRACTICAL GUIDE TO THE INVESTIGATION OF A PATIENT WITH ACUTE GOUT

1. During acute attack, no investigations are indicated other than possible aspiration of synovial fluid to confirm the presence of uric acid crystals – do not measure serum uric acid or do radiographs. You may need to check renal function in relation to use of NSAIDs for treatment.
2. Between acute attacks, check serum uric acid levels and keep an annual check on renal function, also screen for hyperlipidemia.

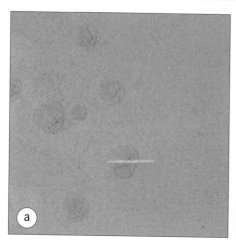
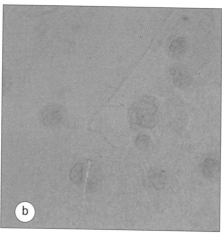

Fig. 16.6. Crystals of monosodium urate monohydrate (the gout culprit) can be visualized by polarized light microscopy because of their birefringence. This results in characteristic color changes when the crystals are aligned in different orientations with respect to the compensator of the microscope. (a, b) A crystal of this type can be seen here, attached to a polymorphonuclear white cell in the synovial fluid.

CHRONIC TOPHACEOUS GOUT

1 TYPICAL CASE: CHRONIC TOPHACEOUS GOUT

Ralph is a 56-year-old man who lost his job 20 years ago, and he subsequently became an alcoholic and homeless man. He has suffered from attacks of gout (which his father also suffered from) for about 15 years, but because of his circumstances has done nothing about it. Over the past few years, he has developed painless, firm swellings over his hands, feet, and elbows. One of the lesions over his hand ulcerated and became infected, which resulted in septicemia, and he was admitted to hospital. On examination he has the classic clinical features of chronic tophaceous gout (Fig. 16.7), and radiographs confirm gout damage to the small joints of his hands and feet (Fig. 16.8).

FEATURES OF CHRONIC TOPHACEOUS GOUT

- Chronic tophaceous gout only appears in people whose acute gout and hyperuricemia have not been treated; it can also manifest in occasional cases of atypical gout with severe hyperuricemia.
- Patients have usually suffered from acute attacks of gout for many years before tophi appear.
- Tophi develop slowly, with the formation of firm, nodular swellings.
- The most common sites are the hands, feet, olecranon bursa of the elbow, and Achilles' tendon; tophi occasionally form in other 'classic' sites such as the helix of the ear.
- Tophaceous development is usually associated with a chronic destructive arthritis of the joints that have suffered attacks of acute gout.
- In the chronic tophaceous stage of the disease, acute attacks may become less common or even disappear completely.
- Tophi can ulcerate and become secondarily infected.

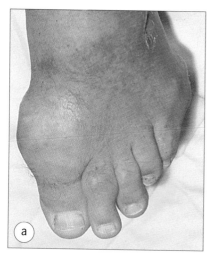
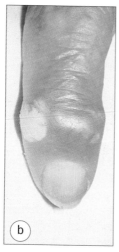
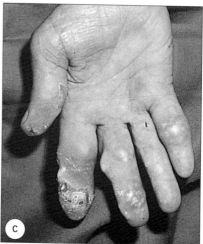
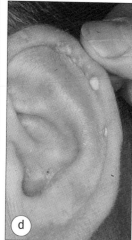

Fig. 16.7 Gouty tophi. (a) Tophi that involve the first, second, and fifth metatarsophalangeal joints with little involvement of overlying skin. (b) An ulcerating tophus of a distal interphalangeal joint with associated redness of the overlying skin. (c) Extensive tophi of all digits. (d) Auricular tophi. (Courtesy of Dr J Webb).

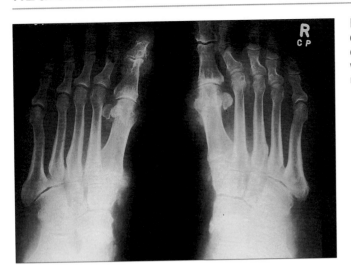

Fig. 16.8 Radiographic changes in the feet characteristic of chronic tophaceous gout. Note the 'punched out' para-articular erosion of the proximal phalanx, with its sclerotic margins, as well as the bony destruction and cyst formation in the first metatarsophalangeal joints.

NATURAL HISTORY AND OTHER CLINICAL FEATURES

By the time chronic tophaceous gout has developed, there is usually evidence of severe joint damage. The course of the condition subsequently depends on the success of treatment with hypouricemic therapy, but it is often difficult to remove all tophi, and damage already done to joints cannot be repaired. Renal disease and renal calculi may also be present. Tophi can develop almost anywhere in the body, including at sites such as the eye, heart, and spine, where they can cause clinical problems and diagnostic confusion.

 ## POINTS TO LOOK OUT FOR

- Renal disease: the combination of hyperuricemia, renal disease, and chronic tophacous gout carries a poor prognosis, and such patients need specialist treatment.
- Ulceration and sepsis: tophi can ulcerate through the skin and may become infected.

DIFFERENTIAL DIAGNOSIS

Chronic tophaceous gout has fairly characteristic features. However, it can mimic nodular rheumatoid arthritis.

 ## MANAGEMENT OF GOUT

The management of gout may involve one of four quite separate issues.
1. Management of the acute attack – principally the management of acute inflammation through rest and anti-inflammatory medications.
2. Prophylactic measures to reduce the risk of further attacks.
3. The management of hyperuricemia through diet or drugs, and the use of agents such as low-dose colchicine or nonsteroidal anti-inflammatory drugs (NSAIDs) in a prophylactic manner.
4. The treatment of asymptomatic hyperuricemia.

Gout is a condition that is relatively easy to manage in primary care, and most patients do not need referral. A small number need specialist input from the rheumatologist.

THE ACUTE ATTACK

Most acute attacks resolve spontaneously. However, they are spectacularly painful, and the severity of the pain as well as the duration of the attack can be reduced by anti-inflammatory therapy.

Provided no contraindication to their use is evident, oral NSAIDs are the treatment of choice. The usual recommendation is to use a 'decrescendo' regime, with an initial high-loading dose, followed by high doses for the first 24–48 hours, after which the drug can quickly be tailed off. Many gout sufferers learn how to manage this themselves, and keep an NSAID with them for immediate dosing as soon as they think an attack is beginning. One of the more potent anti-inflammatory agents, such as indomethacin, should be used.

If NSAIDs are contraindicated, options include a short course of systemic corticosteroids, or a local intra-articular injection of corticosteroids (provided infection is not a risk) or colchicine. However, colchicine is problematic for use with acute attacks, as the dose required to obtain control often produces diarrhea. If corticosteroids are used, dosing should be limited to the first 2–3 days, and patients must be strongly advised against using them for longer periods or on an 'on-demand' basis.

Acutely inflamed gouty joints also benefit from rest. If a large joint, such as the knee, is involved and a tense effusion is present, aspiration to relieve pressure inside the joint (and hence pain) is indicated.

PROPHYLAXIS OF RECURRENT ACUTE ATTACKS

Low-dose colchicine (around 0.6mg twice daily) is the most effective therapy for the prophylaxis of recurrent acute attacks. At this dose level, side effects are uncommon. Regular doses of a nonsteroidal anti-inflammatory agent are an alternative.

CONTROL OF HYPERURICEMIA

In general, hyperuricemia is overtreated. Indications for hypouricemic therapy are relatively few (Fig. 16.9), and (as noted above) many patients prefer to treat the occasional acute attack or to take prophylactic colchicine than to be sentenced to a life-long course of hypuricemic drugs, all of which are occasionally quite toxic.

Many patients who suffer gout have relatively mild hyperuricemia that can be controlled by simple removal of a significant risk factor, such as obesity, alcohol abuse, or drug (such as a diuretic or low-dose aspirin). Dietary means other than the reduction of alcohol and obesity are of little value – a low-purine diet is difficult to adhere to and has only a modest effect on uric acid levels.

If one of the clear indications for treating hyperuricemic (Fig. 16.9) is present, and the patient does not respond to the simple measures outlined above, a hypouricemic drug is needed. If this is agreed, the patient must understand that he/she will probably have to be on the drug therapy for the rest of his/her life, and that in the first few months an increased risk of acute attacks occurs. Hypouricemic therapy should NEVER be started at the time of an acute attack (Fig. 16.10). You should wait for at least one week after an attack has completely resolved before initiating any hypouricemic therapy.

Allopurinol is the drug of choice, and should be given in gradually increasing doses, starting around 100–200mg/day, and increasing at 2–4 weekly intervals to the maintenance level needed to keep uric acid levels well below 0.4mmol/l (6.5mg/dL), which is usually in the 300–600mg/day range. To help deal with the increased risk of acute attacks of gout

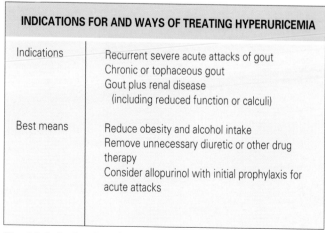

INDICATIONS FOR AND WAYS OF TREATING HYPERURICEMIA	
Indications	Recurrent severe acute attacks of gout Chronic or tophaceous gout Gout plus renal disease (including reduced function or calculi)
Best means	Reduce obesity and alcohol intake Remove unnecessary diuretic or other drug therapy Consider allopurinol with initial prophylaxis for acute attacks

Fig. 16.9 Indications for and ways of treating hyperuricemia.

THE 'NEVER DOs' OF GOUT TREATMENT

- Never introduce hypouricemic therapy during an acute attack – this can turn a simple acute attack into a very severe polyarticular attack of gout and make the patient very sick
- Never start hypouricemic therapy without co-prescribing some form of prophylaxis for acute attacks, either colchicine or a nonsteroidal anti-inflammatory drug
- Never introduce a hypouricemic drug unless you are certain of the diagnosis

Fig. 16.10 The 'NEVER DOs' of gout treatment.

in the first few months of treatment, colchicine 0.5–0.6mg twice daily should be co-prescribed until the allopurinol dosage is settled and uric acid levels are stable.

Patients should initially be monitored with regular checks of uric acid levels to help adjust the drug dosage, and they should all have renal function measured at least once a year.

A small number of patients are unable to tolerate allopurinol because of side effects (severe side effects are particularly likely in elderly patients who have renal disease), in which case a uricosuric drug such as probenecid or sulfinpyrazone might be considered. As with allopurinol, these drugs need to be gradually increased in dose to a level that controls the hyperuricemia, with colchicine cover in the first few months; in addition, a high urine flow must be maintained to reduce the risk of renal calculi. Theoretically, it is logical to treat those patients who are undersecretors of uric acid with a uricosuric agent, and those who are overproducers with allopurinol, which stops uric acid production – but in practice, allopurinol is the drug of first choice for all patients needing pharmacologic treatment for hyperuricemia.

TREATMENT OF ASYMPTOMATIC HYPERURICEMIA

Asymptomatic hyperuricemia, in the absence of renal disease, should not be treated unless levels are consistently very high (>0.7mmol/l [11.4mg/dL]). If renal disease is present, uric acid levels should be controlled (i.e. reduced to <0.4mmol/l [6.5mg/dL] with allopurinol).

POSSIBLE REASONS FOR REFERRAL OF CASES OF GOUT

- Diagnostic uncertainty.
- Severe recurrent attacks not responding to standard therapy.
- Chronic tophaceous gout that is difficult to control.
- Gout with renal disease or calculi.

REGIONAL PAIN AND MONOARTICULAR DISORDERS

17

SEPTIC ARTHRITIS

Septic arthritis is one the few urgent problems in rheumatology, since delay in diagnosis and treatment reduces the likelihood of a successful outcome. The vast majority of cases of septic arthritis present as monoarthritis with pain, tenderness, and loss of function. Septic arthritis can be either acute, typically from bacterial organisms, or chronic caused by mycobacterial, fungal, or parasitic organisms. Analysis and culture of synovial fluid is essential for diagnosis and selection of appropriate antibiotic coverage. With prompt diagnosis and institution of treatment, the majority of patients who suffer septic arthritis recover completely with little or no impairment of joint function.

1 TYPICAL CASE: ACUTE SEPTIC ARTHRITIS

Angus is a 68-year-old retired lobster fisherman seen for a 1-week history of increasing pain and loss of movement of his right shoulder. He has been troubled by 'bursitis' in the shoulder for years, which occasionally caused him difficulty when pulling in the lobster traps.

On physical examination he is afebrile and guards his right shoulder with his arm across his chest. A swelling over the anterior aspect of the shoulder is warm and very tender to touch (Fig. 17.1). Aspiration of the shoulder yields 30ml of

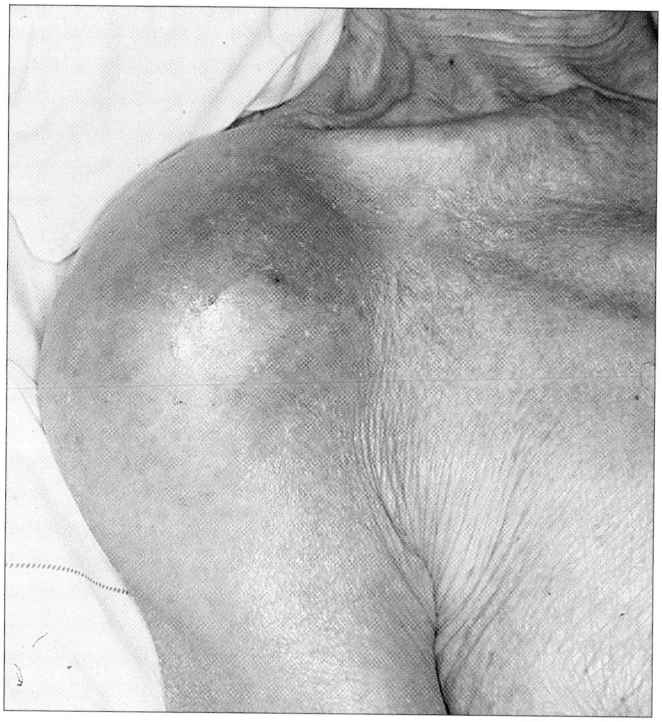

Fig. 17.1 Acute swelling, erythema, and tenderness of the shoulder from septic arthritis.

KEY POINTS

- Infection of the synovial membrane with bacterial, mycobacterial, fungal or other organisms.
- Mostly commonly presents as a monoarthritis, typically of the knee, hip, or shoulder.
- Major risk factors include penetrating injuries to joints, intravenous drug use, human immunodeficiency virus (HIV) infection, prosthetic joints, corticosteroid use, and pre-existing joint disease such as rheumatoid arthritis and other systemic disorders.
- Most cases of septic arthritis are successfully managed medically with appropriate antibiotics, joint drainage, and physical therapy.

FEATURES OF ACUTE SEPTIC ARTHRITIS

- Typically monoarticular and most commonly involves knee, hip, or shoulder.
- Onset is abrupt, with swelling, warmth, tenderness, and inability to move the joint because of pain.
- Fever and shaking chills frequent.
- Major risk factors include penetrating injuries to joints, intravenous drug users, prosthetic joints, HIV infection, and pre-existing joint disease such as rheumatoid arthritis.
- Staphylococcus aureus is the most common infecting organism, except in children <2 years (Haemophilus influenzae more common) and in sexually active young adults (Neisseria gonorrhoeae).
- Other organisms are particularly likly to occur in patients with joint prosthesis and those with predisposing disorders which suppress the immune system.

FEATURES OF CHRONIC SEPTIC ARTHRITIS

- May involve peripheral joints (knees, hips, and wrist most common), sacroiliac joints, or vertebral bodies.
- Insidious onset with nontender swelling of joint or back pain, often causes long delay in diagnosis.
- Joint damage results from erosions by inflamed synovium and infection of bone (osteomyelitis).
- Organisms that cause chronic septic arthritis include mycobacterial infections (Mycobacterium tuberculosis and atypical mycobacterium), invasive fungi (Histoplasma, Blastomyces, Candida, etc.), Brucella, and (rarely) parasitic or protozoal organisms.

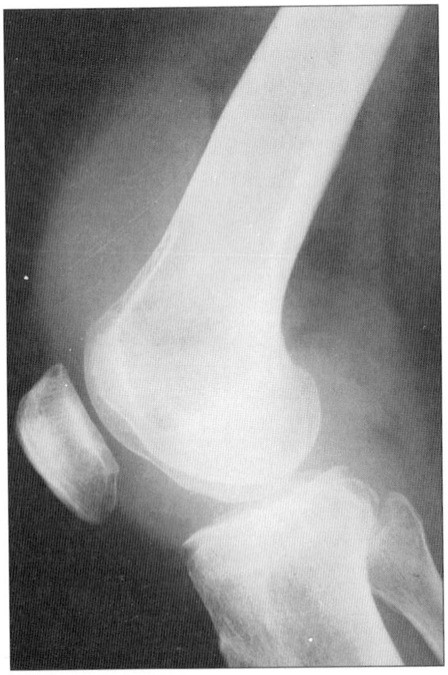

Fig. 17.2 Tuberculosis of the knee. Soft-tissue swelling, blurriness of the subchondral bone, and an anterior marginal erosion of the tibia. (Reproduced with permission from Chapman M, Murray RO, Stoker DJ. Tuberculosis of the bones and joints. Semin Roentgenol. 1979;14:266–82.)

yellow turbid fluid with a white blood cell (WBC) count of 64,000 cells/mm^3 with 90% polymorphonuclear leukocytes. Gram stain of the fluid shows Gram-positive cocci.

2 TYPICAL CASE: CHRONIC SEPTIC ARTHRITIS

Lionel is a 27-year-old, HIV-positive ballet dancer. For the past 6 months he has noted pain in his right knee which he has ascribed to a dancing injury. He is currently in rehearsal for a new ballet and his knee gave way in attempting to lift his partner. On physical examination, the knee appears slightly swollen with no clear effusion or obvious warmth. No instability of the knee is detected. A radiograph of the knee shows soft-tissue swelling and an erosion of the anterior margin of the tibia (Fig. 17.2). Attempts to aspirate fluid from the knee are unsuccessful ('dry tap'). An arthroscopic biopsy of the knee is performed and the synovial tissue shows caseating granuloma and giant cells compatible with tuberculous arthritis (Fig. 17.3).

NATURAL HISTORY AND OTHER CLINICAL FEATURES

Infectious agents may reach the joint by several different routes (Fig. 17.4). An inflammatory reaction within the synovial membrane occurs, with an infiltration of leukocytes, proliferation, and joint effusion, with exudation of infectious organisms, inflammatory cells, and proteolytic enzymes into the synovial cavity. The synovial pannus produces marginal erosions of the joint, and the increased pressure within the joint combined with proteolytic enzymes degrade cartilage surfaces. In addition, the infectious process can spread to involve subchondral bone (to produce osteomyelitis) or extend into tendon sheaths.

! POINTS TO LOOK OUT FOR

- Septic arthritis may be a sign of occult systemic disease, which includes diabetes, chronic liver disease, sickle cell anemia (salmonella arthritis), malignancy, or acquired immunodeficiency syndrome.
- In septic arthritis of the hip, pain is usually referred to the anterior thigh or knee.

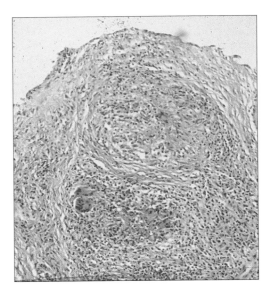

Fig. 17.3 Synovial biopsy from a patient who has tuberculous arthritis showing caseating granuloma and giant cells. (Reproduced with permission from Garcia-Kutzbach A. Tuberculosis arthritis. In: Espinoza LR, Goldenberg DL, Arnett F, Alarcon GS, eds. Infections in the rheumatic diseases. A comprehensive review of microbial relations to rheumatic disorders. New York: Grune & Stratton; 1988:131–8.)

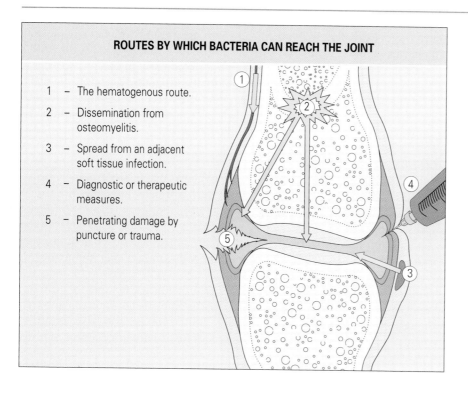

ROUTES BY WHICH BACTERIA CAN REACH THE JOINT

1 – The hematogenous route.

2 – Dissemination from osteomyelitis.

3 – Spread from an adjacent soft tissue infection.

4 – Diagnostic or therapeutic measures.

5 – Penetrating damage by puncture or trauma.

Fig. 17.4 Routes by which bacteria can reach the joint.

- Chronic septic arthritis is often associated with tenosynovitis, commonly of the wrist and hand.
- Gonococcal arthritis is considered in young patients who present with a febrile syndrome of polyarthritis, tenosynovitis, and dermatitis.
- Meningococcemia is considered in patients who have arthritis, rash, and fluctuating neurologic signs.
- In endemic areas, Lyme disease is considered in patients who have characteristic rash and arthritis (see Chapter 18).

ASSOCIATIONS, DIFFERENTIAL DIAGNOSIS, AND INVESTIGATIONS

INVESTIGATIONS

Specialist investigation is mandatory.

Laboratory tests. Synovial fluid analysis and culture are critical in septic arthritis. The synovial WBC count is markedly elevated (typically >50,000 cells/mm^3) with a predominance of polymorphonuclear cells (typically >85%). Gram stain of the synovial fluid reveals organisms in approximately 50% of cases. Synovial fluid should be sent for aerobic and anaerobic cultures. If gonococcal infection is suspected, synovial fluid should be plated at the bedside on chocolate agar or other special medium to avoid drying. In addition, all other body fluids (blood, urine, serosal fluids, etc.), orifices, and clinically apparent foci of suspected infection should similarly be cultured.

The usual nonspecific findings indicative of an infection (such as an elevated, peripheral WBC count, erythrocyte sedimentation rate, or raised C-reactive protein) are usually present.

Imaging. A plain radiograph of the joint is obtained to provide a baseline to monitor treatment and to search for evidence of joint erosions or a contiguous focus of osteomyelitis. In the early stages of acute septic arthritis, only soft-tissue swelling and synovial effusions are present. After 10–14 days of infection, destructive changes of joint space narrowing (which reflect cartilage destruction) and erosions or foci of subchondral osteomyelitis become evident (Fig. 17.5). Gas formation within the joint suggests infection with *Escherichia coli* or

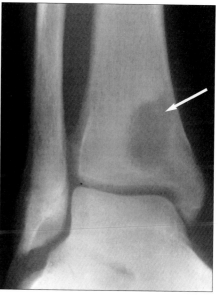

Fig. 17.5 Subacute osteomyelitis (Brodie's abscess). The well-defined oval lucency in the distal tibia shows fading sclerosis along its margins in a pattern typical of a bone abscess. Note the small projection of the upper pole of the lesion pointing to the medial metaphysis, where a subtle periosteal reaction is beginning to form (arrow). This identifies the site where this lesion may ultimately drain.

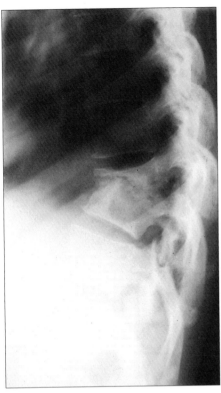

Fig. 17.6 Advanced tuberculosis of the spine. Massive collapse of T9 and T10, with absence of reactive bone sclerosis. (Courtesy of Dr A Keat.)

anaerobes. Destructive radiographic changes are generally obvious in patients who have a chronic septic arthritis (Fig. 17.6).

Radionuclide bone scans may be helpful, particularly in patients suspected to have infection of prosthetic joints or in joints difficult to examine clinically, such as the hip, symphysis pubis, or sacroiliac joint. Technetium phosphate bone scans become abnormal within days, which demonstrates the increased uptake of radioisotope as a result of increased blood flow.

DIFFERENTIAL DIAGNOSIS

Septic arthritis is considered in any patient who has unexplained monoarthritis. Crystalline arthropathies (gout, calcium pyrophosphate dihydrate disease, or apatite deposition) can mimic the clinical and laboratory features of septic arthritis, although these are readily excluded by detection of crystals in the synovial fluid. Rarely, acute septic arthritis and crystal-induced arthritis may coexist, particularly in the setting of multiple myeloma or other immunologically compromising diseases.

The acute onset of most inflammatory arthropathies (rheumatoid arthritis, seronegative spondyloarthropathy, etc.) may resemble acute bacterial arthritis, although cultures of the synovial fluid are negative. Reactive arthritis, particularly with urethritis, may be easily confused with gonococcal arthritis (see Chapter 22).

MANAGEMENT

The principles of successful treatment of septic arthritis include prompt administration of appropriate antibiotics, adequate drainage of the joint space, and active rehabilitation once the inflammation begins to subside.

Drainage of the infected synovial fluid is essential to reduce intra-articular pressure, remove proteolytic enzymes, and facilitate antibiotic actions. In most cases, closed aspiration using a 16-guage (or larger) needle or arthroscopy with lavage once or twice daily for as long as effusions reaccumulate is sufficient. Open surgical drainage is required for drainage and debridement of septic hips, septic joints with coexistent osteomyelitis, and joint infections not controlled after 5 days of antibiotics and closed drainage.

Fig. 17.7 Recommended antibiotic regimens for acute septic arthritis in adults.

RECOMMENDED ANTIBIOTIC REGIMENS FOR ACUTE SEPTIC ARTHRITIS IN ADULTS		
Organism	Drug of choice	Duration (days)
Staphylococcus aureus	Nafcillin or oxacillin, 2–3g i.v. q6h	21–28
S. aureus Methicillin-resistant	Vancomycin, 1g q12h	21–28
Streptococci	Penicillin G, 2 × 10⁶ IU q4–6h i.v.	14
Enterococci	Penicillin G, 2 × 10⁶ IU i.v. q4–6h, plus gentamicin 3–5mg/kg/day i.m. or i.v. q8h	21–28
Neisseria gonorrhoeae	Ceftriaxone 1–2g i.m. or i.v. q24h	7–10
Pseudomonas aeruginosa	Gentamicin, 3–5mg/kg/day q8h, plus piperacillin, 4–5g q6h i.v.	21–28

ANTIBIOTICS

In patients who have suspected septic arthritis, empiric antibiotics should be initiated promptly after appropriate cultures are obtained and before the results of bacteriologic cultures are available. Antibiotics are selected to cover the pathogens most likely to be present or are based on Gram-stain findings. When no bacteria are identified on Gram's stain, a first-generation cephalosporin is recommended, unless the history suggests gonococcal or pseudomonal infection. Antibiotics are given parenterally, which produces therapeutic levels in synovial fluid. Intra-articular injections of antibiotics are unnecessary and may irritate the synovium and produce a chemical synovitis.

Antibiotic regimens are adjusted once culture results are available. Examples of recommended antibiotic regimens for acute septic arthritis in adults are given in Figure 17.7. Antibiotic dosages may need to be changed on the basis of impairments of renal function or other factors, and a longer duration of therapy may be required for patients who have extra-articular infection, osteomyelitis, infected prosthetic joint, or pre-existing structural joint disease.

Infections of prosthetic joints are a major challenge and typically require a much longer course of antibiotic treatment. If the infection persists despite antibiotics, or if there is loosening of the prosthesis, the prosthesis must be removed and the site sterilized with antibiotics for months before replacement of the prosthesis is attempted.

PHYSICAL THERAPY

Physical therapy plays an important role in the management of septic arthritis, to control pain and to maintain joint mobility and muscle strength. Immobilization of the septic joint helps to relieve pain. Once the inflammation begins to subside, passive range of motion exercises are initiated and active exercises begun, as tolerated, to prevent contractures, venous thrombosis, and emboli. For septic joints of the lower extremities, weight bearing is prohibited until all signs of inflammation have cleared.

SURGERY AND OTHER TREATMENT MODALITIES

Surgery may be required to obtain synovial tissue, either by arthroscopy or open biopsy, for diagnostic purposes or for open drainage, lavage, or debridement of the infected joint.

MONITORING PROGRESSION AND OUTCOME

Septic arthritis is easily monitored by changes in the synovial fluid drained from the joint. Within 24–48 hours of starting appropriate antibiotic coverage, synovial WBC counts diminish and aspirated synovial fluid volumes should begin to diminish. If the infection is not responding promptly, synovial fluid bactericidal levels are measured.

The clinical outcome of septic arthritis is dependent on a number of factors, which include duration of symptoms prior to treatment, age of the patient, need for surgical drainage, and presence of pre-existing arthritis of the infected joint. The outcome is generally poor if synovial cultures remain positive for longer than 1 week after antibiotics have been started, or if infection is present, and with Gram-negative infections.

INDICATIONS FOR REFERRAL

Specialty care

Early consultation with a rheumatologist, particularly in patients who have an underlying form of arthritis, or with an infectious disease specialist, particularly for suspected chronic septic arthritis or septic arthritis associated with a poor outcome (i.e. Gram-negative or mixed organisms), is recommended.

Physical therapy

Septic arthritis of large joints, particularly weight-bearing joints of the lower extremities, requires carefully planned passive and active physical therapy and rehabilitation, both during and following antibiotic treatment.

Orthopedic surgery

Patients with suspected infection of a prosthetic joint require prompt referral to an orthopedic surgeon for diagnosis and primary management of the problem. In addition, surgical referral is indicated in the event that an open synovial biopsy or joint drainage or debridement is indicated.

REGIONAL PAIN AND MONOARTICULAR DISORDERS

18

OTHER REGIONAL DISORDERS

TUMORS OR FOREIGN BODIES

IN WHAT CIRCUMSTANCES ARE THESE DISEASES SUSPECTED?

Synovial tumors or foreign body reactions are uncommon. If an isolated swelling of a tendon sheath or joint develops for which no other explanation can be found (i.e. no evidence of a polyarthritis such as rheumatoid disease), and particularly if the condition is chronic, you might suspect a tumor or foreign body.

WHAT ARE THE DIFFERENT DISORDERS THAT CAN OCCUR ?

PIGMENTED VILLONODULAR SYNOVITIS

Pigmented villonodular synovitis is a benign, slowly progressive synovial tumor that can occur at almost any age, and most frequently presents as an isolated swelling in the hand or foot, but can also occur in any joint (Fig. 18.1). Magnetic resonance imaging can be useful in diagnosis (Fig. 18.2).

SYNOVIAL OSTEOCHONDROMATOSIS

Synovial osteochondromatosis is an uncommon benign, tumorous condition characterized by the formation of cartilage and bone in the synovium. It usually presents as monoarticular pain and swelling and can occur at almost any site, but most often affects the knee joint (Fig. 18.3).

KEY POINTS

Definition
- Uncommon synovial disorders are tumors or foreign bodies in the synovium.

Clinical features
- Painful swellings of bursae or joints.
- Isolated to one site.
- No other obvious cause.

Diagnosis
- Imaging may help.
- Often requires synovial biopsy to establish the diagnosis.

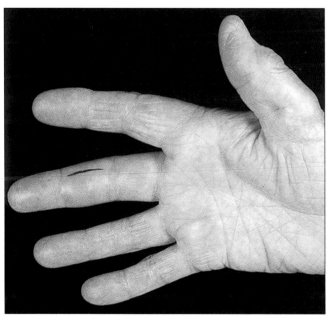

Fig. 18.1 Villonodular tenosynovitis. Swelling over the middle phalanx attached to the flexor tendon.

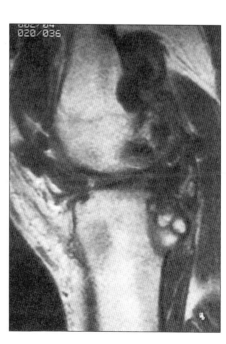

Fig. 18.2 Pigmented villonodular synovitis. Magnetic resonance imaging is a useful procedure to diagnose pigmented villonodular synovitis.

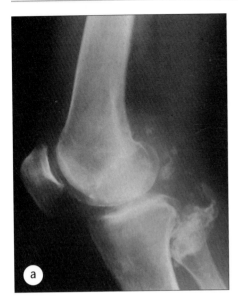

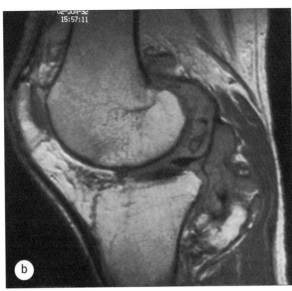

Fig. 18.3 Synovial osteochondromatosis.
(a) Radiograph showing numerous ossific bodies within the knee joint.
(b) Magnetic resonance image showing the synovial hypertrophy in which the new bone is forming.

SYNOVIAL SARCOMAS

Synovial sarcomas are rare, malignant tumors of the synovium, most likely to occur in adolescents and young adults, and are usually seen around joints, rather than within them.

FOREIGN BODY SYNOVITIS

Foreign body synovitis is an uncommon condition in which a fragment of plant thorn, wood, silica glass, or sea urchin spine is embedded in a joint in the fingers, wrists, or knees. After a period of initial inflammation, symptoms subside, only to be followed by the subsequent development of a painful monoarthritis with swelling.

HEMARTHROSIS/BLEEDING DISORDERS

KEY POINTS

Definition
- Hemarthroses are bleeds into a joint or its synovial cavity.

Clinical features
- Acute pain and swelling of a joint.
- Other features depend on the cause.

Diagnosis
- Aspirate from the joint is heavily blood stained.
- Other investigations depend on the likely cause.

IN WHAT CIRCUMSTANCES ARE THESE CONDITIONS SUSPECTED?

In established hemophilia, any acute pain or swelling of a joint is likely to be caused by a hemarthrosis (Fig. 18.4).

WHAT PATTERNS OF DISEASE OCCUR?

Hemophilias are associated both with episodes of acute hemarthrosis and with the development of a chronic destructive arthropathy, secondary to repeated intra-articular bleeding (Fig. 18.5).

Rx MANAGEMENT

An acute hemarthrosis causes a very painful, hot, swollen joint. Ice packs, rest, and analgesia are appropriate in the acute phase, followed by graded mobilization, physical therapy, and rehabilitation. Aspiration is only required if a very tense effusion occurs, or if the diagnosis is uncertain.

The key to successful management of any hemarthrosis is prophylaxis and treatment of the cause, be it through factor replacement in hemophilia, removal of an anticoagulant, or the specific treatment of rarer causes such as synovial tumors and scurvy.

POSSIBLE CAUSES OF A HEMARTHROSIS	
In young people	In older people
Hemophilias	Trauma/fractures
Other bleeding disorders	Pseudogout
Trauma/fractures	Tumors
Anticoagulant therapy	Scurvy
Tumors/hemangiomas	Milwaukee shoulder

Fig. 18.4 Possible causes of a hemarthrosis.

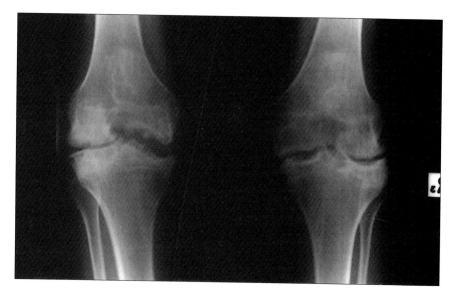

Fig. 18.5 Anteroposterior knee radiographs of a patient who has chronic hemophilic arthropathy. The characteristic severe destructive changes in the joint are shown, with ragged erosion of bone on both sides of the joint space.

NEUROPATHIC ARTHROPATHY (CHARCOT JOINTS)

IN WHAT CIRCUMSTANCES IS NEUROPATHIC ARTHROPATHY SUSPECTED?

The main causes of neuropathic arthropathy are diabetes (complicated by sensory neuropathy), syringomyelia, tabes dorsalis, and leprosy, and other rare neurologic disorders such as congenital sensory neuropathy. A destructive arthritis in association with one of these diseases raises the suspicion of neuropathic arthropathy.

WHAT PATTERNS OF DISEASE ARE TYPICAL OF NEUROPATHIC ARTHROPATHY?

The pattern of involvement is characteristic, depending on the neurologic cause (Fig. 18.6).

WHAT IS MOST LIKELY TO BE SEEN IN CLINICAL PRACTICE?

Diabetic osteoarthropathy of the hindfoot or midfoot, with gross destruction and subluxation of the foot, in association with diabetic sensory peripheral neuropathy (see Figs 18.7 & 18.8). The differential diagnosis is septic arthritis and osteomyelitis.

KEY POINTS

Definition
- Neuropathic arthropathy is a progressive destructive joint disease associated with a neurologic (sensory) deficit.

Main clinical features
- Bony and soft-tissue swelling, with gross deformity and instability of the affected joints.
- Pain may be relatively mild for the degree of damage.

Diagnosis
- Association of severe joint damage with neurologic deficit, confirmed by characteristic radiographic features that include a mixture of destruction and heterotopic new-bone formation.

PATTERNS OF DISEASE TYPICAL OF NEUROPATHIC ARTHROPATHY	
Joint pattern	Associated disorder
Upper limb disease (shoulder, elbow, wrist)	Syringomyelia
Knee and ankle involvement	Tabes dorsalis Congenital neuropathy
Ankle and foot	Diabetes Leprosy

Fig. 18.6 Patterns of disease typical of neuropathic arthropathy.

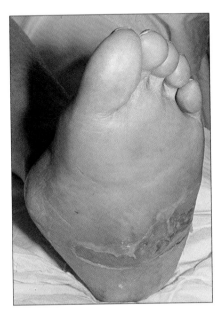

Fig. 18.7 Diabetic neuropathy and vasculopathy. Gross (and originally painless) distortion of the foot anatomy has occurred. Pressure has resulted in an ulcer in the midfoot, which has become infected.

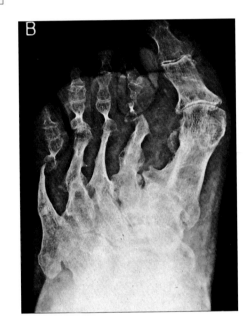

Fig. 18.8 End-stage diabetic osteoarthropathy. Radiograph showing a deformed, widened, diabetic foot with pointed metatarsals after long-standing, mutilating arthropathy and spontaneous fractures.

REFLEX SYMPATHETIC DYSTROPHY (ALGODYSTROPHY)

KEY POINTS

Definition
- Reflex sympathetic dystrophy is a symptom complex characterized by severe pain, swelling, autonomic vasomotor dysfunction, and impaired mobility of the affected joint area.

Main clinical features
- An uncommon disorder that can occur following trauma, or as a complication of a variety of other disorders; sometimes it develops spontaneously.
- Most common in the hand or foot, but can occur in the hip, knee or other sites.
- Progresses through three stages of evolution:
  In stage 1 (hypertrophic), pain and swelling occur, which usually develop quickly, associated with vasomotor changes (which include edema, color changes, and sweating) – the pain is 'causalgic' and is often described as 'tearing' (Fig. 18.9).
  In stage 2 (atrophic), atrophy of the skin and subcutaneous tissues and muscles develops, with the development of marked osteopenia (Fig. 18.10).
  In stage 3, contracture of the skin and joints may occur.
- The condition usually resolves completely after a few years
- A special form of the condition can occur in pregnancy, when it affects the hip (Fig. 18.11).

Diagnosis
- The clinical picture is characteristic, blood tests are normal, but patchy osteoporosis usually develops, which helps diagnosis.

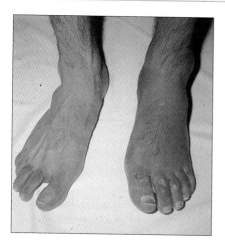

Fig. 18.9 Early reflex sympathetic dystrophy of the foot. Note the edema and redness of the left foot, which was warm.

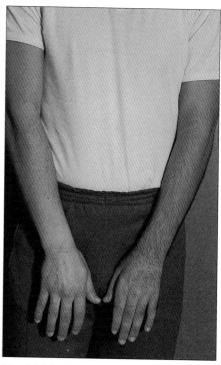

Fig. 18.10 Established reflex sympathetic dystrophy of the upper limb. Note the color change, and hair growth of the left upper limb, which was cool.

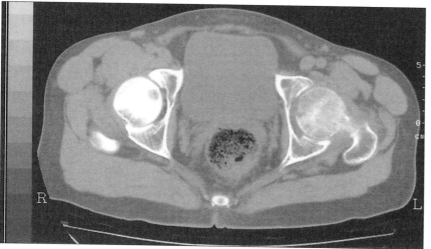

Fig. 18.11 Painful osteoporosis of the hip in pregnancy (MRI). This is an uncommon special form of reflex sympathetic dystrophy, which presents as severe hip pain in pregnancy, usually on the left hip.

IN WHAT CIRCUMSTANCES IS REFLEX SYMPATHETIC DYSTROPHY SUSPECTED?

The condition is most often seen after trauma or immobilization of a limb, and the development of unusual pain and swelling in a hand or foot in these circumstances is very suggestive of the diagnosis, particularly if accompanied by vasomotor changes.

The diagnosis is much more difficult when the condition affects a central joint, such as the hip or knee, or when it occurs without preceding trauma, but it should be suspected in cases of unusual joint pain of no known cause.

 MANAGEMENT

The earlier the condition is diagnosed and treated the better, and atrophic changes and contractures can be avoided by early aggressive therapy.

Nonsteroidal anti-inflammatory drugs or short courses of corticosteroids may help in the early stages, but are often insufficient for pain control. Calcitonin injections can provide excellent pain relief. If this is not effective, sympathetic nerve blockade should be considered.

Physical therapy is important, it being crucial to keep the limb moving and to be as active as possible to help prevent late atrophy and contractures.

LYME DISEASE

KEY POINTS

Definition
- Lyme disease is a tick-borne infection by the spirochete Borrelia burgdorferi that causes systemic inflammatory lesions of the skin, joints, nervous system, and/or heart.

Main clinical features
- Characteristic expanding erythematous, annular lesion with sharply demarcated border (erythema migrans) typically found on the groin, buttock, axilla, and popliteal fossa (Fig. 18.12).
- Most patients develop brief, recurrent attacks of monoarticular or oligoarticular inflammatory arthritis that involve the large joints, particularly the knee; joint effusions may be massive.
- Systemic manifestations may include carditis, particularly heart block, and neurologic features, particularly meningitis or Bell's palsy.

Diagnosis
- The rash of erythema migrans is nearly pathognomonic for Lyme disease and diagnosis is confirmed by documentation of a serologic immune response to B. burgdorferi (Fig. 18.13).

IN WHAT CIRCUMSTANCES IS LYME DISEASE SUSPECTED?

Lyme disease is transmitted by ticks of the *Ixodes ricinus* complex; it is the most common vector-borne disease in the USA and occurs widely throughout Europe. Endemic regions in the USA are the northeast, upper midwest, and Pacific coast regions. A seasonal variation is present and most cases begin in the spring and summer months. Only one-third of patients with Lyme disease recall being bitten by a tick. The interval between tick bite and erythema migrans (EM) varies from a few days to a month. A flu-like illness with severe malaise, fatigue, lethargy, headache, fever and chills, arthralgia, and myalgia is common early in the disease course. Symptoms fluctuate rapidly and vary from day to day. Most patients progress to develop systemic disease manifestations. Most patients also have

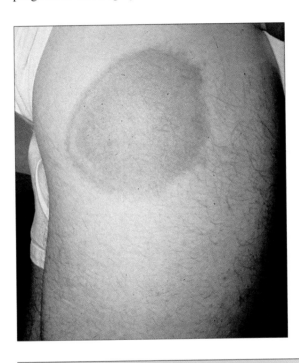

Fig. 18.12 Erythema migrans. A typical annular, flat, erythematous lesion with a sharply demarcated border and partial central healing. (Courtesy of S. Luger)

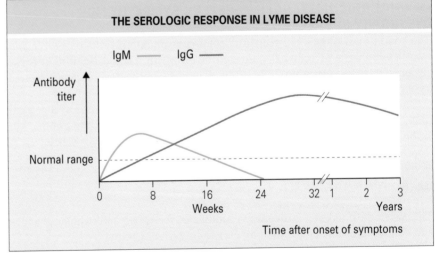

THE SEROLOGIC RESPONSE IN LYME DISEASE

Fig. 18.13 The usual serologic response in Lyme disease. Specific IgM becomes detectable 1–2 weeks after symptom onset and the appearance of erythema chronicum migrans. The later appearance of IgG is frequently concurrent with systemic manifestations. IgG is nearly always elevated in late disease. Typically, and even in untreated patients, IgM falls over 4–6 months; persistence for longer than this predicts later manifestations.

migratory musculoskeletal pain, which begins with EM and persists for weeks or months before the appearance of overt arthritis. Polyarthritis is decidedly uncommon, and the majority of patients have recurrent attacks of monoarthritis or oligoarthritis that last a few days to a few weeks. Approximately 20% of patients develop a chronic arthritis.

HOW IS LYME DISEASE MANAGED?

Antibiotic regimens for Lyme disease are chosen based on the stage of illness and organ involvement (Fig. 18.14). Despite antibiotic treatment, some patients experience delayed resolution of systemic symptoms (headache, musculoskeletal pain, fatigue), which may persist for months after completion of therapy. These symptoms usually resolve spontaneously and do not indicate continued infection that requires further antibiotic treatment.

Fig. 18.14 Suggested antibiotic regimens for Lyme disease.

SUGGESTED ANTIBIOTIC REGIMENS FOR LYME DISEASE	
Early disease	• Doxycycline, 100mg p.o., q12h for 21 days, or • Amoxicillin (with or without probenecid) 500mg, q8h for 21 days, or • Erythromycin, 250–500mg p.o., q6h for 21 days or • Azithromycin 500mg every day for 7 days, or • Cefuroxime axetil, 500mg p.o., q12h for 21 days. Shorter courses may suffice for localized early disease. Erythromycin and azithromycin are less effective than other choices.
Lyme arthritis	Initial treatment: • Doxycyline, 100mg p.o., q12h for 30 days, or • Amoxicillin and probenecid, 500mg each, p.o., q6h for 30 days. If initial treatment fails: • Penicillin G, 20×10^6 IU i.v., daily in divided doses for 14 days, or • Ceftriaxone sodium, 2g i.v., daily for 14 days.
Neurologic manifestations	For facial nerve paralysis alone: • Doxycycline, 100mg p.o., q12h for 21–30 days, or • Amoxicillin, 500mg p.o., q8h for 21–30 days.
Additional signs (e.g. Lyme meningitis, radiculopathy, encephalitis)	• Ceftriaxone, 2g i.v., daily for 30 days, or • Penicillin G, 20×10^6 IU i.v., daily in divided doses for 30 days. Possible alternatives: • Cefotaxime sodium, 2g i.v., q8h for 30 days, or • Doxycycline, 100mg p.o., q12h for 14–30 days, or • Chloramphenicol, 1g i.v., q6h for 14–30 days.
Lyme carditis	• Ceftriaxone, 2g i.v., daily for 14 days, or • Penicillin G, 20×10^6 IU i.v., daily in divided doses for 14 days. Possible alternatives: • Doxycycline, 100mg p.o., q12h for 21 days, or • Amoxicillin, 500mg p.o., q8h for 21 days.
During pregnancy	Localized, early disease: • Amoxicillin, 500mg p.o., q8h for 21 days. Other manifestations: • Penicillin G, 20×10^6 IU i.v., daily in divided doses for 14–30 days, or • Ceftriaxone, 2g, daily for 14–30 days.

SECTION 3

POLYARTICULAR DISORDERS

AN INTRODUCTION TO POLYARTICULAR DISORDERS

Most forms of polyarthritis can be readily diagnosed from a careful history and physical examination with particular attention to the predominant joints affected (see algorithm). Categorization of the arthritis into one of three common joint patterns helps to narrow the diagnostic possibilities – distal interphalangeal (DIP) joints; wrist, metacarpophalangeal (MCP); and metatarsophalangeal (MTP); and hips, knees, or ankles.

DISTAL INTERPHALANGEAL JOINTS

Generalized osteoarthritis is, by far, the most common form of polyarthritis in this group (Fig. 1). It is readily recognized by bony hard swellings (Heberden's nodes), which occasionally become red, warm, and very tender. In addition, patients frequently develop arthritis of the hip or knee, which may be unilateral or bilateral.

Psoriatic arthritis is the only other common form of polyarthritis that affects the DIP joints. Many patients develop nail changes (pitting, onycholysis, etc.) that provide a clue to diagnosis, which is usually readily confirmed by the presence of typical psoriatic plaques on the skin. Most patients who have psoriatic arthritis also develop other signs of peripheral arthritis that affects joints of the lower extremities, hands and feet (see below), or the lumbosacral spine.

WRIST, METACARPOPHALANGEAL, AND METATARSOPHALANGEAL JOINTS

A spectrum of systemic inflammatory, infectious, and endocrine disorders produce polyarthritis of the wrists, hands, and feet (Fig. 2). At the very onset of this pattern of arthritis, to determine the exact cause is often difficult. The search for clues from extra-articular signs and symptoms (see below) is important, but in many patients watchful waiting to see what happens is the best course of action. Most patients who have viral arthritis have prominent joint pain with few physical findings, and the arthritis is completely gone within a month.

Rheumatoid arthritis is the most common of the group, and typically presents in young to middle-aged women. The bilateral, and mostly symmetric nature of the arthritis, combined with the persistence of arthritis on a daily basis for a month or more, suggests the diagnosis. The detection of subcutaneous nodules over the elbows or other pressure points, prolonged stiffness when first rising out of bed in the morning, or eliciting a family history of rheumatoid arthritis makes the diagnosis easy.

HIPS, KNEES, AND ANKLES

Arthritis of the large joints of the lower extremities is characteristic of a family of inflammatory arthropathies that involve inflammation at tendinous insertions (enthesopathy) and back pain from sacroiliitis and the involvement of the lumbosacral spine (Fig. 3). Often referred to as the spondyloarthropathies, these include reactive arthritis, ankylosing spondylitis, inflammatory bowel disease (e.g. ulcerative colitis and Crohn's disease), and psoriatic arthritis. A careful history and physical examination to detect evidence of a recent infection (particularly urethritis or gastroenteritis) should be carried out, and such infection, rashes, a family history of any of the spondyloarthropathies, back or buttock pain, or heel pain at the insertion of the Achilles' or plantar tendons, are likely to be found alone or in any combination.

CAUSES OF ARTHRITIS

To determine what else is wrong with the patient, from both the review of systems and from the physical examination, helps to suggest certain causes for the polyarthritis (Fig. 4).

Specific questions that often help to categorize polyarthritis are described below.

IS THE ONSET OF THE ARTHRITIS ACUTE OR GRADUAL?

Most forms of polyarthritis begin gradually, such that the patient is somewhat vague as to precisely when the condition started to develop. In acute polyarthritis, in which the patient can usually remember the day and often the hour when the problem began, consider gonococcal arthritis, acute rheumatic fever, crystalline arthropathy, or reactive arthritis.

DIAGNOSTIC ALGORITHM FOR POLYARTICULAR DISORDERS

Pattern of joint involvement

Distal interphalangeal joints

Fig. 1 Osteoarthritis of the distal interphalangeal (DIP) joints. This patient has the typical clinical findings of advanced osteoarthritis of the DIP joints, which include large, firm swellings (Heberden's nodes), some of which are tender and red because of associated inflammation of the periarticular tissues as well as of the joint.

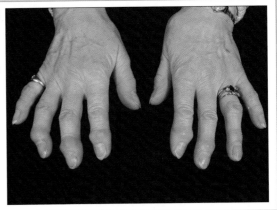

Generalized osteoarthritis (Ch. 42)

Psoriatic arthritis (Ch. 20)

Wrist, metacarpophalangeal, and metatarsophalangeal joints

Fig. 2 Deforming symmetrical polyarthritis with involvement of wrists and metacarpophalangeal joints is characteristic of rheumatoid arthritis.

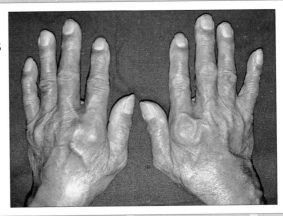

Psoriatic arthritis (Ch. 20)

Gonococcal arthritis (Ch. 23)

Rheumatic fever (Ch. 19)

Palindromic rheumatism (Ch. 23)

Rheumatoid arthritis (Ch. 19)

Crystalline arthropathy (Ch. 10)

Endocrine arthropathy (Ch. 23)

Inflammatory osteoarthropathy (Ch. 23)

Systemic rheumatic disease (see algorithm p.220)

Viral arthritis (Ch. 21)

Hips, knees, and ankles

Fig. 3 Patient with a 6-month history of pain and swelling in both knees. Psoriatic plaques are evident on both knees. The knees are warm and tender to palpation with small joint effusions.

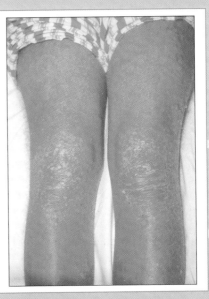

Reactive arthritis (Ch. 22)

Ankylosing spondylitis (Ch. 26)

Psoriatic arthritis (Ch. 20)

Sarcoidosis (Ch. 23)

Intermittent hydrarthrosis (Ch. 23)

'POLYARTHRITIS PLUS': ASSOCIATIONS OF OTHER DISORDERS WITH ARTHRITIS	
Polyarthritis plus	Potential diagnosis
Abdominal pain	Polyarteritis nodosa
Abortions	Primary antiphospholipid syndrome
Alopecia	Systemic lupus erythematosus
Butterfly rash	Systemic lupus erythematosus
Calcinosis	Dermatomyositis, scleroderma
Cardiac failure	Too nonspecific
Clubbing	Hypertrophic osteoarthropathy
Coma	Systemic lupus erythematosus
Confusional state	Systemic lupus erythematosus
Diarrhea	Reactive arthritis
Digital vasculitis	Rheumatoid arthritis
Deep vein thrombosis	Primary antiphospholipid syndrome
Dysphagia	Scleroderma
Fits	Systemic lupus erythematosus
Headaches	Temporal arteritis
Hemolysis	Systemic lupus erythematosus
Hypertension	Systemic lupus erythematosus, polyarteritis nodosa
Malabsorption	Scleroderma
Mononeuritis multiplex	Polyarteritis nodosa, rheumatoid arthritis
Neuropathy	Rheumatoid arthritis, polyarteritis nodosa
Neutropenia	Drugs, Felty's syndrome, systemic lupus erythematosus
Pericarditis	Rheumatoid arthritis, systemic lupus erythematosus, juvenile chronic arthritis
Pleural effusion	Rheumatoid arthritis, systemic lupus erythematosus
Pneumonitis	Systemic lupus erythematosus
Proteinuria	Systemic lupus erythematosus, drugs
Pulmonary fibrosis	Rheumatoid arthritis, scleroderma, methotrexate
Purpura	Systemic lupus erythematosus, drugs
Raynaud's phenomenon	Scleroderma, systemic lupus erythematosus, rheumatoid arthritis
Renal failure	Systemic lupus erythematosus, drugs
Thrombocytopenia	Systemic lupus erythematosus, drugs
Urethritis	Reactive arthritis

Fig. 4 Polyarthritis plus: associations of other disorders with arthritis.

ARE RASHES OR OTHER SKIN FINDINGS PRESENT?

A number of polyarthritis syndromes are associated with skin findings that provide clues to the diagnosis, such as:
- thickened skin (scleroderma, acromegaly, hyperthyroidism);
- nodules (rheumatoid arthritis, rheumatic fever, sarcoidosis, erythema nodosum, gout); and
- rashes (psoriatic arthritis, lupus, dermatomyositis, rheumatic fever, reactive arthritis, Still's disease).

IS THE COURSE OF THE ARTHROPATHY CHRONIC, PERSISTENT OR RELAPSING, REMITTING ?

In most forms of polyarthritis, day-to-day fluctuations occur in the intensity and distribution of the arthritis, but the arthritis is always present to some degree or other. Truly relapsing, remitting attacks of arthritis in which the patient has no signs or symptoms of arthritis between attacks is unusual and suggests a systemic rheumatic disease (like lupus), crystalline arthropathies (like gout or chondrocalcinosis), intermittent hydrarthrosis, or palindromic rheumatism.

INVESTIGATIONS

Laboratory and imaging studies in polyarthritis are most helpful in instances in which a tentative clinical diagnosis can be made from the history and physical examination and appropriate studies are tailored to the patient. Ordering a radiograph simply because the joints are swollen, or screening for rheumatoid factor, antinuclear antibody, etc., rarely, if ever, helps to clarify a difficult problem and only adds unnecessary costs to the work-up. Minimal work-up should include acute phase reactants (erythrocyte sedimentation rate or C-reactive protein) and a complete blood count as objective measures for the presence or absence of inflammation. Joint aspiration and analysis of synovial fluid usually help to discriminate between inflammatory (rheumatoid arthritis, reactive arthritis, etc.) and noninflammatory (osteoarthritis, endocrine arthropathy) polyarthritis, and are mandatory if crystals or infectious arthritis are a consideration. In patients who have chronic (i.e. more than 6 weeks of symptoms) arthritis, radiographs often provide important clues to the diagnosis in terms of distribution and nature of erosive changes or the presence or absence of new bone formation.

POLYARTICULAR DISORDERS

19

RHEUMATOID ARTHRITIS

Rheumatoid arthritis (RA) is the most common form of inflammatory joint disease and is found in up to 1% of the population. It affects at least twice as many women as men, with a peak onset in the fourth and fifth decades of life. The disease is characterized by symmetric polyarthritis that over time leads to destruction of joint cartilage and bone, and to deformities of the joint. Most patients develop prominent impairments of joint function and recent evidence suggests RA may be associated with a shortened life span. The clinical course of RA can be divided into early, late, and systemic forms.

 TYPICAL CASE: EARLY RHEUMATOID ARTHRITIS

Carrie, a 34-year-old mother of two small children, presents with a 2-month history of pain in her hands and feet. She notes that her symptoms are much worse in the morning and cause her some difficulty dressing and preparing breakfast for her family. On physical examination, tender, symmetric swelling is detected in her proximal interphalangeal (PIP) joints, metacarpophalangeal (MCP) joints, and wrists (Fig. 19.1). A pea-sized, non-tender nodule is noted in the right olecranon bursae. Laboratory studies reveal an erythrocyte sedimentation rate (ESR) of 100mm/h and a positive rheumatoid factor (RF; titer 1:320).

KEY POINTS

- Chronic inflammatory disorder of the synovium, bursae, and tendon sheaths.
- Key clinical features include symmetric polyarthritis, morning stiffness, and subcutaneous nodules.
- Synovitis (pannus) leads to erosions of juxta-articular bone and cartilage.
- Most patients develop antibodies to gammaglobulin (rheumatoid factor).
- May be associated with serious, systemic complications such as vasculitis, pulmonary fibrosis, or Felty's syndrome.

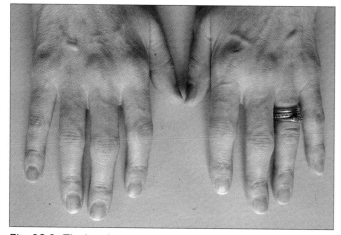

Fig. 19.1 The hand in early rheumatoid arthritis (RA). Symmetrical swelling of the metacarpophalangeal and proximal interphalangeal (PIP) joints. Fusiform swelling of the PIP joints is typical of RA and is associated with morning stiffness, difficulty in making a fist, reduced grip strength, and tenderness of the affected joints.

FEATURES OF EARLY RHEUMATOID ARTHRITIS

- Symmetric polyarthritis, typically beginning in the wrists, small joints of the hands (metacarpophalangeal and proximal interphalangeal joints), and balls of the feet (metatarsophalangeal joints).
- Stiff joints in the morning that last an hour or more.
- Subcutaneous nodules over pressure areas such as the elbows, sacrum, occiput, and Achilles' tendon.
- Laboratory studies with mild anemia, elevated acute phase reactants (erythrocyte sedimentation rate and C-reactive protein), and positive rheumatoid factor (80%).
- Minimal bone or cartilage destruction evident on joint radiographs.

- Characterized by joint destruction with impairments of joint functions and/or structures in close proximity to the joint – examples include:
- Hand deformities with radial deviation of the wrist, ulnar deviation of the metacarpophalangeal joints, and subluxations of the proximal interphalangeal joints (Fig. 19.5).
- Instability of the cervical spine with neurologic impairments (Fig. 19.3).
- Deformities of the forefoot with cock-up toes and subluxation of the metatarsal heads (Fig. 19.6).
- Tendon ruptures – most commonly seen in the extensor tendons of the hand (Fig. 19.7).

2 TYPICAL CASE: LATE RHEUMATOID ARTHRITIS

Jo Ann is 63-year-old sales clerk with a 20-year history of seropositive RA who is seen for evaluation of occipital headaches, heaviness of the arms and legs, and tingling and numbness in the hands (Fig. 19.2). Neurologic examination revealed a spastic paresis of both arms and the right leg, a positive Babinski sign, and impaired vibration sense in both legs. Radiographs of the cervical spine showed a subluxation of C1 on C2 of 15mm in flexion (Fig. 19.3). Magnetic resonance imaging (MRI) of the cervical spine revealed an anteroposterior slip of C1 on C2, obliteration of the subarachnoid space, and compression of the cervical cord by the posterior arch of C1 (Fig. 19.4).

ALARM SIGNS OF SPINAL CORD DAMAGE IN RHEUMATOID ARTHRITIS

Severe neck pain, often radiating to the occiput

Diminished motor power in arms and legs

Tingling of the fingers and feet, or only numbness

A 'marble' sensation in the limbs and trunk

Jumping legs, as a consequence of spinal automatism

Disturbed bladder function, varying from incontinence to urinary retention

Fig. 19.2 Alarm signs of spinal cord damage in rheumatoid arthritis.

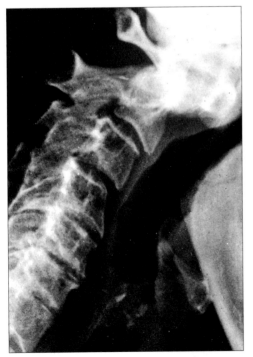

Fig. 19.3 Instability of the cervical spine. The slip of C1–C2 distance between atlas and ventral-side odontoid process exceeds 15mm.

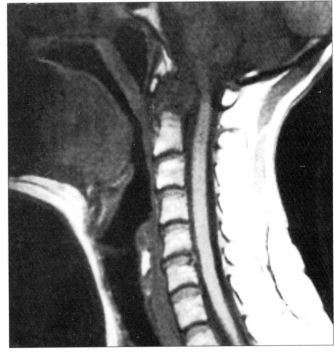

Fig. 19.4 Magnetic resonance image of the unstable cervical spine (T1-weighted). There is compression of the cervical region of the spinal cord by pannus along the posterior margin of the odontoid. (Courtesy of John L Sherman, Washington Imaging Center, Washington DC.)

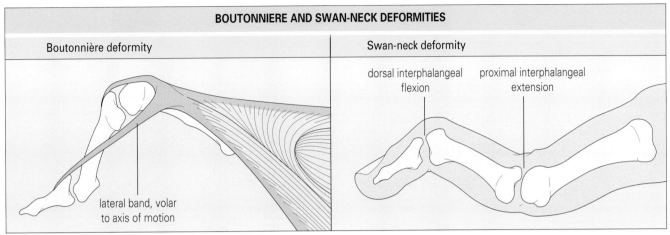

BOUTONNIERE AND SWAN-NECK DEFORMITIES

Boutonnière deformity	Swan-neck deformity

lateral band, volar to axis of motion

dorsal interphalangeal flexion   proximal interphalangeal extension

Fig. 19.5 Proximal interphalangeal (PIP) joint deformities in rheumatoid arthritis. The boutonnière deformity – PIP flexion and dorsal interphalangeal (DIP) hyperextension – results from relaxation of the central slip, with 'button-holing' of the PIP joint between the lateral bands. The swan-neck deformity – metacarpophalangeal (MCP) flexion, PIP hyperextension, and DIP flexion – may be mobile, snapping, or fixed. Its pathogenesis may be related primarily to PIP or MCP involvement. (Adapted with permission from Hastings DE, Walsh RP. Surgical reconstruction of the rheumatoid hand. Toronto: Orthopaedic Medical Management Corporation; 1979).

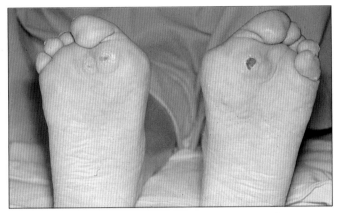

Fig. 19.6 Rheumatoid forefoot. Plantar view of the feet in a patient with rheumatoid arthritis. Hallux valgus, metatarsophalangeal subluxation, and bursal swelling under weight-bearing areas are seen. Subluxation of the metatarsal head is associated with clawing of the toes, cock-up digital deformities, and over-riding of the toes. The ulcerated bursae under the left metatarsal head has resulted from a chronic synovial fistula with secondary infection.

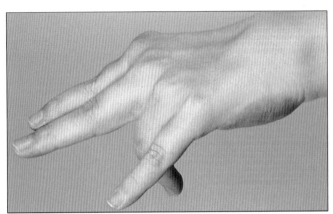

Fig. 19.7 Extensor tendon rupture of the fourth finger. Synovitis of the wrist combined with erosive changes of the carpus have led to rupture of the extensor tendon.

3 TYPICAL CASE: SYSTEMIC RHEUMATOID ARTHRITIS

Sadie is 58-year-old patent attorney with a 15-year history of severe, progressive, seropositive, nodular RA. She has been troubled by persistent swelling in most joints with little improvement from drugs, including daily corticosteroids (which she has taken for the past 10 years) and most second-line drugs, most recently a combination of methotrexate (15mg weekly) and cyclosporine (4mg/kg daily). About 6 months previously she began to complain of numbness in both feet. She accidentally bumped her right shin on a chair leg 3 months ago and developed a small bruise that did not heal properly, and over the previous 10 days the skin on the leg has broken down (Fig. 19.8).

FEATURES OF SYSTEMIC RHEUMATOID ARTHRITIS

- Typically occurs in the setting of severe, seropositive, nodular rheumatoid arthritis – examples include:
- Felty's syndrome – splenomegaly, leukopenia, bacterial infections, skin ulcers.
- Systemic vasculitis with peripheral neuropathy, mononeuritis, or leg ulcers (Fig. 19.8).
- Pulmonary nodules, interstitial fibrosis, or pleural effusions (Fig. 19.9).
- Pericarditis, myocardial dysfunction, valvular abnormalities.
- Keratoconjunctivitis sicca and scleritis (Fig. 19.10).

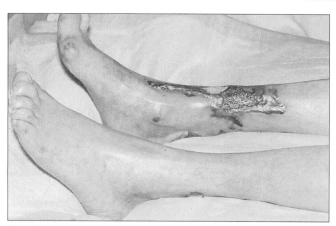

Fig. 19.8 Severe ulcers of the lower leg caused by necrotizing vasculitis in rheumatoid arthritis.

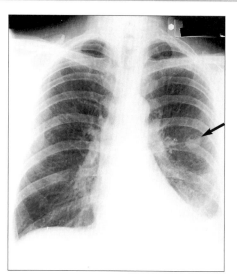

Fig. 19.9 Pleural effusion and rheumatoid nodule (arrow) in rheumatoid arthritis.

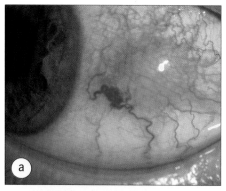

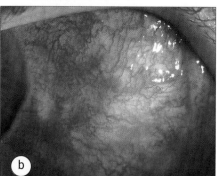

Fig. 19.10 Scleritis in rheumatoid arthritis. (a) Nodular episcleritis. (b) Anterior scleritis. (c) Necrotizing scleritis; it may expose the underlying uvea. Here it is associated with marginal corneal melting.

She was placed on bed rest, with elevation of the legs, and wet-to-dry dressings applied daily. She was treated with oral cyclophosphamide 100mg daily. Healing of the ulcers took place within 6 weeks, along with some improvement in her peripheral neuropathy.

NATURAL HISTORY AND OTHER CLINICAL FEATURES

The clinical course of RA follows an onset of disease that may be either abrupt and acute or gradual and insidious. A generally held view is that an acute onset forecasts a favorable prognosis, whereas an insidious onset heralds a worse outcome. Although the onset is predominantly articular, most patients note weakness, anorexia, weight loss, or fever. In some patients, fatigue alone or diffuse, nonspecific aching, or extra-articular features (such as pulmonary disease) may herald the onset of polyarthritis by weeks or months.

The most common presentation at onset is a gradual one that affects the small peripheral joints, such as the wrists, MCP joints, PIP joints, ankles, or metatarsophalangeal (MTP) joints. Patients are often unclear as to when the disease actually started and can only date symptoms to the nearest month. The distribution of the arthritis is usually symmetric and the patient complains of difficulty in making a fist, poor strength in the hands, and pain in the feet when rising from sleep in the morning. Morning stiffness that lasts minutes to hours is usually present.

Less commonly, RA presents as an acute or slowly progressive arthritis that affects the larger joints such as shoulders or knees. Although symptoms may remain confined to one or two joints for weeks or months, most patients go on to develop an additional, symmetric polyarthritis over the days and weeks following onset of the disease. A variation of the abrupt onset of monoarthritis is known as intermittent hydrarthrosis or, in the instance of polyarthritis, palindromic rheumatism. Here, variable episodes of arthritis suddenly affect one or more large and/or peripheral joints, last a few hours or a few days, and spontaneously subside, only to recur weeks or months later. The patient is entirely well between attacks with no signs of rheumatic disease. These short-lived episodes often occur with increased frequency and severity, and may herald the onset of persistent polyarthritis. At least one third of such patients show evolution into typical RA.

No matter what the onset or presentation, the patient's subsequent progress follows several different patterns (Fig. 19.11):

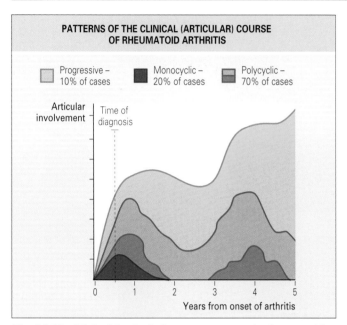

PATTERNS OF THE CLINICAL (ARTICULAR) COURSE
OF RHEUMATOID ARTHRITIS

Progressive –
10% of cases

Monocyclic –
20% of cases

Polycyclic –
70% of cases

Articular
involvement

Time of
diagnosis

Years from onset of arthritis

Fig. 19.11 Clinical (articular) course patterns in rheumatoid arthritis (RA). Articular patterns in 50 patients with RA. [Data from Masi AT, Feigenbaum SL, Kaplan SB. Articular patterns in the early course of rheumatoid arthritis. Am J Med. 1983;75(Suppl. 6A):16–26.]

FACTORS IN RHEUMATOID ARTHRITIS INDICATING AN UNFAVORABLE PROGNOSIS
Accumulated joint damage rate Uncontrolled polyarthritis Structural damage and deformity Functional disability
Presence of extra-articular features Local and/or systemic
Psychosocial problems
Rheumatoid factor seropositivity Presence of immune complexes
Immunogenetic testing for ≥1 HLA-DR4 cluster of rheumatoid arthritis susceptibility genes (DRB1* 0401, 0404, 0405)

Fig. 19.12 Clinical evaluation of rheumatoid arthritis – prognostic factors. The greater the number of factors present, the more unfavorable the outlook.

- Monocyclic pattern – a single cycle with remission for at least 1 year, seen in 20% of patients;
- Polycyclic pattern – seen in 70% of patients with either intermittent or continuous subtypes.
- Progressive pattern – with increasing joint involvement seen in about 10% of patients; patients with malignant and systemic RA generally follow this pattern.

With continuous disease activity, the patient's daily activities and functional capacity are affected to a greater or lesser extent. A number of factors have been associated with a poor outcome in RA (Fig. 19.12).

 POINTS TO LOOK OUT FOR

- Carpal tunnel syndrome.
- Pressure ulcers – commonly occur at sites exposed to repeated trauma, such as the elbow or tops of the toes (Fig. 19.13).
- Acute synovial rupture – most commonly occurs in knees (ruptured Baker's cyst); presents with calf swelling and tenderness (Figs 19.14 & 19.15), and is readily confused with thrombophlebitis.
- Septic arthritis – monoarticular flare of arthritis is unusual in RA and suggests joint infection.
- Neurologic signs – may indicate vasculitis or spinal cord damage (see Fig. 19.2)
- Tendon ruptures – result from invasion of synovial lining of tendons or abrasions cause by tendons rubbing over eroded bony surfaces; most commonly involve tendons of dorsum of wrist and hand (see Fig. 19.7).
- Dry eyes and/or dry mouth – Sjögren's syndrome, common in RA.
- Red, painful eye – scleritis (see Fig. 19.10b) may lead to corneal thinning with ulceration.
- Leukemia – lymphoproliferative (i.e. non-Hodgkin's lymphoma) and T-cell leukemia (large granular lymphocyte) in patients with Felty's syndrome.

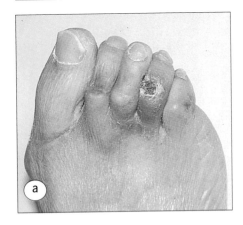

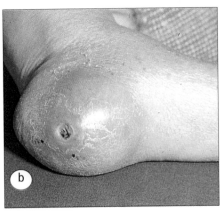

Fig. 19.13 Pressure ulcers. Ulceration over the surface of (a) the proximal interphalangeal joints of the toe and (b) the olecranon bursa.

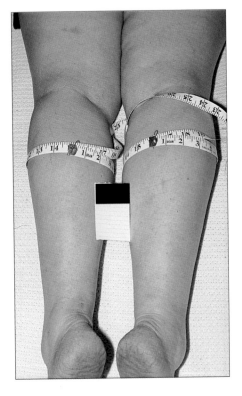

Fig. 19.14 Swelling of the calf following acute synovial rupture of the knee in rheumatoid arthritis.

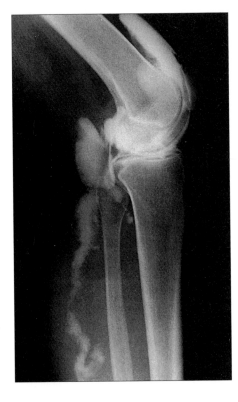

Fig. 19.15 Contrast arthrogram following acute synovial rupture of the knee.

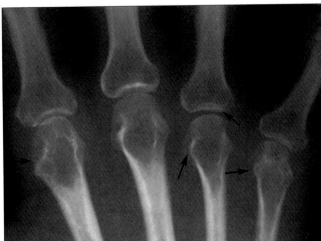

Fig. 19.16 Early erosions in the 'bare' areas of the metacarpal heads in rheumatoid arthritis. The erosions are the disruption of continuity of the white cortical line (arrows).

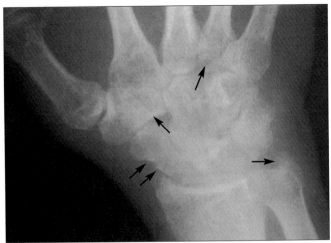

Fig. 19.17 Posteroanterior view of the wrist demonstrating advanced erosive changes in rheumatoid arthritis. Erosions are present at the waist of the scaphoid, the waist of the capitate, the ulnar styloid, the radial styloid, and the base of the fourth metacarpal (arrows).

INVESTIGATIONS

LABORATORY TESTS

In patients with suspected RA, a complete blood count, acute phase reactants [ESR or C-reactive protein (CRP)], and RF should be ordered. Anemia, typically with microchromic, microcytic indices, is common. Elevations of ESR or CRP parallel the degree of inflammation and are often used to follow the course of RA (see below). RF is found in the majority of patients, but it is also present in other arthropathies and thus is not diagnostic of RA *per se*.

IMAGING

The presence of characteristic erosions of the hands (Fig. 19.16), wrists (Fig. 19.17), and feet (Fig. 19.18) helps to confirm the diagnosis of the disease. However, these changes typically occur only after weeks or months of arthritis, and early radiographs typically show soft-tissue swelling only. In late RA, radiographs show evidence of destructive changes (Fig. 19.19), which are typically of little practical clinical utility. However, radiographs are of particular importance in sorting out complications associated with RA, such as joint infection (Fig. 19.20), stress fracture (Fig. 19.21), or rupture of a synovial cyst (using an arthrogram, see Fig. 19.15). An important role is played by MRI in the assessment of cervical spine complications of RA in patients with neurologic symptoms (Fig. 19.22).

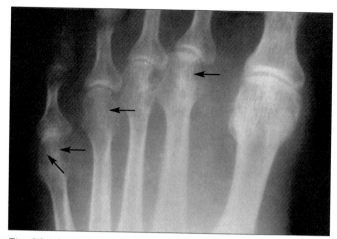

Fig. 19.18 Anteroposterior view of the forefoot in rheumatoid arthritis. Erosions of the 'bare' areas of bone (areas not covered by cartilage) in the metatarsal heads are demonstrated (arrows).

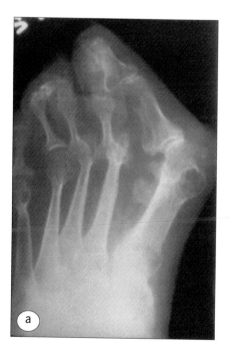
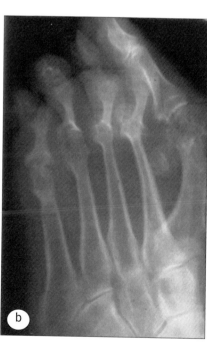

Fig. 19.19 Late changes of rheumatoid arthritis. (a) Anteroposterior and (b) oblique view of the forefoot showing osteoporosis, dramatic erosive changes, and subluxation that involves the metatarsal heads. Also shown is fibular subluxation of the proximal phalanges in relation to the metatarsal heads.

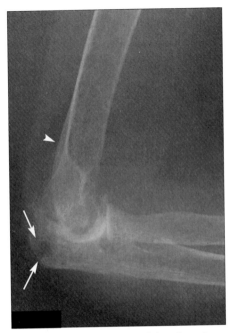

Fig. 19.20 Lateral view of the elbow in rheumatoid arthritis with infection. The joint space is completely destroyed. A posterior fat pad is demonstrated (arrowhead), which results from the presence of pus, and there is extensive erosion of the olecranon (arrows).

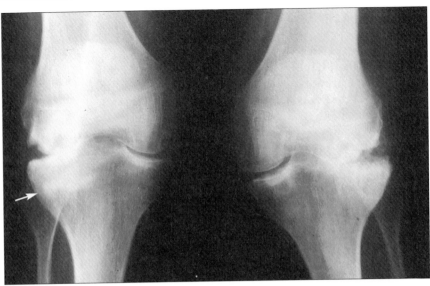

Fig. 19.21 Anteroposterior view of the rheumatoid knee with stress fracture. Narrowing of the medial compartments and total loss of the lateral compartments have occurred. The line of sclerosis just distal to the lateral tibial plateau of the right knee (arrow) represents the stress fracture.

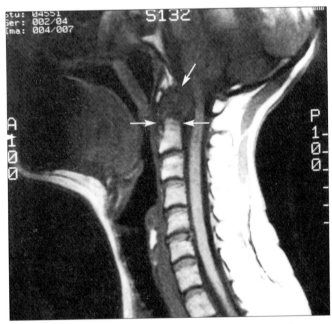

Fig. 19.22 A T1-weighted sagittal magnetic resonance image of the unstable cervical spine. Replacement of the odontoid process by abnormal, decreased soft-tissue intensity has occurred, compatible with rheumatoid pannus (arrows). Stenosis of the canal and compression of the spinal cord can be seen. (Courtesy of John L Sherman, Washington Imaging Center, Washington DC.)

DIFFERENTIAL DIAGNOSIS

In the very earliest (days or weeks) stages of arthritis, to differentiate RA from infection, particularly viral infection (see Chapter 21), and from systemic rheumatic diseases such as lupus, reactive arthritis (see Chapter 22), or spondyloarthropathy that present with peripheral arthritis, is difficult if not impossible. The presence of bilateral arthritis that affects the wrists, or MCP or MTP joints is highly suggestive of RA. The persistence of polyarthritis, particularly in a symmetric distribution, combined with a positive RF and the eventual development of erosive changes on joint radiographs, confirms the diagnosis (Fig. 19.23).

A relapsing and remitting course of arthritis with the patient entirely well between attacks is distinctly unusual in RA and suggests a systemic rheumatic disease, palindromic rheumatism, or a crystalline arthropathy such as polyarticular gout or chondrocalcinosis. In most patients with RA, radiographs of the hands or feet show clear evidence of erosions after 1–2 years of arthritis, and failure to find such erosions suggests other causes of polyarthritis such as the systemic rheumatic diseases or endocrine arthropathies. Patients with lupus can develop hand deformities that are virtually identical to those of RA – so-called Jaccoud's arthropathy (Fig. 19.24).

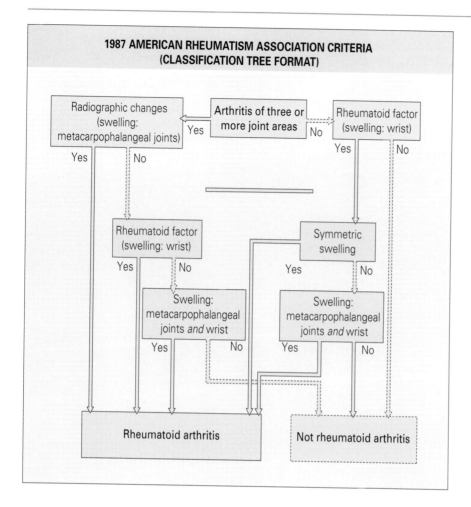

1987 AMERICAN RHEUMATISM ASSOCIATION CRITERIA (CLASSIFICATION TREE FORMAT)

Fig. 19.23 1987 American Rheumatism Association criteria (classification tree format). Variables in parentheses can be used when data on the first-listed variable are not available. (Reproduced with permission from Arnett FC, Edworthy SM, Bloch DA, et al. The American Rheumatism Association 1987 revised criteria for the classification of rheumatoid arthritis. Arthritis Rheum. 1988;31:315–24; and MacGregor AJ. Classification criteria for rheumatoid arthritis. Baillière's Clin Rheumatol. 1995;9:287–304.)

R̲x̲ MANAGEMENT

The treatment needs of a patient with RA typically change over time and commonly require input from a multidisciplinary team (Fig. 19.25). In most instances, the rheumatologist co-ordinates care provided by the different disciplines. Control of joint inflammation to prevent progressive joint damage is a basic premise throughout the entire course of the disease. Other management strategies are highly individualized depending on the needs of the patient and vary with the stage of the disease (Fig. 19.26).

PATIENT EDUCATION AND SELF-HELP

Education is extremely important in RA and most patients have questions about the disease, its course, treatment options and their side effects, and consequences of the disease and how to cope with these. A wealth of information is available to the patient over the Internet or from professional organizations (Arthritis Foundation, Arthritis Society, Arthritis and Rheumatism Council, etc.). Similarly, the professional organizations sponsor structured programs to teach self-help and to develop coping skills to deal with chronic illness (see Self-Help Leaflet, page 342).

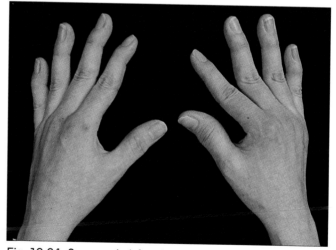

Fig. 19.24 Swan-neck deformities in a patient with systemic lupus erythematosus (Jaccoud's arthropathy).

MEMBERS OF THE MULTIDISCIPLINARY TEAM
Rheumatologist
Nurse
Occupational therapist
Physical therapist
Social worker
Psychologist/psychiatrist
Neurologist
Orthopedic surgeon
General physician
Podiatrist

Fig. 19.25 Members of the multidisciplinary team involved in the care of patients with rheumatoid arthritis.

THE ROLE OF THERAPEUTIC REGIMENS IN THE MANAGEMENT OF RHEUMATOID ARTHRITIS RELATED TO THE STAGE OF DISEASE		
Therapeutic regimen	Early and established disease	End-stage disease
Conservative therapy		
Patient education	+++	+
Rest		
Systemic/therapeutic	+	+
Local/protective	++	++
Physical therapy		
Maintenance range of motion	++	+
Prevention of disuse atrophy of muscle, support of condition	+	++
Occupational therapy		
Joint protection	++	+
Adaptation	+	++
Drug therapy		
Nonsteroidal anti-inflammatory drugs	++	++
Second-line drugs	++	+
Corticosteroids (systemic)	+	±
Intra-articular therapy	++	+
Surgical intervention		
Therapeutic (synovectomy)	+	−
Reconstructive	+	++
Joint replacement	−	+++

Fig. 19.26 The role of therapeutic regimens in the management of rheumatoid arthritis related to the stage of disease.

PHYSICAL AND OCCUPATIONAL THERAPY

In early RA, physical therapy plays an important role in the assessment of functional limitations caused by the arthritis, and in developing a physical therapy program to preserve joint range of motion and prevent muscle atrophy. The main features of a traditional physical therapy program are isometric and range-of-motion exercises, rest and relaxation techniques, physical conditioning, and maintenance of a good posture. Hydrotherapy or the use of resting splints (Fig. 19.27) often helps to relieve pain and joint swelling. Placement of a metatarsal bar in the shoes to transfer weight from painful metatarsal heads helps with the patient's ability to walk. Teaching patients 'joint protection' by accomplishing everyday tasks with minimal stresses across joints helps to prevent joint deformities (Fig. 19.28).

In late RA, goals of physical therapy emphasize techniques to improve function and maintain activities of daily living through the use of ambulation devices such as canes or walkers and the use of aids or appliances such as special grips, raised toilet seat, and other household adaptations.

DRUG THERAPY

Nonsteroidal anti-inflammatory drugs (NSAIDs), corticosteroids, and so-called second-line agents (SLAs) are used in the drug treatment of RA (Fig. 19.29).

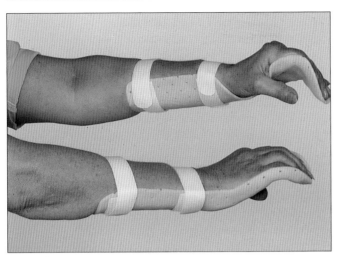

Fig. 19.27 Wrist and hand splint.

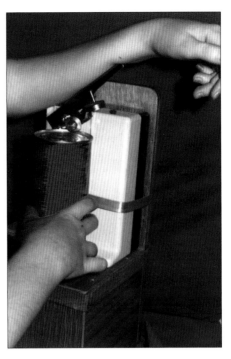

Fig. 19.28
Joint protection.
Sparing of the joints to open a can reduces stresses across wrist and finger joints.

Whereas in the past patients with newly diagnosed RA were maintained on NSAIDs alone for weeks or months, a recent trend is to start SLAs very early in the disease, especially in patients with a poor prognosis (see Fig. 19.12). In general, decisions about the drug management of RA, including provisions to monitor for drug toxicities, are coordinated by the rheumatologist.

Fig. 19.29 A pharmacologic approach to inflammatory rheumatoid arthritis.

A PHARMACOLOGIC APPROACH TO ACTIVE INFLAMMATORY RHEUMATOID ARTHRITIS
Active inflammatory rheumatoid arthritis
Nonsteroidal anti-inflammatory drugs (NSAIDs) Often more than one has to be tried before the right NSAID is found for the individual patient If disease activity is insufficiently suppressed consider adding second-line agent

Second-line agent (SLA)
First choice – fast mode of action, e.g. sulfasalazine or methotrexate
In case of adverse reactions or inefficacy, second choice of SLA
(in alphabetic order) depends on disease severity
  Antimalarial
  Azathioprine
  Gold (oral, intramuscular)
  D-Penicillamine
If response is inadequate or absent, try combining SLAs instead of substitution.
Low-dose oral corticosteroids can be combined with an NSAID or SLA

Treatment of flares or bridge therapy
Intramuscular methylprednisolone injections (120mg every month) or bolus infusions (500–1000mg)
Acute inflammation of a single joint
Intra-articular nonabsorbable corticosteroid injections If response is inadequate – synoviorthesis, or arthroscopic or surgical synovectomy

RECOMMENDATIONS FOR REFERRAL

Subspecialty
- Early referral of patients with rheumatoid arthritis to a rheumatologist to stage the disease, develop a treatment plan and coordinate care by a multidisciplinary team is recommended. Primary care of patients with chronic, progressive disease is generally provided by the rheumatologist.

Physical therapy/rehabilitation
- Patients with functional limitations caused by the arthritis (acute or chronic) should be referred to physical therapy/rehabilitation.

Orthopedic surgery
- Patients with severe pain, functional limitation, or joint instability associated with destructive rheumatoid arthritis should be referred to orthopedic surgeons with expertise in management of arthritis.

SURGERY AND OTHER TREATMENT MODALITIES

Surgery has an important role in the management of complications of both RA and end-stage joint disease. Examples of complications that require surgical interventions include decompression of resistant carpal tunnel syndrome, synovectomy (particularly of the wrist or knee), and repair of tendon ruptures. Wrist fusion or correction of hand deformities with tendon realignments and the placement of sialastic MCP implants helps to improve hand function. Total joint replacement to relieve pain and improve function in end-stage joint disease is possible for most peripheral joints, although this is most commonly carried out on the knees and hips.

DIET AND COMPLEMENTARY TECHNIQUES

The failure of current medical therapies to completely relieve pain in RA prompts many patients to seek alternative approaches to treatment, which are often used unbeknown to the physician. Diet, vitamin, and herbal therapies are particularly popular, although little evidence indicates that they have any true influences on RA, except for fish oil capsules (eicosanoids), which have been clearly shown to reduce inflammation in RA.

RECOMMENDATIONS FOR REFERRAL

Rheumatoid arthritis is a serious rheumatic disease, usually requiring expert management from a multidisciplinary care team. In patients with mild, slowly progressive arthritis, most of the monitoring of the patient can take place in a primary care setting with periodic review by a rheumatologist.

POLYARTICULAR DISORDERS

20

PSORIATIC ARTHRITIS

Psoriatic arthritis is one of the more common forms of inflammatory arthritis. The overall population prevalence is around 0.1% and it occurs in some 5–8% of patients with psoriasis. The sex incidence is roughly equal and the peak age of onset is between 20 and 40 years.

Five main subtypes or clinical patterns of the disease are recognized, four of which are relatively common (Fig. 20.1).

The condition is often confused with other inflammatory disorders, particularly rheumatoid arthritis, reactive arthritis, and ankylosing spondylitis.

CLASSIFICATION OF PSORIATIC ARTHRITIS

Classic psoriatic arthritis confined to distal interphalangeal joints of hands and feet

Arthritis mutilans

Symmetric polyarthritis similar to rheumatoid arthritis

Asymmetric oligoarthritis with dactylitis

Ankylosing spondylitis with or without peripheral joint involvement

---

Fig. 20.1 The main clinical patterns seen in psoriatic arthritis. Arthritis mutilans is pathognomonic of the condition, but rare.

1 TYPICAL CASE: ASYMMETRIC OLIGOARTHRITIS WITH DACTYLITIS

Ralph is a 28-year-old plumber with a 3-year history of mild psoriasis, who first presented with a 1-week history of a painful left knee and right foot. On examination you note a few plaques of psoriasis, a large effusion in the left knee (Fig. 20.2), and dactylitis of the second right toe (Fig. 20.3).

FEATURES OF PSORIATIC, ASYMMETRIC OLIGOARTHRITIS WITH DACTYLITIS

- The most common form of psoriatic arthritis.
- Commonly affects the lower limbs.
- Recurrent, large effusions in the knees.
- Intermittent dactylitis of toes or fingers.
- The psoriasis is often mild.
- Variable course with unpredictable exacerbations and remissions.
- Variable outcome, but often leads to disability in the long term.

KEY POINTS

Definition
- An inflammatory arthritis associated with psoriasis.
- Usually rheumatoid factor negative.

Clinical features
- Any form of psoriasis or a history compatible with psoriasis (arthritis occasionally precedes skin disease).
- Peripheral arthritis – variable types.
- Inflammatory disease of distal interphalangeal joints.
- Asymmetric spondylitis and sacroiliitis.
- Dactylitis.
- Enthesitis (especially of Achilles' tendon insertion).
- Occasionally arthritis mutilans or joint ankylosis.
- Very variable course with exacerbations and remissions.
- No relationship between activity of skin and joint features.

Management
- The basic principles are the same as those for rheumatoid arthritis or ankylosing spondylitis.
- Attention needs to be paid to drugs and other factors that might either exacerbate or help the skin lesions as well as joints.

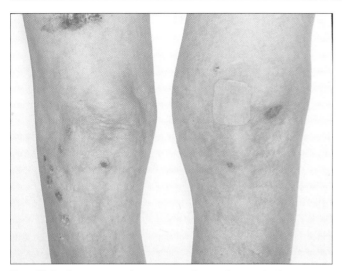

Fig. 20.2 A patient with psoriatic oligoarthritis who has a large, warm swelling of the left knee.

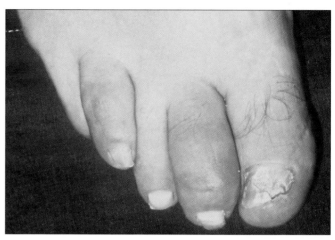

Fig. 20.3 Dactylitis of the second toe in a patient with psoriatic oligoarthritis. Dactylitis is characterized by inflammation of all joints in a digit and of the tendon sheaths, which results in the whole toe (or finger) becoming red, swollen, and painful ('sausage' toe).

FEATURES OF PSORIATIC POLYARTHRITIS THAT MIMICS RHEUMATOID ARTHRITIS

- May be impossible to distinguish from seronegative rheumatoid arthritis.
- Features that suggest the diagnosis include:
- Presence of psoriasis.
- Persistent seronegativity and absence of other organ involvement.
- Distal interphalangeal joint involvement.
- Asymmetric involvement in hands and feet.
- New bone formation around radiologic erosions.
- A tendency to ankylosis of the joints.
- Enthesitis or dactylitis can occur.
- Has a better prognosis than rheumatoid arthritis, but can still cause severe problems.

You treat him with a course of nonsteroidal anti-inflammatory drugs (NSAIDs) and after 3 weeks he has recovered completely. However, he subsequently develops recurrent attacks with large effusions in the knees, interrupted by further periods when he is completely normal. As the attacks are severe and disruptive you refer him to a rheumatologist.

2 TYPICAL CASE: POLYARTHRITIS MIMICKING RHEUMATOID ARTHRITIS

Martha is a 33-year-old woman with a long-standing history of psoriasis who presents with the gradual onset of pain and stiffness in her hands, feet, and knees. On examination you find a symmetric polyarthritis that resembles rheumatoid arthritis, as well as widespread skin psoriasis.

The rheumatoid factor (RF) is negative, and you presume that this is a case of psoriatic arthritis rather than seronegative rheumatoid disease. Martha subsequently develops some distal interphalangeal (DIP) joint disease along with 'typical' rheumatoid deformities (Fig. 20.4). She also develops painful feet

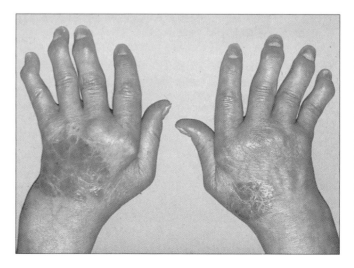

Fig. 20.4 The hands of a woman with symmetric polyarthritis. Initially, this was indistinguishable from rheumatoid disease, but note the distal interphalangeal joint involvement, which is uncommon in rheumatoid arthritis, as well as the skin psoriasis.

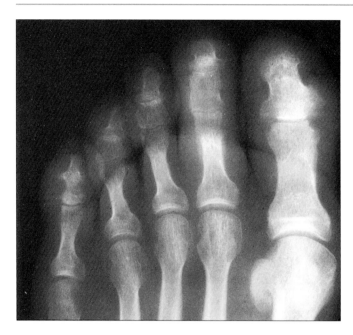

Fig. 20.5 Anteroposterior view of the forefoot in a patient with psoriatic arthritis. Juxta-articular osteoporosis is present and erosive changes accompany bone-productive changes at the interphalangeal joint of the big toe. Soft-tissue swelling and periostitis are visible along the proximal phalanx of the second digit. (Reproduced with permission from Brower AC, Colon E. Spondyloarthropathies. Postgrad Radiol. 1989;9:203–20.)

and the radiographs show new bone growth around the erosions (Fig. 20.5), which help to confirm your diagnosis.

You refer Martha to a rheumatologist, who treats her with methotrexate and physical measures, but in spite of this some of her finger joints become ankylosed a few years later, and she becomes severely disabled.

3 TYPICAL CASE: PSORIATIC SPONDYLITIS

Mark is a 39-year-old economist with a family history of severe psoriasis who presents with a rash, a stiff neck and a painful heel. On examination you find severe scalp psoriasis, a cervical spine that hardly moves at all, stiffness of the lumbar spine, and Achilles' insertional tendinitis (Fig. 20.6).

Radiographs confirm the diagnosis of spondylitis, but show that the sacro-iliitis is asymmetric (Fig. 20.7).

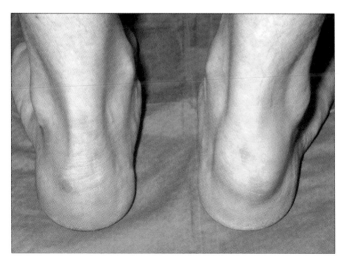

Fig. 20.6 Achilles' insertional tendinitis.

FEATURES OF PSORIATIC SPONDYLITIS

- Sacroiliitis is common in patients with psoriasis, but it is often asymptomatic.
- When spondylitis develops it is clinically indistinguishable from ankylosing spondylitis.
- Radiologically, asymmetric sacroiliitis and other differences occur, contrasting with the changes seen in ankylosing spondylitis.
- Severe cervical disease is common in those with bad scalp psoriasis.
- Peripheral enthesitis, particularly at the insertion of the Achilles' tendon, is common.
- Other peripheral features, such as asymmetric peripheral joint oligoarthritis or dactylitis, may occur.

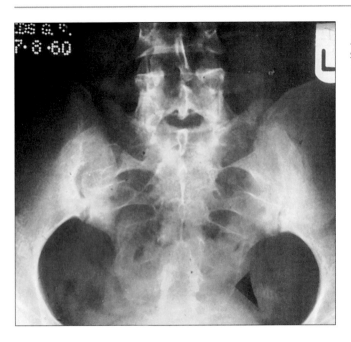

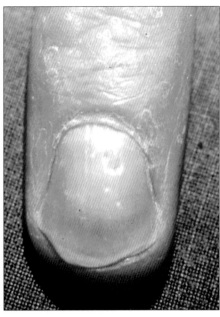

Fig. 20.7
Asymmetric
sacroiliitis.
(Same patient as
in Fig. 20.6)

Fig. 20.8 Pitting of the nails in a patient
with psoriatic arthritis.

FEATURES OF PSORIATIC ARTHRITIS OF THE DISTAL INTERPHALANGEAL JOINTS

- Common and distinctive feature of psoriatic arthritis.
- More common in men than in women.
- Skin disease may or may not be obvious, but there is always some involvement of the nails on the affected digits.
- A variable course; it may be quite benign, but can lead to severe deformity (Fig. 20.9).

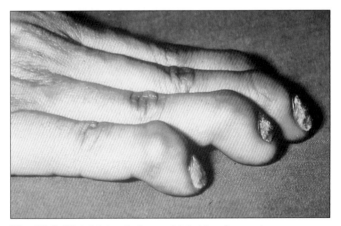

Fig. 20.9 Distal interphalangeal joint involvement.

4 TYPICAL CASE: PSORIATIC DISTAL INTERPHALANGEAL ARTHRITIS

John is 42 years old, has a family history of psoriasis, and presents with painful swelling of the DIP joints of his hands. He denies ever having had any skin problems, but on examination you note pitting of his nails (Fig. 20.8), as well as the DIP joint problems.

You diagnose psoriatic arthritis, treat him with NSAIDs alone, and he develops few long-term problems.

NATURAL HISTORY AND OTHER CLINICAL FEATURES

The activity of the inflammation in psoriatic arthritis is notoriously variable, with extreme exacerbations and remissions of the condition that occur without any apparent cause. There is no association between the activity of the joint disease and the activity of the skin condition. In the majority of patients, skin psoriasis is present for months or years before joint disease develops, but in roughly 15% the two develop together and in some patients the arthritis precedes the skin disease.

The long-term prognosis and outcome is also variable, and in general is better than that for patients with rheumatoid disease. However, recent studies show that most patients do become disabled with time. Factors that appear to predict a worse prognosis include a younger age at onset, polyarticular involvement, and possibly extensive skin involvement.

A rare but highly characteristic feature of late psoriatic arthritis is the development of arthritis mutilans, with osteolysis and shortening of the phalanges (Fig. 20.10). Joints may also become ankylosed.

Psoriatic arthritis is not a multisystem disorder, but occasionally patients develop eye inflammation, which includes conjunctivitis and uveitis, and aortic insufficiency can occur.

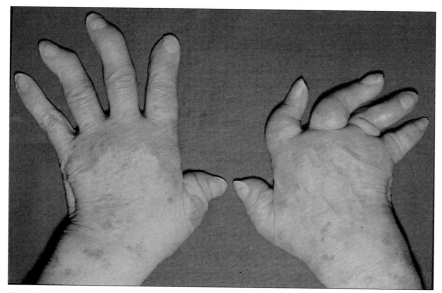

Fig. 20.10 Arthritis mutilans.

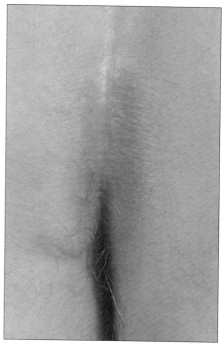

Fig. 20.11 Psoriasis in the natal cleft of a patient who presented with arthritis. No other evidence of skin disease was found.

! POINTS TO LOOK OUT FOR

- Psoriatic arthritis sine psoriasis. Arthritis can precede the onset of any skin disease. More commonly, the skin disease is occult, and only a careful search of flexure sites, the scalp, and the nails reveals the evidence of skin disease, and helps to determine the cause of an arthritis (Fig. 20.11).
- Development of ankylosed joints. Ankylosis of peripheral joints is rare in other forms of inflammatory arthritis, but relatively common in psoriasis, and maintaining the mobility and range of motion of affected joints is therefore particularly important.
- Severe exacerbations of the disease. Severe exacerbations can occur spontaneously, and may also be precipitated by the human immunodeficiency virus in patients with this condition. Severe skin and/or joint disease may require hospital admission for treatment.
- Arthritis mutilans.

INVESTIGATIONS

Investigations may help with the difficult problem of differential diagnosis (see below). The RF is usually negative and when the disease is well established, the radiographs show differences from the type of lesions seen in either ankylosing spondylitis or rheumatoid disease, with features such as DIP joint erosion (Fig. 20.12), asymmetric sacroiliitis (see Fig. 20.7), and new bone growth around peripheral erosions.

As in rheumatoid disease, serologic measures of the acute phase response (such as the erythrocyte sedimentation rate and C-reactive protein) can be used to assess disease activity when treatment is monitored.

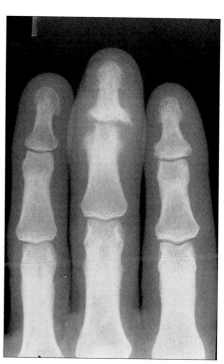

Fig. 20.12 Typical erosive arthritis caused by psoriasis. Note the new bone growth around the erosions of the distal interphalangeal joint, which differentiates this from rheumatoid erosive changes.

DIFFERENTIAL DIAGNOSIS

Differential diagnosis clearly depends on the clinical subtype. Since DIP joint disease is relatively distinct, problems only arise when a single joint is involved, in which case the presence of nail changes should lead to the correct diagnosis. The other three common clinical subtypes create major problems of differential diagnosis, as follows:

- Oligoarthritis may be indistinguishable from a reactive arthritis (see Chapter 22).
- Polyarthritis may be indistinguishable from rheumatoid arthritis (see Chapter 19).
- Spondylitis may be indistinguishable from ankylosing spondylitis (see Chapter 26).

In addition, arthritis that occurs in patients with severe acne can be confused with psoriatic arthritis.

A further problem is that the skin disease in these patients may be occult, and a thorough search may be needed to find it (see Fig. 20.11).

It is important to try to establish the correct diagnosis, because of the differences in clinical course (more variable in psoriatic arthritis than in other diseases) and outcome (more favorable, although very variable). Clinical clues have already been mentioned, and radiographs are the other major aid to diagnosis.

Rx MANAGEMENT

AIMS

The overall aims of management are similar to those of other inflammatory arthropathies:

- Education and support in adjusting to having arthritis.
- Suppression of disease activity (inflammation).
- Prevention of joint deformity and disability.
- Preservation of optimal musculoskeletal function.

In addition, patients with psoriatic arthritis may need expert help with the skin disease, although it is important to understand that treatment of the skin disease may have little or no effect on the arthritis and vice-versa.

These aims can be achieved through a combination of approaches (Fig. 20.13).

PATIENT EDUCATION AND SELF-HELP

As in other forms of arthritis, a good understanding of the condition, which includes the wide swings in activity, is often very helpful in itself. Patients should be taught the rudiments of joint protection and particular emphasis needs to be given to the maintenance of range of motion in view of the tendency for this condition to lead to late joint ankylosis.

Issues of great concern to patients include factors that might be responsible for the exacerbations, which can include stress, some drugs, infections (particularly streptococcal infections), and possibly trauma. Drugs known to have this effect include lithium, β-blockers, and antimalarials.

PHYSICAL THERAPY

The recommended regime clearly depends on the pattern of psoriatic arthritis, those with spinal disease being treated in a similar way to those with ankylosing spondylitis, and those with the oligoarticular or polyarticular patterns being treated in a similar way to those with rheumatoid arthritis. Physical measures can help in the resolution of an inflamed joint (rest and local applications), to maintain joint mobility, to preserve joint function, and to improve functional capabilities.

THERAPEUTIC MEASURES IN THE TREATMENT OF PSORIATIC ARTHRITIS
Pharmacologic measures
Nonsteroidal anti-inflammatory drugs Disease-modifying drugs Photochemotherapy with psoralen Miscellaneous
Surgical measures
Synovectomy Joint arthroplasty
Rehabilitative measures
Aggressive active and passive physical therapy Dynamic strengthening exercises Contact sports and heavy physical activity should be discouraged

Fig. 20.13 Therapeutic measures in the treatment of psoriatic arthritis.

DRUG THERAPY

As with other inflammatory arthropathies, NSAIDs have an important role in controlling symptoms, but they have no effect on the natural history of the disease.

The variable nature and outcome of the disease can make the timing of any decision to use additional drugs to suppress the condition difficult. Increasingly, the emphasis is on the early use of disease-modifying drugs in the majority of cases, save for patients with disease confined to the DIP joints or those with minimal signs and symptoms.

Approaches with disease-modifying drugs are similar to those used in rheumatoid arthritis or ankylosing spondylitis, but selection is also based on the severity of the skin disease, which is sometimes exacerbated by gold or hydroxychloroquine but suppressed by methotrexate and azathioprine.

Methotrexate is the current drug of choice for patients with predominant peripheral arthritis, particularly those with severe skin disease, whereas sulfasalazine is preferred for patients with spondylitis.

SURGERY AND OTHER TREATMENT MODALITIES

Surgery is reserved for patients with significant joint damage, deformity, and functional impairment, and the main role of surgery is reconstructive in late disease. In general, reconstructive surgery of the hips and knees gives a better functional result than surgery on the upper extremities.

A number of other experimental and new approaches are being used in psoriasis and psoriatic arthritis, some of which are targeted at both skin and joint disease, such as derivatives of vitamins A (retinoids).

DIET

Dietary supplementation with polyunsaturated ethyl ester lipids and fish oil has been reported to have some benefits. Although relatively little is understood about the pathogenesis of psoriatic arthritis, no current evidence indicates that diet is of great importance.

RECOMMENDATIONS FOR REFERRAL

Patients with mild psoriatic arthritis or arthritis confined to the distal interphalangeal joints are appropriately managed in a primary care setting.

RECOMMENDATIONS FOR REFERRAL

Subspecialty
- Patients in whom there is diagnostic difficulty, and anyone with significant pain and disability arising from their arthritis, should be referred to a rheumatologist for help with diagnosis and the development of a management plan, and to aid access to coordinated multidisciplinary care, which may need to include a dermatologist.

Physical therapy/rehabilitation
- Patients with functional limitations caused by the arthritis (acute or chronic) should be referred to physical therapy/rehabilitation.

Orthopedic surgery
- Patients with severe pain, functional limitation, or joint instability associated with destructive rheumatoid arthritis should be referred to orthopedic surgeons with expertise in management of arthritis.

POLYARTICULAR DISORDERS

21

VIRAL ARTHRITIS

Musculoskeletal symptoms such as arthralgias and myalgias are a common and disabling feature of most self-limited febrile illnesses attributed to viral infections. Of the many viruses know to cause polyarthritis (Fig. 21.1), for all practical purposes only five forms of viral arthritis are seen with any frequency in Western countries – human immunodeficiency virus (HIV), parvovirus B19, rubella, and hepatitis B and C. These are important to recognize since they may be easily confused with other acute polyarthritis syndromes, particularly rheumatoid arthritis (RA) and reactive arthritis.

VIRUS INFECTIONS WITH PROMINENT ARTHRITIS	
Erythrovirus	
Parvovirus B19	Symmetric polyarthralgia/polyarthritis lasting days to weeks. Prolonged in about 12% of cases, lasting months to years
Togaviruses	
Rubella virus	Morbilliform rash and symmetric polyarthritis in women and children following natural infection or immunization
Chikungunya virus	Explosive onset fever, polyarthralgia/polyarthritis, and rash, in epidemics in Africa and Asia
O'nyong-nyong virus	Epidemic fever, polyarthralgia/polyarthritis, and rash, in Africa
Igbo-ora virus	An epidemic of fever, myalgia, arthralgia, and rash, in the Ivory Coast
Ross River virus (epidemic polyarthritis)	Fever, rash, and polyarthritis, in Australia, New Zealand, New Guinea, and the Pacific islands, in sporadic and epidemic occurrence
Sindbis virus	Epidemic rash and arthritis in Sweden, Finland, and the Karelian isthmus
Mayaro virus	Epidemic febrile polyarthritis in South American rain forest
Hepadnavirus	
Hepatitis B virus	Urticarial rash and small- and large-joint arthritis preceding icterus
Flavivirus	
Hepatitis C virus	Acute polyarthritis in acute infection. Cryoglobulinemia in chronic infection, including essential mixed cryoglobulinemia
Retroviruses	
Human T-lymphocyte leukemia virus 1	Nodular rash and oligoarthritis associated with abnormal cellular infiltrates
Human immuno-deficiency virus	Reactive and psoriatic arthritis, spondyloarthropathy Sjögren-like syndrome

KEY POINTS

Definitions
- A host of different viruses may cause arthritis through various pathogenetic mechanisms, which include direct infection of synovial cells and immune complex formation.
- The most common arthritogenic viruses in North America and Western Europe include parvovirus B19, rubella, and hepatitis B, while a variety of mosquito-borne viruses cause epidemics of polyarthritis in Africa, the Western Pacific and South America.

Clinical features
- The majority of virally caused arthritides are acute and self-limited illnesses, usually accompanied by fever, distinctive cutaneous manifestations, hematologic abnormalities (especially B19 infection), and other clinical features.
- Chronic polyarthritis that mimics rheumatoid arthritis may occur, especially in adults with parvovirus B19 infection, but also with several other types of infection.
- Diagnosis requires knowledge of the epidemiology of these viral infections and laboratory investigations of the disease processes.

Fig. 21.1 Viruses that cause illness with prominent joint involvement.

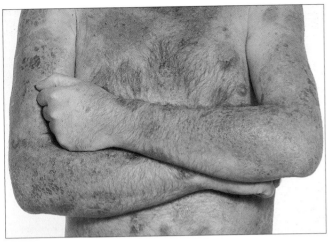

Fig. 21.2 Psoriasiform rash on the trunk and arms of a patient who presented with arthritis and myalgia. He was subsequently shown to be HIV positive.

1 TYPICAL CASE: VIRAL ARTHRITIS

Norman is a 46-year-old, highly successful playwright admitted with a 3-month history of progressive low back pain associated with morning stiffness. During the previous month he had developed a psoriasiform rash on his legs, arms, and trunk (Fig. 21.2).

Over the past 2 weeks he has developed acute pain and swelling in the right ankle, which has progressed to the left knee and left elbow. On questioning you learn that he is bisexual, has multiple partners, and occasionally has unprotected sex.

On physical examination, the left knee is markedly swollen, warm, and tender and there is some limitation in movement of his lumbar spine. Fluid aspirated from the knee shows a white blood cell count of 15,000 cells/mm^3 and cultures of the fluid are negative. An erythrocyte sedimentation rate (ESR) is 120mm/h. A Western blot antibody test for HIV is reported to be positive.

FEATURES OF HUMAN IMMUNODEFICIENCY VIRUS ARTHRITIS

- Parenteral, sexual, and transplacental transmission.
- A number of rheumatic syndromes occur with human immunodeficiency virus (HIV) infection.
- Arthralgias and myalgia are common, particularly in late stages of the disease.
- Reactive arthritis (Reiter's syndrome), psoriatic arthritis (Fig. 21.3), or undifferentiated spondyloarthropathy may develop.
- Septic arthritis should be considered with monoarthritis in an HIV-infected patient.
- Parotid gland enlargement and sicca complaints (pseudo-Sjögren's syndrome) may develop.
- Muscle weakness may develop as a result of HIV-associated inflammatory myopathy, pyomyositis, or zidovudine myopathy.

HUMAN IMMUNODEFICIENCY VIRUS ARTHRITIS

LABORATORY TESTS

An enzyme-linked immunosorbent assay is recommended for initial screening – positive tests must be confirmed with a Western blot. Patients with connective tissue diseases, particularly systemic lupus, may develop false-positive HIV serologies.

PARVOVIRUS B19 ARTHRITIS

LABORATORY TESTS

Serologic diagnosis is possible by detection of immunoglobulin (Ig) M anti-B19 antibodies, which are elevated for approximately 2 months following acute infection. A high prevalence of anti-B19 IgG antibodies occurs in adults, but this is not useful for the diagnosis.

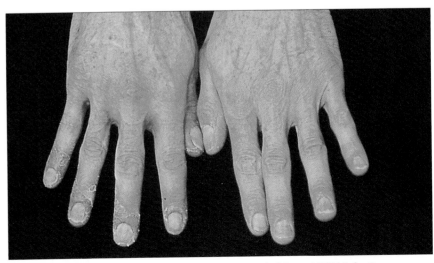

Fig. 21.3 The hands of a patient with psoriatic arthritis and HIV infection.

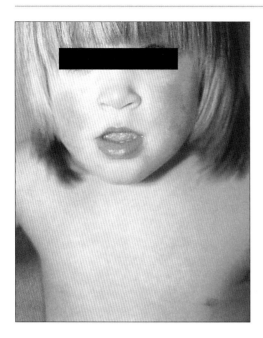

Fig. 21.4 Classic 'slapped cheeks' of a child with erythema infectiosum, caused by parvovirus B19. A lacy, macular erythematous eruption is also present on the trunk. (With permission from Feder HM Jr. Fifth disease. New Engl J Med. 1994;331:1062. Copyright Massachusetts Medical Society, 1994.)

FEATURES OF PARVOVIRUS B19 ARTHRITIS

- Transmission by respiratory tract secretions; incubation period of 7–10 days.
- Fever, sore throat, headache, cough, anorexia, and gastrointestinal symptoms.
- Outbreaks in late winter and spring.
- Characteristic 'slapped-cheek' rash (Fig. 21.4) and blotchy rash on trunk and extremities (much more common in children than in adults).
- Symmetric polyarthritis (similar to rheumatoid arthritis) with morning stiffness (much more common in adults than in children).
- Majority of patients have self-limited course of arthritis of 10–14 days' duration.
- Small number of patients (10%) have chronic, nonerosive arthritis.

RUBELLA VIRUS ARTHRITIS

LABORATORY TESTS

Antirubella IgM and IgG are usually present at the onset of joint symptoms. Since IgM antibody peaks 8–21 days after onset of symptoms and is undetectable after 5 weeks, antirubella IgM positivity indicates recent infection. A diagnosis of rubella infection based on IgG serology can only be made with paired acute and convalescent sera.

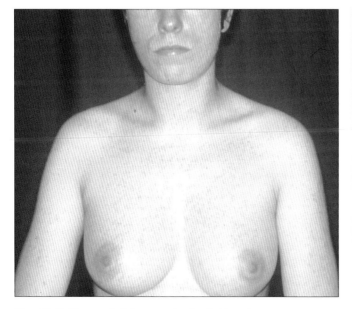

Fig. 21.5 The morbilliform rash of rubella infection.

FEATURES OF RUBELLA VIRUS ARTHRITIS

- Transmission by nasopharyngeal secretions (incubation period of 14–21 days) or following vaccination.
- Peak incidence in late winter and spring.
- Morbilliform rash (Fig. 21.5), low-grade fever, coryza, and lymphadenopathy.
- Arthralgia much more common than arthritis and occurs 1 week before or after the rash.
- Joint symptoms typically resolve over 7–10 days; rarely, symptoms may persist for months or years.
- Children may develop a brachial radiculopathy that causes arm and hand pain ('arm syndrome') or a lumbar radiculopathy ('catcher's crouch' syndrome; Fig. 21.6).

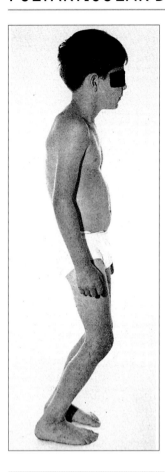

Fig. 21.6 Catcher's crouch syndrome in a child following rubella immunization. (With permission from Kilroy AW, Schaffner W, Fleet WF Jr, Lefkowitz LD, Karzon DT, Fenichel GM. Two syndromes following rubella immunization. Clinical observations and epidemiological studies. JAMA. 1970;214:2287–92).

HEPATITIS B VIRUS ARTHRITIS

LABORATORY TESTS

Elevated transaminase and bilirubin levels typically present when arthritis appears. At the time of arthritis onset, serum hepatitis B surface antigen, hepatitis B e antigen, and anti-hepatitis B core antigen IgM antibodies are typically present.

HEPATITIS C VIRUS ARTHRITIS

LABORATORY TESTS

Serologic diagnosis is possible by detection of IgM anti-B19 antibodies, which are elevated for approximately 2 months following acute infection. The high prevalence of anti-B19 IgG antibody in adults is not useful to the diagnosis.

NATURAL HISTORY AND OTHER CLINICAL FEATURES

In the vast majority of patients, acute non-HIV viral arthritis is a self-limited process of 10–14 days' duration with complete resolution of symptoms. Chronic, nonerosive arthropathy has rarely been described with rubella and hepatitis B virus, and systemic vasculitis syndromes may be a late complication (see below). The arthropathies and rheumatic manifestations associated with HIV infection are chronic and, in instances of reactive and psoriatic arthritis or spondylo-arthropathy, have a similar disease course to that observed with idiopathic forms.

Several other specific viral arthropathies, in addition to those discussed above, are worth noting. Mononucleosis associated with Epstein–Barr virus is frequently accompanied by polyarthralgia, but frank arthritis is uncommon. Adults who develop mumps occasionally develop small- or large-joint synovitis that lasts several weeks; arthritis may precede or follow parotitis by up to 4 weeks. In rare instances, children with varicella have been reported to develop brief monoarticular arthritis or pauciarthritis.

! POINTS TO LOOK OUT FOR

- Henoch–Schönlein purpura, pancytopenia, and vasculitis with parvovirus B19.
- Polyarteritis nodosa (PAN) with chronic hepatitis B viremia.
- A syndrome of mixed cryoglobulinemia with weakness, arthritis, and palpable purpura (Fig. 21.7) with hepatitis C virus.

DIFFERENTIAL DIAGNOSIS

Acute viral polyarthritis typically affects large and small joints in a symmetric distribution similar to that of RA. The presence of characteristic rashes, upper respiratory or gastrointestinal symptoms, or liver enzyme elevations helps to identify viral arthropathies. Abrupt, acute polyarthritis is an uncommon (10–25%) presentation of adult RA and occurs mostly in elderly patients. Differentiation of this form of RA from viral arthritis at presentation is difficult, with a clear diagnosis possible when the arthritis fails to resolve after several weeks. In children, juvenile chronic polyarthritis is much more of a diagnostic problem since it is commonly associated with fever, rashes, respiratory or gastrointestinal symptoms, and liver enzyme abnormalities (see Chapter 36).

FEATURES OF HEPATITIS B VIRUS ARTHRITIS

- Transmission by parenteral and sexual routes; 45–120 day incubation period.
- Fever, myalgia, malaise, anorexia, nausea, and vomiting.
- Prominent urticaria with or without jaundice.
- Acute, symmetric polyarthritis (similar to rheumatoid arthritis) with morning stiffness.
- Arthritis typically limited to preicteric prodrome; recurrent or chronic arthritis possible with chronic hepatitis B viremia or chronic active hepatitis.

gastrointestinal symptoms, and liver enzyme abnormalities (see Chapter 36). Arthropathies associated with HIV are considered principally in patients who present with pauciarticular arthritis of the lower extremities.

MANAGEMENT

Management of viral arthritis is symptomatic with an emphasis on rest, fluid replacement, and antipyretics.

DRUG THERAPY

The control of musculoskeletal symptoms is helped by NSAIDs. Although not well studied, the rheumatic syndromes associated with HIV do not appear to respond to treatment with antiviral drug therapy such as zidovudine. Disease-modifying antirheumatic drugs, particularly sulfasalazine and hydroxychloroquine, are used in HIV patients with chronic arthritis. Both methotrexate and corticosteroids are generally avoided in HIV patients since there have been rare reports of severe exacerbations of disease with these agents. Interferon-α and immunosuppressive therapy have a role in patients with complications of hepatitis virus, such as PAN and cryoglobulinemia.

RECOMMENDATIONS FOR REFERRAL

Most patients with acute viral arthritis have a self-limited disease process that can be managed in a primary care setting.

RECOMMENDATIONS FOR REFERRAL

Subspecialty
Patients with suspected viral arthritis who fail to show the expected improvement and resolution should be referred to rheumatology for reconsideration of the diagnosis and exclusion of other forms of polyarthritis. Referral is particularly warranted in patients who develop long-term or delayed systemic complications of viral arthritis (i.e. vasculitis, chronic hepatitis, and so on).

FEATURES OF HEPATITIS C VIRUS ARTHRITIS

- Transmission by parenteral route.
- Majority of infections are asymptomatic.
- Acute, symmetric polyarthritis (similar to rheumatoid arthritis) with morning stiffness.

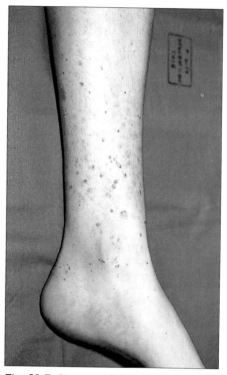

Fig. 21.7 Purpura of the lower extremities in a patient with mixed cryoglobulinemia and hepatitis C virus.

POLYARTICULAR DISORDERS

22

REACTIVE ARTHRITIS

Reactive arthritis (Reiter's syndrome) refers to a syndrome of inflammatory arthritis triggered by an infection, most commonly of the genitourinary or gastro-intestinal tracts. The arthritis typically develops 2–4 weeks following the infection and, in contrast to septic arthritis, cultures of synovial fluid and synovial tissues are negative. Most patients experience often-profound constitutional symptoms (fever, anorexia, and fatigue) as part of the acute illness and develop extra-articular manifestations (affecting eyes, skin, mucous membranes, and heart) during the course of the disease (Fig. 22.1).

1   TYPICAL CASE: REACTIVE ARTHRITIS

Duncan is a 23-year-old sailor in the merchant marine, who has a 6-week history of pain and swelling that involves his right knee and both ankles. Roughly 3 months ago he developed a discharge from his penis and was treated for gonorrhea with ceftriaxone. He has continued to have a slight discharge and has recently noted a sore on the tip of the penis.

On physical examination the right knee is warm and markedly swollen (Fig. 22.2) and a serpiginous, shallow ulcer with an erythematous border is seen on the glans of the penis (Fig. 22.3).

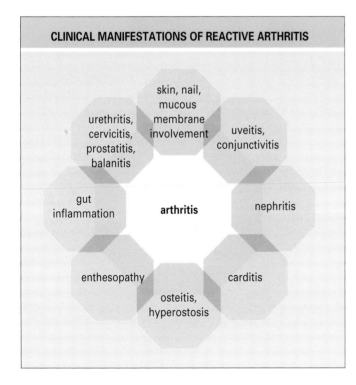

Fig. 22.1 Clinical manifestations of reactive arthritis.

KEY POINTS

Definitions

- A sterile joint inflammation that develops after a distant infection.
- The disease is systemic and not limited to the joints, in spite of its name.
- Triggering infections most commonly originate in the throat, urogenital organs, or gastrointestinal tract.
- The disease also occurs with no obvious preceding infection, for example in association with inflammatory bowel disease.

Clinical features

- Arthritis, enthesopathy, tendinitis, tenosynovitis, osteitis, and muscle pains.
- Skin and mucous membrane lesions are frequent.
- Eye inflammations, for example uveitis and conjunctivitis.
- Visceral involvement, such as nephritis or carditis, is relatively rare.
- Severity ranges from mild arthralgia to disabling disease.
- Spontaneous recovery is common and the prognosis is, in general, good.
- Later, many patients suffer arthralgias and recurrences.
- Susceptibility to the disease is strongly linked to possession of the HLA-B27 antigen.

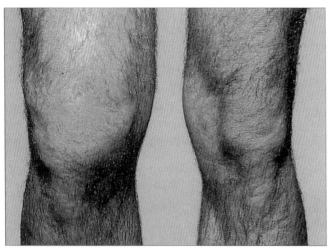

Fig. 22.2 Swelling of the right knee in a patient with reactive arthritis.

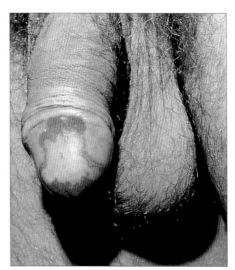

Fig. 22.3 Circinate balanitis in a man with reactive arthritis. (Courtesy of Professor VK Havu, Department of Dermatology, University of Turku.)

FEATURES OF REACTIVE ARTHRITIS

- Constitutional signs – fever, fatigue, and anorexia.
- Asymmetric migratory mono- or oligoarthritis of the weight-bearing joints – knees, ankles, and hips.
- Inflammation and swelling of an entire toe or finger ('dactylitis'; Fig. 22.4).
- Low back or buttock pain.
- Hyperkeratotic skin lesion ('keratoderma blennorrhagicum') on the palms or soles (Fig. 22.5).
- Acute conjunctivitis or anterior uveitis.
- Marked elevation of erythrocyte sedimentation rate.

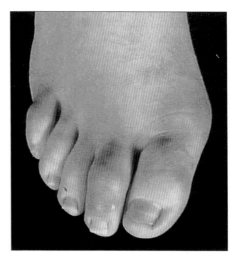

Fig. 22.4 Dactylitis of the second toe ('sausage' toe) in a man with reactive arthritis.

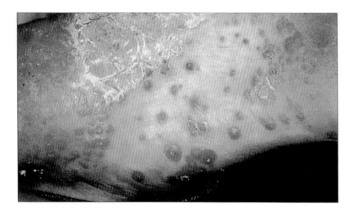

Fig. 22.5 Skin lesions (keratoderma blennorrhagicum) on the sole of a patient with reactive arthritis.

NATURAL HISTORY AND OTHER CLINICAL FEATURES

Reactive arthritis is considered in patients who present with a seronegative, asymmetric polyarthritis of the lower extremities. A history of an antecedent diarrheal illness or venereal exposure (Fig. 22.6) adds weight to the diagnosis, but is often absent. In most patients, reactive arthritis is a self-limited disease process that lasts 4–6 months; a small minority of patients develop a chronic, relapsing course of destructive peripheral arthropathy, typically of the knees and ankles, or ankylosing spondylitis.

 POINTS TO LOOK OUT FOR

- Carditis with aortic insufficiency or atrioventricular (AV) block.
- Proteinuria secondary to IgA nephropathy or amyloidosis.
- Cranial or peripheral neuropathies or other central nervous system lesions.

INVESTIGATIONS

LABORATORY TESTS

A complete blood count and differential count, rheumatoid factor (RF) assay, and measurement of acute phase reactants are routinely carried out in all patients with suspected reactive arthritis. A modest leukocytosis is commonly present and patients are seronegative for RF. Acute phase reactant indicators such as erythrocyte sedimentation rate (ESR) or C-reactive protein are usually markedly elevated, and are measures often used to monitor the activity of the arthritis over the course of the disease.

IMAGING

Radiographic studies are rarely indicated in acute reactive arthritis. Standard joint radiographs reveal only soft-tissue swelling with no abnormalities of bone or cartilage. In scintigraphy with technetium-99m methylene diphosphonate, increased uptake of the isotope may be demonstrated in involved joints, a finding that may on occasion be useful in patients with suspected sacroiliac involvement. In patients with recurrent or chronic reactive arthritis, characteristic radiographic features may be seen. These include bone formation at sites of osseous erosions, which lead to subchondral sclerosis and eburnation (Fig. 22.7), and calcification and ossification of the enthesis, which causes spur formation.

MICROBIOLOGY

Cultures of synovial fluid and sites of potential infection, which includes swabs of the cervix, urethra, and rectum, are taken. The detection of organisms from other sites, particularly those known to be commonly associated with reactive arthritis, provides confirmation of the diagnosis. However, in many patients, even those with a clear antecedent infection, all cultures are negative at the time of the arthritis. In such patients, serologic studies for organisms associated with reactive arthritis may help to document a recent infection. Since patients infected with the human immunodeficiency virus (HIV) virus have been reported to develop a Reiter's-like syndrome, serologic studies for HIV are obtained in all patients.

OTHER STUDIES

A baseline electrocardiogram is obtained as part of the initial evaluation to detect AV conduction delays.

TRIGGERING INFECTIONS IN REACTIVE ARTHRITIS
Urogenital tract
Chlamydia trachomatis   *Ureaplasma urealyticum*
Gastrointestinal tract
Yersinia enterocolitica   *Yersinia pseudotuberculosis*   *Salmonella* spp.   *Shigella* spp.   *Campylobacter* spp.
Respiratory tract
Chlamydia pneumoniae

Fig. 22.6 Triggering infections in reactive arthritis.

LESS COMMON FEATURES OF REACTIVE ARTHRITIS INCLUDE
• Enthesitis – most commonly with plantar fasciitis or Achilles' tendinitis.   • Sterile urethritis.   • Oral ulcers.

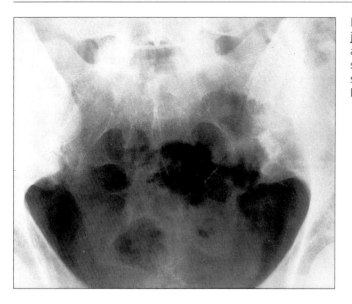

Fig. 22.7 Anteroposterior Ferguson view of the sacroiliac joints in a patient with reactive arthritis. There is bilateral, asymmetric involvement, and bone repair is present on the right side. A large erosion is visible on the inferior aspect of the left sacroiliac joint. (Reproduced with permission from Brower A. Disorders of the sacroiliac joint. Radiology. 1978;1:3–26.)

DIFFERENTIAL DIAGNOSIS

In most patients, it is important to exclude septic arthritis, so synovial fluid must be aspirated for cell count, Gram stain, and cultures. The cell count may be high (10,000–50,000 cells/mm^3). The differential shows predominantly polymorphonuclear leukocytes in the early stages of the illness followed by a lymphocyte predominance late in the disease course. In patients with urogenital involvement, it is very important to exclude infection with *Neisseria gonorrhoeae* and appropriate cultures need to be obtained. The finding of bloody or prolonged diarrhea is distinctly unusual in reactive arthritis and suggests the possibility of inflammatory bowel disease, ulcerative colitis, or some other bowel pathology as a cause of the arthritis. In such instances, ileocolonoscopy or radiographic studies may be required to differentiate these diseases.

Reactive arthritis may occur in patients with HIV infection (see Chapter 21), presumably as a consequence of the high rate of venereal or enteric infections seen in HIV disease.

 ## MANAGEMENT

The primary goals of therapy of the acute illness are to:
• Suppress joint inflammation with the use of anti-inflammatory drugs;
• Provide local management of various extra-articular manifestations;
• Institute a program of physical therapy to relieve symptoms and prevent or minimize functional impairments.

PHYSICAL THERAPY

Physical therapy is tailored to the needs of the individual patient. Most patients benefit from bed rest or from immobilization of affected joints by splinting. However, passive range of motion exercises by an experienced therapist must be used during this time to prevent joint contractures and muscle wasting. Local applications of heat or cold often help to relieve joint or periarticular pain. In patients with arthritis of the forefoot, ankle or subtalar joints, custom-made orthotics can reduce pain and enable the patient to remain ambulatory. Once joint inflammation has subsided the patient must begin active, rehabilitative exercises to restore full motion within the joint.

DRUG THERAPY

Drugs are an important part of the management of patients with reactive arthritis (Fig. 22.8). Nonsteroidal anti-inflammatory drugs (NSAIDs) are the mainstay of drug treatment for joint symptoms in reactive arthritis; systemic corticosteroids have little or no role in management. It may be necessary to give courses of several different NSAIDs in maximum doses before settling on an optimal therapy. Initiation of therapy with, for example, indomethacin at 100mg/day divided into four doses and taken with food is a widely used and often effective regimen. Increases in the dose of indomethacin beyond these levels often causes intolerable headaches and lightheadedness.

Intra-articular or periarticular injections of corticosteroids are often beneficial in patients with refractory arthritis limited to a single joint or in patients with severe tendinitis or enthesitis. Long-acting corticosteroid preparations such as triamcinolone hexacetonide are preferred in doses of 5–10mg for small joints and injections into tendon sheaths, and in doses of 20–40mg for large joints. In the instance of infiltration of tendon sheaths or entheses, meticulous care must be taken to avoid injection directly into the tendon itself.

Drug therapy in patients with chronic arthritis is similar to approaches used in rheumatoid arthritis and involves the use of disease-modifying or second-line antirheumatic drugs (see Chapter 9). Sulfasalazine (500–3000mg/day), because of its known efficacy in treating inflammatory bowel disease and its potential antibacterial role, is increasingly used in patients with chronic forms of reactive arthritis. Low-dose oral methotrexate (7.5–15mg/week) or azathioprine (50–150mg/day) are popular alternative options. It is important to exclude HIV infection before starting either of these drugs, since severe exacerbations of reactive arthritis have been reported in HIV-positive patients treated with them.

Antibiotic treatment with a tetracycline is indicated only in patients with an acute *Chlamydia*-triggered reactive arthritis. The efficacy of long-term antibiotic therapy in patients with reactive arthritis, to prevent relapses of the disease, has not been established and cannot be recommended.

Dilating eye-drops are recommended in patients with uveitis for relief of pain induced by spasm of the ciliary muscles and to prevent synechiae formation. Systemic corticosteroids or immunosuppressive agents may be indicated for patients with very severe uveitis associated with visual loss.

MONITORING PROGRESSION AND OUTCOME

Clinical signs and symptoms and ESR provide useful guides by which to monitor the disease course.

RECOMMENDATIONS FOR REFERRAL

Most patients with reactive arthritis can typically be diagnosed and successfully managed with NSAIDs in a primary care setting.

RECOMMENDATIONS FOR REFERRAL

Subspecialty

- Patients with reactive arthritis failing to respond to treatment with an NSAID or who present with multisystem disease should be referred to a rheumatologist for confirmation of diagnosis and treatment recommendations. Patients with chronic reactive arthritis often require care by a multidisciplinary team, coordinated by the rheumatologist. Patients with suspected inflammatory bowel disease should be referred to a gastroenterologist for evaluation and treatment recommendations.

Physical therapy/rehabilitation

- Physical therapy/rehabilitation assumes an important role in patients with chronic reactive arthritis to improve/preserve musculoskeletal function.

Other

- Patients with uveitis should be referred to an ophthalmologist for a thorough eye examination and for treatment recommendations.

DRUGS USED IN ACUTE REACTIVE ARTHRITIS

Antibiotics if infection is still present

Nonsteroidal anti-inflammatory drugs

Intra-articular corticosteroids

Second-line antirheumatic drugs

Fig. 22.8 Drugs used in reactive arthritis.

OTHER POLYARTICULAR DISORDERS

SARCOIDOSIS

IN WHAT CIRCUMSTANCES IS SARCOIDOSIS SUSPECTED?

Sarcoidosis is suspected in patients (particularly African–American women) with arthritis accompanied by erythema nodosum, hilar or peripheral lymphadenopathy, and pulmonary signs and symptoms.

HOW IS SARCOIDOSIS MANAGED?

Most patients with acute musculoskeletal manifestations of sarcoidosis respond well to nonsteroidal anti-inflammatory drugs (NSAIDs); colchicine may also help in acute arthritis. The chronic, persistent form of arthritis generally responds to treatment with corticosteroids; second-line antirheumatic drugs such as methotrexate or cyclosporine may be indicated in treatment-resistant cases.

KEY POINTS

Definition

- Sarcoidosis is a chronic, systemic granulomatous disease most commonly seen in young (20–40 years old) women.
- Granuloma formation in synovial tissues, bone, and muscle may lead to rheumatic symptoms.

Main clinical features

- Patients with sarcoidosis commonly present with pulmonary symptoms (dry cough, dyspnea, chest pain), constitutional symptoms (fever, weight loss, fatigue), bilateral hilar adenopathy, and rheumatic complaints.
- Acute polyarthritis most commonly occurs in the knees and ankles and is typically associated with erythema nodosum (Fig. 23.1) and bilateral hilar adenopathy.
- Chronic polyarthritis may result from granulomatous infiltration of synovial tissues (Fig. 23.2) and a sausage-like swelling of the digit (dactylitis) from cyst formation on the phalanges (Fig. 23.3).
- Uveitis, sinusitis, parotitis, and myositis are rare features of sarcoidosis and may cause diagnostic confusion with other rheumatic syndromes (Fig. 23.4).

Diagnosis

- Diagnosis depends on a compatible clinical picture and the detection of noncaseating granulomas of affected tissues.
- Cells in the sarcoid granuloma produce angiotensin-converting enzyme (ACE) and 1,25-dihydroxyvitamin D, which leads to hypercalcemia, hypercalcuria, and increased serum ACE levels.
- The Kveim test is rarely performed in the US for diagnostic purposes (Fig. 23.5).

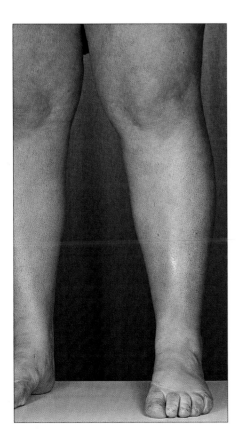

Fig. 23.1 Erythema nodosum. This patient presented with an arthropathy of knee joints associated with bilateral hilar lymph node enlargement. Symptoms (extreme lassitude, with pain and stiffness of large joints) were unusually persistent, and failed to resolve spontaneously or respond to treatment with nonsteroidal anti-inflammatory drugs. The patient is shown after 3 weeks of treatment with prednisolone.

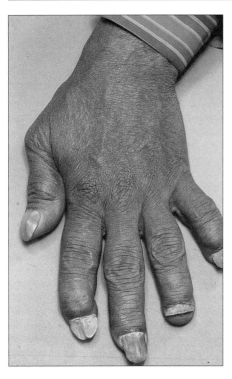

Fig. 23.2
Chronic
polyarthritis.
This patient with
long-standing
pulmonary
sarcoidosis and
granulomatous
skin lesions
developed
polyarthritis of
the
interphalangeal
joints.

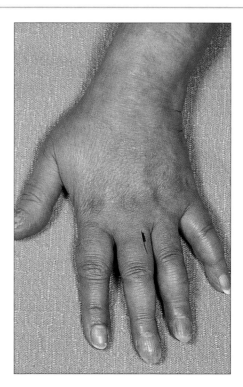

Fig. 23.3
Sarcoid
dactylitis. Soft-
tissue swelling
of the digits is
seen in this
patient with
long-standing
sarcoidosis.

Fig. 23.4 Differential diagnosis of
sarcoidosis.

DIFFERENTIAL DIAGNOSIS OF SARCOIDOSIS		
Sign	Frequency in sarcoidosis (%)	Differential rheumatic diagnosis
Uveitis	20	Spondyloarthropathies, Behçet's syndrome
Arthritis	15	Rheumatoid arthritis, systemic lupus erythematosus, spondylo arthropathies, reactive arthritis
Parotid gland enlargement	5	Sjögren's syndrome
Upper airway disease	5	Wegener's granulomatosis
Myositis	5	Idiopathic inflammatory myopathy

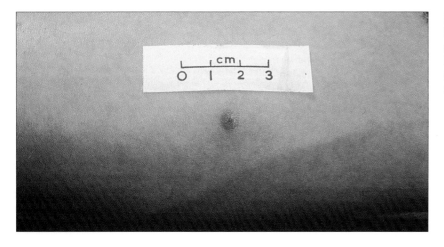

Fig. 23.5 Classic Kveim papule. The
histology of the lesion showed noncaseating,
epithelioid, and giant cell granulomas.
However, there is a 4–6 week delay before
test interpretation and a 20% false-negative
rate.

PALINDROMIC RHEUMATISM AND INTERMITTENT HYDRARTHROSIS

IN WHAT CIRCUMSTANCES ARE PALINDROMIC RHEUMATISM AND INTERMITTENT HYDRARTHROSIS SUSPECTED?

Palindromic rheumatism and intermittent hydrarthrosis are considered in patients with intermittent joint swelling. The main differential diagnoses are connective tissue diseases, crystalline arthropathies such as gout (see Chapter 10) or calcium pyrophosphate arthropathy (see Chapter 44), or (in the instance of recurrent knee effusions) mechanical injuries. Although connective tissue disorders such as lupus typically have relapsing and remitting arthropathies, patients invariably develop signs and symptoms that reflect the systemic nature of the disease. Crystalline arthropathies typically have marked signs of inflammation and can be readily identified by the finding of crystals on microscopic analysis of synovial fluid. Effusions from mechanical damage to the joint, such as a partially torn meniscus of the knee, typically form after vigorous use of the knee.

HOW ARE PALINDROMIC RHEUMATISM AND INTERMITTENT HYDRARTHROSIS MANAGED?

Some relief of joint symptoms is provided by NSAIDs, but they do not reliably prevent attacks. Patients with recurrent attacks of palindromic rheumatism are managed with the same drugs as used in rheumatoid arthritis (RA).

KEY POINTS

Definition
- Palindromic rheumatism and intermittent hydrarthrosis are syndromes of recurrent, brief, self-limited attacks of arthritis or joint effusions followed by periods of remission.

Main clinical features
- Rapid development of painful joint effusions with little or no evidence of inflammation or systemic signs or symptoms.
- Knees or other large joints most commonly involved.
- Arthritis of the small joints of the hands and feet (as well as periarticular attacks or transient nodules) may be seen in palindromic rheumatism.
- Attacks last 2–5 days and resolve completely, only to recur weeks or months later.
- Episodes may be life-long without producing damage to the joint.
- Approximately one third of patients show evolution of disease into typical rheumatoid arthritis.

Diagnosis
- Relapsing, remitting course and pattern of arthropathy is sufficient for diagnosis.

HYPERTROPHIC OSTEOARTHROPATHY

KEY POINTS

Definition
- Hypertrophic osteoarthropathy (HOA) is a syndrome characterized by digital clubbing, periostosis of the distal extremities, and joint effusions.
- Although it may occur as a rare primary disorder (hereditary pachydermoperiostosis), most cases are 'secondary' to pathology in other organs, most commonly the lungs and gastrointestinal tract.

Main clinical features
- Clubbing of the fingers (Fig. 23.6) and toes is the hallmark of HOA. The nail becomes convex (watch-crystal nail), and the skin that overlies its base becomes thin and shiny with the disappearance of the normal nail crease.
- Periostosis may lead to complaints of shin or forearm pain and marked bony tenderness on palpation.
- Joints adjacent to bones with periostosis may develop joint effusions, most commonly seen in the knees, ankles, and wrists.

- In cases of secondary HOA, clinical signs of the underlying pathology are typically evident such as abdominal pain and diarrhea in inflammatory bowel disease, exophthalmos and pretibial edema in Graves' disease, or jaundice or ascites in liver cirrhosis.

Diagnosis
- In the majority of patients, digital clubbing is the only manifestation of the syndrome.
- Plain radiographs of the extremities show typical periosteal elevations and thickening of the distal tibia (Fig. 23.7), femur, and radius and ulna (Fig. 23.8).
- Secondary forms of HOA are categorized on the basis of whether findings are localized or generalized (Fig. 23.9).
- Evaluation is generally dictated by the suspected cause of HOA from clues found in the history and physical examination, but the association of HOA with primary and metastatic tumors of the lungs requires chest radiographs for every patient.

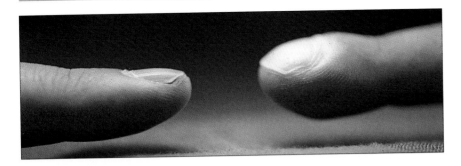

Fig. 23.6 Clubbing deformity of hypertrophic osteoarthropathy. The finger on the right is clubbed compared with the normal finger shape on the left.

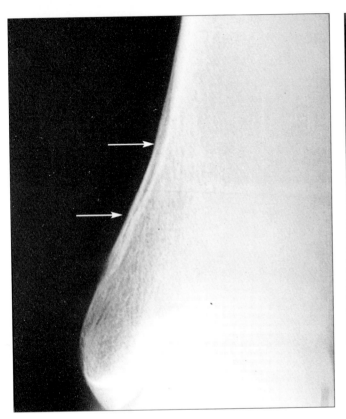

Fig. 23.7 Monolayer periostosis. Typical location of the early periosteal changes (arrows) of hypertrophic osteoarthropathy. A monolayer type of periostosis is seen in this anteroposterior view of the ankle of a 20-year-old woman with Fallot's tetralogy.

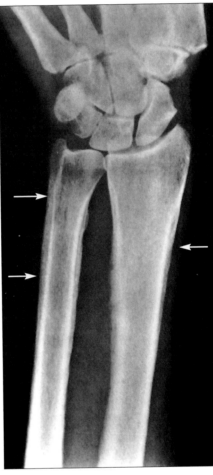

Fig. 23.8 Hypertrophic osteoarthropathy. The wrist radiograph shows periostosis at the distal ends of the radius and ulna (arrows). The coarse, layered appearance is most evident along the diaphyses. The relative sparing of the former epiphyses is characteristic.

IN WHAT CIRCUMSTANCES IS HYPERTROPHIC OSTEOARTHROPATHY SUSPECTED?

Hypertrophic osteoarthropathy (HOA) should be suspected in patients who complain of pain in the long bones of the extremities, particularly the shins, or in patients with unexplained, noninflammatory (synovial fluid white count <500 cells/mm^3) effusions in the knees, ankles, or wrists. Digital clubbing is generally completely asymptomatic and in mild cases only detected by a careful clinical examination.

HOW IS HYPERTROPHIC OSTEOARTHROPATHY MANAGED?

Some relief of bone pain and arthritis is provided by NSAIDs. In secondary forms, the syndrome resolves with treatment of the underlying illness. For example, resection of a lung tumor, correction of heart malformation, or successful antibiotic treatment of bacterial endocarditis is associated with regression of all features of the syndrome.

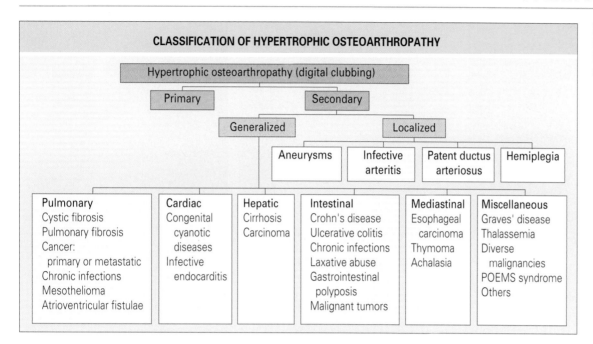

CLASSIFICATION OF HYPERTROPHIC OSTEOARTHROPATHY

Hypertrophic osteoarthropathy (digital clubbing)

Primary — Secondary

Secondary: Generalized — Localized

Localized: Aneurysms | Infective arteritis | Patent ductus arteriosus | Hemiplegia

Pulmonary	Cardiac	Hepatic	Intestinal	Mediastinal	Miscellaneous
Cystic fibrosis	Congenital	Cirrhosis	Crohn's disease	Esophageal	Graves' disease
Pulmonary fibrosis	cyanotic	Carcinoma	Ulcerative colitis	carcinoma	Thalassemia
Cancer:	diseases		Chronic infections	Thymoma	Diverse
primary or metastatic	Infective		Laxative abuse	Achalasia	malignancies
Chronic infections	endocarditis		Gastrointestinal		POEMS syndrome
Mesothelioma			polyposis		Others
Atrioventricular fistulae			Malignant tumors		

Fig. 23.9 Classification of hypertrophic osteoarthropathy.

ENDOCRINE ARTHROPATHIES

IN WHAT CIRCUMSTANCES ARE ENDOCRINE ARTHROPATHIES SUSPECTED?

Patients with endocrine diseases often first seek medical help because of rheumatic complaints. Diffuse aches and pains, fatigue, or complaints of muscle weakness are particularly common and readily confused with fibromyalgia or systemic rheumatic diseases. In addition, complaints may be localized to joints, which include both the spine or small and large peripheral joints and suggest frank arthritis such as RA or a spondyloarthropathy. On rare occasions, the physical appearance of the patient allows for immediate diagnosis of the problem (Figs 23.10–23.12).

WHAT PATTERNS OF DISEASE ARE TYPICAL OF ENDOCRINE ARTHROPATHIES?

Patterns of disease typical of endocrine arthropathies are given in Figure 23.13.

KEY POINTS

Definition
- Endocrine arthropathies are musculoskeletal manifestations that occur with endocrine disease and include diabetes mellitus, hypo- and hyperthyroidism, hyperparathyroidism, acromegaly, and Cushing's syndrome.

Main clinical features
- Rheumatic syndromes vary with endocrine disease (see Fig. 23.13).
- Common clinical features include proximal muscle weakness, soft-tissue changes (carpal tunnel syndrome, tendinitis, etc.), and bone and cartilage abnormalities.

Diagnosis
- Diagnosis rests on laboratory documentation of appropriate endocrine abnormalities.

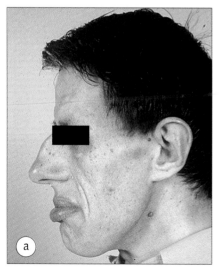
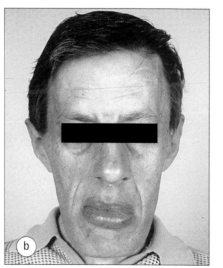

Fig. 23.10 Characteristic facial appearance in acromegaly.

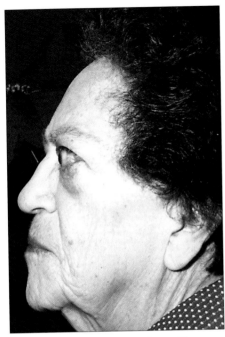

Fig. 23.11 Profile of a patient with hyperthyroidism who developed thyroid acropachy. The exophthalmos that was present is demonstrated.

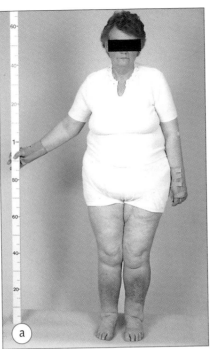
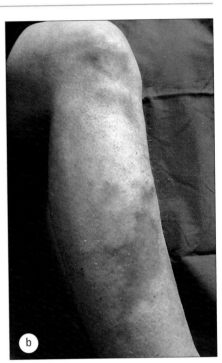

Fig. 23.12 Hypothyroidism. This patient presented with (a) carpal tunnel syndrome (note the wrist splints) and typical facial and other features of hypothyroidism and (b) pretibial myxedema.

PATTERNS OF DISEASE TYPICAL OF ENDOCRINE ARTHROPATHIES

Disease	Endocrine arthropathies
Diabetes mellitus	A number of rheumatic syndromes are seen in diabetic patients – the most important being the diabetic hand syndrome detected by the 'prayer sign' on physical examination (Fig. 23.14) and destructive lytic bone changes most commonly seen in the feet (Fig. 23.15) Other rheumatic complications commonly seen in diabetic patients include frozen shoulder, reflex sympathetic dystrophy, and diffuse skeletal hyperostosis
Hypo-thyroidism	In infants, may be associated with growth retardation and skeletal and dental abnormalities (cretinism) Adults with severe hypothyroidism may develop knee pain, swelling and stiffness Synovial fluid is noninflammatory and very viscous
Hyper-thyroidism	Musculoskeletal manifestations are common in patients with hyperthyroidism, including proximal muscle weakness, carpal tunnel syndrome, and premature osteoporosis Patients with Graves' disease develop a peculiar, painless soft-tissue swelling of fingers and toes with clubbing and periostitis ('thyroid acropachy'; Fig, 23.16) Acute thyroiditis (Hashimoto's) occurs with connective tissue diseases (systemic lupus erythematosus, Sjögren's, etc.), as well as rheumatoid arthritis
Hyperpara-thyroidism	Mainly bone-related problems caused by bone resorption from increased levels of parathyroid hormone Osteitis fibrosa cystica (Fig. 23.17) produces nonspecific hand pain often localized to the proximal interphalangeal joints Other rheumatic complications include proximal muscle weakness, generalized osteoporosis, and chondrocalcinosis
Acromegaly	Arthropathy results from effects of growth hormone on cartilage – may involve large joints (knees, shoulders, hips), cervical and lumbar spine, or hands Radiographs show widening of joint space early (Fig. 23.18) and degenerative changes late in the disease course (Fig. 23.19) Other rheumatic complications seen in acromegaly include carpal tunnel syndrome (50% of cases), Raynaud's phenomenon (30%), proximal muscle weakness (30%), and chondrocalcinosis (rare)
Cushing's syndrome	Characterized by proximal myopathy, osteonecrosis, and premature osteoporosis Electromyograph and serum levels of muscle enzymes normal; muscle biopsy shows atrophy of type 2b fibers

Fig. 23.13 Patterns of disease typical of endocrine arthropathies.

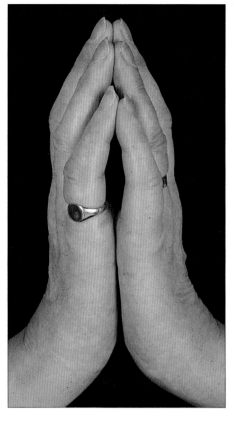

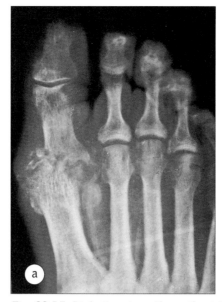

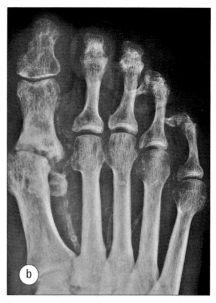

Fig. 23.15 Diabetic osteoarthropathy. (a) Fragmentation and severe osteolysis on the articular surfaces of the first metatarsophalangeal joint. (b) The process has healed with moderate deformation of the articular surfaces.

Fig. 23.14 Diabetic hand syndrome. The patient is unable to press both hands together ('prayer' sign).

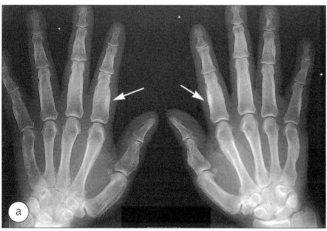

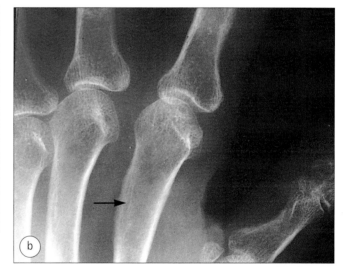

Fig. 23.16 Thyroid acropachy. Arrows show (a) periosteal new bone formation and (b) longitudinal striation within the cortex.

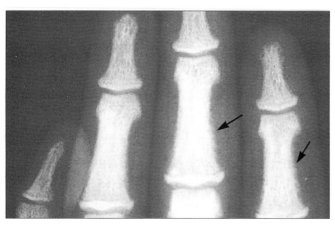

Fig. 23.17 Part of the hand radiograph of a patient with hyperparathyroidism showing the characteristic subperiosteal resorption of the phalanges and lace-like trabecular pattern. This patient also had lytic lesions ('brown tumors') in the long bones.

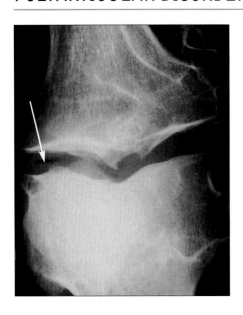

Fig. 23.18 Radiograph of the knee in acromegaly. Widening of the articular joint space – the 'vacuum' sign is visible (arrow).

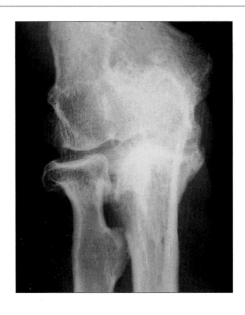

Fig. 23.19 Deformation of the epiphysis and progressive osteophytosis, seen late in the disease course of acromegaly.

HOW ARE ENDOCRINE ARTHROPATHIES MANAGED?

Therapy should be directed primarily at correction or control of endocrine disease, which generally results in resolution or improvement of rheumatic complaints. Management is much more complex in instances where structural damage of musculoskeletal tissues has occurred – diabetic or acromegalic osteoarthropathy, osteoporosis, etc – and generally requires subspecialty care from rheumatologists, physical therapists, and orthopedic surgeons.

INFLAMMATORY OSTEOARTHRITIS

KEY POINTS

Definition
- Inflammatory osteoarthritis is the onset of interphalangeal joint osteoarthritis in middle-aged people, with inflammatory features.

Main clinical features
- Most common in perimenopausal women.
- Onset of pain and swelling in interphalangeal joints of the hands – the distal or proximal interphalangeal joints (Fig. 23.20), or both.
- A family history of osteoarthritis may be found.
- Blood tests are generally normal, and radiographs may also be normal in the early stages.

Diagnosis
- It may be difficult to distinguish this entity from other inflammatory polyarthropathies such as rheumatoid arthritis.
- A wait-and-watch policy, with frequent checks on radiographs, erythrocyte sedimentation rate and rheumatoid factor may be necessary – the diagnosis becomes obvious with time.

IN WHAT CIRCUMSTANCES IS INFLAMMATORY OSTEOARTHRITIS SUSPECTED?

Any polyarthritis of the hands in middle-aged people (especially women) could result from inflammatory osteoarthritis (OA). Clinical features that help to distinguish inflammatory OA from rheumatoid disease include the usual absence of any involvement of the metacarpophalangeal joints of wrists (although the thumb base may be affected) in

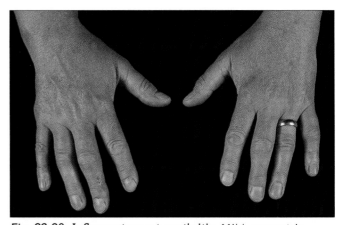

Fig. 23.20 Inflammatory osteoarthritis. Mild, symmetric swellings of the proximal interphalangeal joints at presentation.

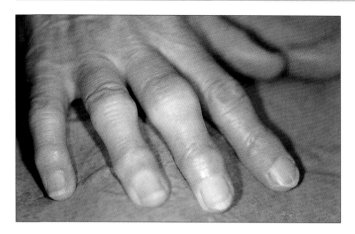

Fig. 23.21 Clinical assessments of process and outcome in osteoarthritis (OA). This hand shows the swelling and redness of a patient with active interphalangeal joint OA. Heat and redness could be used as process measures, and the swelling, deformity, stability, and movement of the joint are potential outcome measures. However, the usefulness of these clinical measures is hampered by high inter- and intraobserver variation and lack of sensitivity to change.

inflammatory OA, the firm nature of the swelling around the joints (rather than soft-tissue swelling) (Fig. 23.21), and normal blood tests. However, this condition can also mimic psoriatic arthritis of the interphalangeal joints. The diagnosis generally becomes obvious with time.

 ## MANAGEMENT

A wait-and-watch diagnostic policy is a necessary part of the management to avoid the damaging physical and psychologic consequences of an incorrect diagnosis of and treatment for RA.

In the early phases, NSAIDs can help. The condition generally has a fairly benign course and outcome – it tends to become less active with time; it leaves patients with the characteristic Heberden's and Bourchard's nodes, but with relatively little pain or disability unless a large joint becomes affected with OA.

GONOCOCCAL ARTHRITIS

DEFINITION

- Gonococcal arthritis is a syndrome of polyarthritis, tenosynovitis, and dermatitis caused by the Gram-negative diplococcus Neisseria gonorrhoeae.

Main clinical features
- The clinical spectrum of gonococcal arthritis ranges from an early bacteremic form to a resultant more-traditional septic arthritis (Fig. 23.22).
- The bacteremic stage is characterized by fever, migratory or additive polyarthritis, painful tenosynovitis, and dermatitis.
- Tenosynovitis is most common over the dorsum of the hand (Fig. 23.23), wrist, knee, or ankle.
- Skin lesions appear on the extremities or trunk and consist of tiny papules, pustules, or vesicles with an erythematous base (Fig. 23.24).

- Approximately two thirds of patients develop a septic arthritis that typically involves the knee, ankle, elbow, or wrist.

Diagnosis
- Gram stain of the synovial fluid or other mucosal surfaces (endocervix, urethra, rectum, or pharynx) reveals Gram-negative diplococci (Fig. 23.25).
- The organism is fragile and difficult to culture.
- Cultures are plated at the bedside on special media (Thayer–Martin).
- Approximately 50% of patients have positive blood and synovial fluid cultures, and 80% a positive culture.

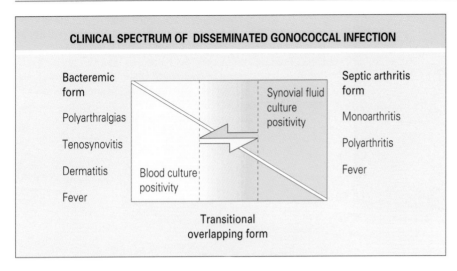

CLINICAL SPECTRUM OF DISSEMINATED GONOCOCCAL INFECTION

Bacteremic form

Polyarthralgias

Tenosynovitis

Dermatitis

Fever

Blood culture positivity

Synovial fluid culture positivity

Septic arthritis form

Monoarthritis

Polyarthritis

Fever

Transitional overlapping form

Fig. 23.22 Clinical spectrum of disseminated gonococcal infection.

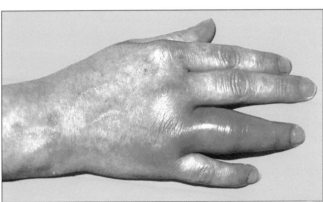

Fig. 23.23 Gonococcal arthritis. Dactylitis of the ring finger caused by tenosynovitis in a 24-year-old woman. (Courtesy of Dr S E Thompson.)

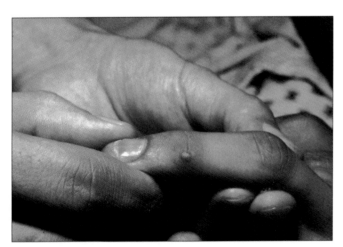

Fig. 23.24 Disseminated gonoccal infection skin lesion. Hemorrhagic vesicle over a distal interphalangeal joint. (Courtesy of Dr Peter Schlessinger.)

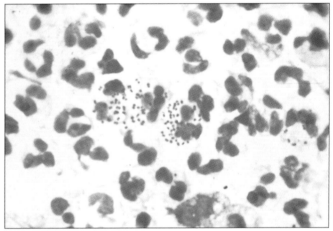

Fig. 23.25 Neisseria gonorrhoeae. Gram stain of urethral exudate in gonorrhea showing intracellular Gram-negative reniform diplococci. (Courtesy of Dr S E Thompson.)

IN WHAT CIRCUMSTANCES IS GONOCOCCAL ARTHRITIS SUSPECTED?

Gonococcal arthritis is suspected in all sexually active adults who present with fever and poly- or monoarthritis. The differential diagnosis during the bacteremic stage includes viral infections (hepatitis B, parvovirus B19, etc.), rheumatic fever, bacterial endocarditis, reactive arthritis, and Lyme disease. In the septic arthritis stage, gonococcal arthritis must be differentiated from other forms of joint infection.

HOW IS GONOCOCCAL ARTHRITIS MANAGED?

As with other forms of septic arthritis, infected joints are aspirated daily to remove all purulent material – a saline lavage may be helpful. The recommended treatment for gonococcal arthritis is parenteral ceftriaxone (1–2g/day) plus doxy-cycline 100mg twice daily for 7–10 days. If the patient has improved after 2–3 days of parenteral therapy, treatment is completed with oral cefixime 400mg twice daily or ciprofloxacin 500mg twice daily. If the infecting strain is known to be penicillin sensitive, therapy can be changed to intravenous penicillin G (10 million units/day) or amoxicillin (500mg four times a day), either drug being used with probenecid 1g/day. As gonorrheal infections are often associated with other sexually transmitted diseases, patients are also tested for chlamydial infection and syphilis, and treated with tetracycline or doxycycline (7 days) or with either of these regimens plus azithromycin (single 1g oral dose). For pregnant women, erythromycin (500mg four times a day) or amoxicillin (500mg three times a day) for 10 days are used. Repeat testing for syphilis is performed 4–6 weeks later. In addition, the patient's sexual partner(s) for the 30 days prior to symptoms must be examined and treated to prevent reinfection and spread to other partners. Patient education also includes advice to use a condom and a spermicide as the most effective means of spread prevention.

SPINAL DISORDERS

AN INTRODUCTION TO SPINAL DISORDERS

Pain in the spine is a huge problem in Western societies, and one which remains ill-understood by the medical profession. It has reached endemic proportions, with some 70% of us experiencing some significant form of low back or neck problem in our lives.

Risk factors appear to include poor posture, occupational issues such as working positions and work-related injuries, and psychosocial factors, which often complicate chronic low back or neck pain.

The regions of the vertebral column are shown in Figure 1.

The dorsal (thoracic) spine is the least mobile and the most rigid section, and as a result mechanical pain in this segment is relatively uncommon; it is, however, the segment most prone to compression fractures in osteoporosis in older people.

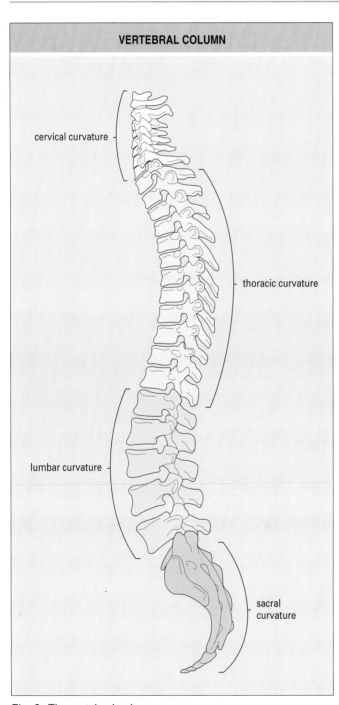

VERTEBRAL COLUMN

cervical curvature

thoracic curvature

lumbar curvature

sacral curvature

Fig. 1 The vertebral column.

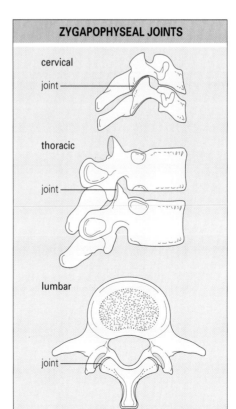

ZYGAPOPHYSEAL JOINTS

cervical

joint

thoracic

joint

lumbar

joint

Fig. 2 The zygapophyseal joints. Regional differences in joint orientation are evident.

The more mobile cervical and lumbar regions are the most vulnerable to mechanical lesions, particularly at the points of greatest mobility and stress, which are in the lower cervical region (C5-7) and the low lumbar region (L3-5).

By far, most neck and low back pain is mechanical in type (related to movement and activities and relieved by rest) and the exact anatomic or pathologic cause is impossible to define in almost all cases. Trauma and occupational factors frequently contribute. Investigations are rarely helpful and radiographs in particular are overused in primary care.

Joint disease can affect either the synovial zygapophyseal joints (Fig. 2) or the intervertebral discs (Fig. 3). The apophyseal joints are most vulnerable in the neck, and the discs in the low lumbar spine, but disc herniation via rupture of the anulus fibrosus and extrusion of the nucleus pulposus can occur at either level. Because of the proximity of the discs to the spinal cord and nerve roots (Figs 4 & 5), compression of roots or the cord can follow. Root lesions are commoner than cord lesions, and symptoms and signs then accord to dermatomes (Fig. 6).

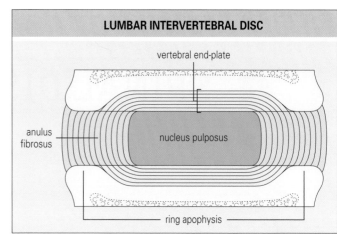

Fig. 3 The lumbar intervertebral disc: schematic sagittal section.

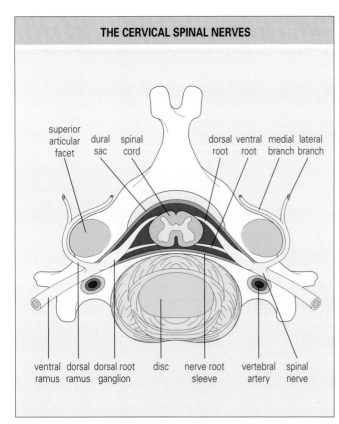

Fig. 4 Schematic transverse section showing the cervical spinal nerves with their ventral and dorsal roots and rami. It is apparent that they are vulnerable to any posterior bulging or protrusion of the intervertebral disc and to pressure from bony overgrowth.

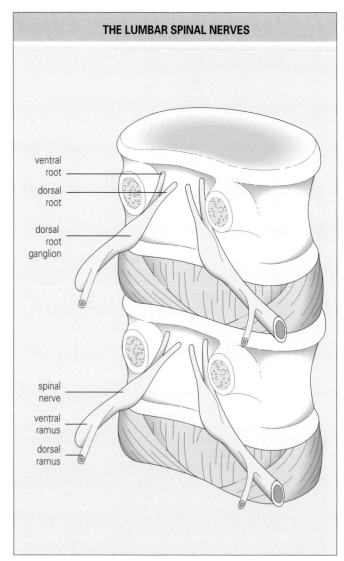

Fig. 5 The lumbar spinal nerves. The spinal nerve is formed by the junction of the dorsal and ventral roots immediately below the pedicle. The spinal nerve and roots lie behind the lower part of the vertebral body, not behind the disc.

Occasional cases are due to other causes, which can include inflammatory joint diseases (spondylitis), osteoarthritis (spondylosis), infections, tumors and rare disorders.

Psychosocial factors often complicate chronic spinal disorders and may lead to exaggeration, but malingering or pure psychogenic pain is rare.

This has led us to adopt, for this book, the pragmatic classification of low back pain and neck pain into the following five main categories:

1. **Mechanical/nonspecific** – pain related to activity and movement, of no diagnosable cause.
2. **Inflammatory** – pain with morning stiffness, due to inflammatory joint disease.
3. **Neurogenic** – pain associated with pressure on nerve roots or the spinal cord.
4. **Systemic/sinister** – pain caused by a serious condition such as infection or tumor.
5. **Psychogenic**.

Management needs to be conservative in most cases, with an emphasis on self-help and empowerment through facilitation of an understanding of the mechanical and other factors that are contributing to the problem.

The algorithm that follows stresses the need to differentiate inflammatory and systemic disorders from other forms of back pain.

Fig. 6 The dermatomes.

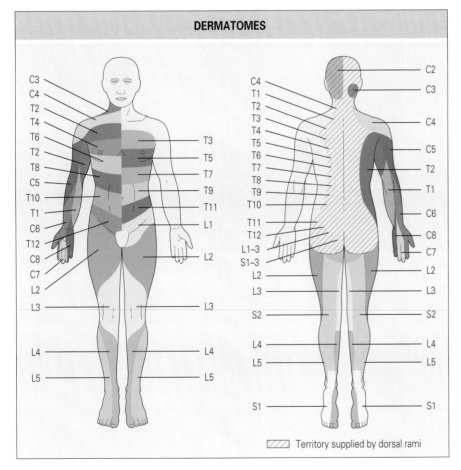

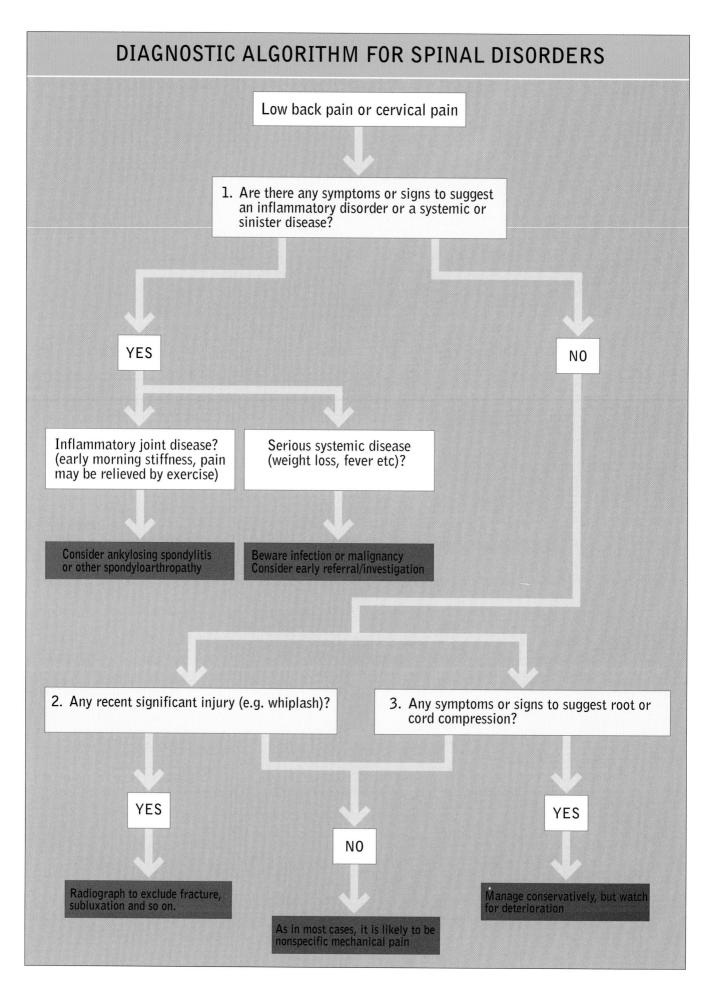

DIAGNOSTIC ALGORITHM FOR SPINAL DISORDERS

Low back pain or cervical pain

1. Are there any symptoms or signs to suggest an inflammatory disorder or a systemic or sinister disease?

YES

NO

Inflammatory joint disease? (early morning stiffness, pain may be relieved by exercise)

Serious systemic disease (weight loss, fever etc)?

Consider ankylosing spondylitis or other spondyloarthropathy

Beware infection or malignancy Consider early referral/investigation

2. Any recent significant injury (e.g. whiplash)?

3. Any symptoms or signs to suggest root or cord compression?

YES

NO

YES

Radiograph to exclude fracture, subluxation and so on.

As in most cases, it is likely to be nonspecific mechanical pain

Manage conservatively, but watch for deterioration

SPINAL DISORDERS

24

LOW BACK PAIN

Low back pain is a ubiquitous health problem and the second most frequent cause of illness to humankind after the common cold. In the USA it is said to be responsible for 2.8% of all physician office visits, and it is one of the most common causes of pain and impairment in adults.

Low back pain often presents as an acute episode, and is most common in the age range 30–50 years. The natural history of such attacks concludes with resolution – some 90% of cases resolve after 8 weeks, irrespective of any interventions. However, a small percentage of people have repeated acute attacks, or develop chronic low back pain, and it is this minority who account for the huge economic burden in terms of work loss and medical resource usage.

The vast majority of patients have mechanical low back pain, and do not require any investigations or specific treatment. The responsibilities of the primary care physician are to identify the minority with other, more serious or potentially treatable causes, and to protect the majority from undergoing unnecessary and potentially harmful investigations and treatment.

COMMON CAUSES OF LOW BACK PAIN

The pragmatic approach outlined below categorizes five main patterns of low back pain, which can be differentiated from the history.

MECHANICAL LOW BACK PAIN
Mechanical low back pain is characterized by pain related to movement and relieved by rest (although prolonged sitting or standing also brings on the pain). The onset is often associated with a specific physical task or minor injury. The pain is usually maximal in the low back area, but may radiate to the leg, as far as the knee. Muscle and ligament strains and spondylosis are probably the main causes.

NEUROGENIC PAIN
Neurogenic pain is characterized by lancing, shooting, or burning pain that radiates to the leg in the distribution of the affected nerve roots (Fig. 24.1). Muscle spasms and paresthesia may be associated. Intervertebral disc herniation is the most common cause, but neurogenic pain can also result from spinal stenosis, fractures, infections, or neoplasms.

INFLAMMATORY LOW BACK PAIN
Inflammatory low back pain features early morning stiffness and pain that is relieved by exercise. The most common cause is ankylosing spondylitis (see Chapter 26).

SYSTEMIC/SINISTER CAUSES OF BACK PAIN
Back pain may result from infections of the bones or disc spaces, primary or secondary tumors, or (rarely) be caused by other sinister conditions such as an expanding abdominal aneurysm. If one of these sinister disorders is the cause, the onset is likely to be insidious, and the pain may be accompanied by systemic

KEY POINTS

- Low back pain is one of humankind's commonest health problems.
- Back pain can be differentiated into five patterns on the basis of the history: mechanical, neurogenic, inflammatory, sinister and exaggerated types; the commonest forms are acute mechanical low back pain, sciatica and chronic low back pain.
- Investigations are rarely necessary and no tests should be done routinely.
- Most acute attacks resolve spontaneously.
- Prolonged rest should be avoided, and patients with back pain should be encouraged to return to normal activities as soon as possible.

PRAGMATIC, HISTORY-BASED CATEGORIZATION OF LOW BACK PAIN

- Mechanical (over 90%) – e.g. muscle or ligamentous strain
- Neurogenic (about 5%) – e.g. intervertebral disc herniation
- Inflammatory (about 1%) – e.g. ankylosing spondylitis
- Systemic/sinister causes (about 1%) – e.g. spinal metastasis
- Psychogenic (rare)

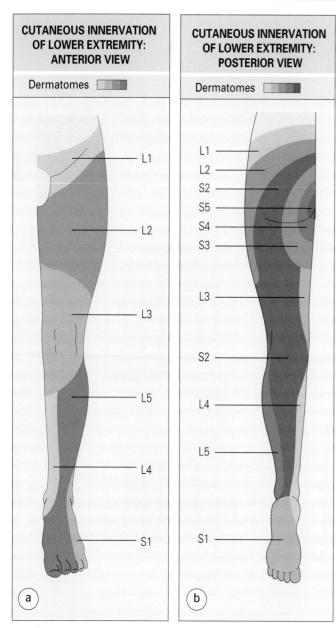

| CUTANEOUS INNERVATION OF LOWER EXTREMITY: ANTERIOR VIEW | CUTANEOUS INNERVATION OF LOWER EXTREMITY: POSTERIOR VIEW |

Dermatomes

Dermatomes

a

b

Fig. 24.1 Cutaneous dermatomes of the lower extremity. (a) Anterior and (b) posterior, both showing the areas that are affected by paresthesia or sensory loss if pressure is applied to specific nerve roots (L4, L5, and S1 are most frequently affected).

features of ill-health such as fever or weight loss. First onset of severe back pain before 30 or over 50 years of age should also raise suspicion, as should severe, local bony tenderness, or pain that is not relieved by resting supine.

EXAGGERATED AND PSYCHOGENIC BACK PAIN

Back pain occurs at some stage of the life of most people. The severity is often exaggerated by the patient, either consciously or unconsciously – for example, to avoid work for a few days. The pain may be made worse by psychosocial factors such as depression, and psychologic problems may present with back pain. True psychogenic back pain is rare. Exaggerated or psychogenic pain is characterized by symptoms that are disproportionate to the apparent impairment and disability, and by a variety of spurious physical signs such as tenderness to superficial touch or pain in the back to pressure on the top of the head. The history and examination findings may contain inconsistencies and distraction may change them. Obvious features of depression or some form of major psychosocial problem may be apparent.

THE HISTORY

Clearly, the first step in resolving the nature of back pain is a careful history, which helps place the type of pain within the suggested categories outlined above. In addition, a careful inquiry is made of any antecedent injury, as well as of postural or occupational factors that might be of relevance to the back pain. The history also needs to include some questions on psychosocial status, as well as the impact of the pain on the patient's activities. The patient's use (or abuse) of drugs and over-the-counter medications should also be ascertained.

The primary care physician needs to be mindful of the 'red flags' that might suggest a serious problem (Fig. 24.2).

EXAMINATION

- *Look.* The back should be inspected with the patient standing, undressed, and facing away from the physician. Note any asymmetry or deformities of the spine (Fig. 24.3), and look for asymmetric iliac spines or skin folds, and for any evidence of muscle spasm to one side of the spine.
- *Feel.* The spine can be palpated with the patient bending over a table, supported by their arms on the table. Feel for any localized tenderness, for muscle spasm in the long extensors of the spine, and for any palpable 'step' in the vertebrae, which suggest a spondylolisthesis (an abnormal step between two vertebrae, see Fig. 24.8).
- *Move.* Examine for spinal movements, as shown in Figure 24.4.

'RED FLAGS' FOR BACK PAIN	
History	**Possible diagnosis**
Pain and stiffness, worst in the morning and relieved by exercise	Ankylosing spondylitis
Pain made worse by walking and by hyperextension of the spine	Spinal stenosis
Acute severe pain for no reason	Abdominal aneurysm Compression fracture Disc herniation
Pain that radiates below the knee, made worse by coughing or sneezing, and described as shooting or burning	Nerve root compression
Radiation of pain into both legs	Central disc herniation Tumor
First episode of severe pain below 30 or above 50 years of age	Infection Tumor Metabolic disease
Fever, weight loss, or other systemic features	Infection Tumor
Bowel or bladder problems	Spinal stenosis Cauda equina syndrome Tumor
Recent severe trauma	Fracture Spondylolisthesis
Prolonged corticosteroid usage	Compression fracture
Drug abuse	Infection
Pain not relieved by lying with legs flexed or persistent pain for >2 months	Infection Tumor

Fig. 24.2 'Red flags' for back pain. Shown are features of the history that should alert the physician to a serious cause.

SPINAL DEFORMITIES

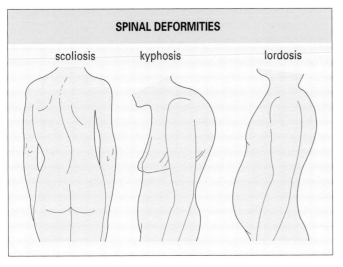

scoliosis   kyphosis   lordosis

Fig. 24.3 Spinal deformities. These are best observed from behind and from the side, with the patient in the erect posture.

- *Neurologic.* Any suspicion of neurogenic pain, requires a neurologic examination, to seek a positive sciatic or femoral stretch test (Fig. 24.5), numbness in the affected dermatomes (see Fig. 24.1), abnormal reflexes, or muscle weakness (Fig. 24.6).
- The abdomen should also be examined for evidence of conditions such as aortic aneurysm or kidney infections which can present with back pain.

INVESTIGATIONS

BACK PAIN SHOULD NOT NORMALLY BE INVESTIGATED.

- *Radiographs* are not only of no use in common mechanical low back pain, they can be positively misleading through the reporting of irrelevant findings such as osteophytes or reduced vertebral density. No association has been found between the presence of radiographic features of disc disease or spinal osteoarthritis ('spondylitis') and pain. Radiographs provide no help in the diagnosis of herniated discs. The only need for radiographs in low back pain is to diagnose compression fractures, spondylolisthesis, Paget's disease and some tumors, as well as to detect established sacroiliitis in ankylosing spondylitis and associated disorders (Chapter 26) (Fig. 24.7). Disc herniation and uncommon conditions such as spinal stenosis and cauda equina compression can only be visualized by more advanced imaging modalities such as computed tomography or magnetic resonance imaging, and these should only be undertaken if a surgical option is being considered in a secondary care setting.
- *Blood tests* should only be considered if a systemic or sinister cause of back pain is suspected, in which case the erythrocyte sedimentation rate (ESR) may be elevated. Blood tests have no place in the majority of cases, and tests for calcium or other metabolic investigations are of no value, although acid phosphatase levels may be helpful in diffuse prostatic cancer with spinal metastases. Consideration may need to be given to a urine examination, particularly in young women.

EXAMINATION OF THE SPINE

Lumbar spine

Lumbar flexion

normal   abnormal

Maneuver	For ankylosing spondylitis, also include overall spinal movement (C7 to line between dimples of venus), Schober index, and finger–floor distance
Assessment	Note the distance between the fingertips and the floor
Normal angle	–
Active/passive	Active

The patient stands in the erect posture, with his/her back to the examiner. The patient is asked to bend forward as if trying to touch his/her toes. Note is made of the range of movement, the presence of spasm of the erector spinae muscles, pain on movement, deviation to one or other side (sciatic scoliosis) or the induction of sciatica (indicating nerve root compression). The last two conditions listed are found in herniated intervertebral disc.

Hypermobility

Maneuver	Try to place hands flat on floor while knees are extended
Assessment	Adds 1 to Beighton score if hands are placed flat on floor
Normal angle	–
Active/passive	–

The patient stands in the erect posture, with their back to the examiner. The patient is then asked to bend forward and try to place his/her hands flat on the floor without bending his/her knees. If successful, the patient is deemed to have a hypermobile spine.

Right/left lateral flexion

Maneuver	Bend to sides
Assessment	Estimate angle
Normal angle	30° to right – 30° to left
Active/passive	Active

The patient stands in the erect posture with his/her back to the examiner. The patient is asked to bend to the right, then to the left, as if trying to edge his/her fingers as far as the knee. Note is made of the range of movement. Reduction of lateral flexion is typically seen in ankylosing spondylitis, while in disc prolapse lateral flexion is characteristically relatively well preserved.

Lumbar extension

Maneuver	Bend backward
Assessment	Estimate angle
Normal angle	30°
Active/passive	Active

The patient stands in the erect posture, with his/her back to the examiner. The patient is then asked to bend backward, trying to arch his/her back as much as possible. Note is made of restricted range. Pain on extension is encountered in facet joint syndrome but may also be seen in herniated intervertebral disc.

The spinal examination is completed by careful palpation of each individual spinous process in order to detect tenderness, thereby indicating the site of a lesion (but not, of course, its nature). This may be most effectively achieved with the patient in a prone position. A similar process is adopted for the facet joints (in facet joint syndrome) by palpating 3cm from the midline on both sides at each vertebral level.

The lumbar spine houses the lumbar spinal nerve roots and the cauda equina. These nerve roots and their sheaths are thus liable to come under tension or be affected by compression, affecting adjacent spinal structures. The examination of the lumbar spine is completed by a complete neurologic examination of the lower limbs and the performance of tests to detect the presence of tension affecting the nerve roots in either the femoral or sciatic nerves.

Fig. 24.4 Examination of the spine.

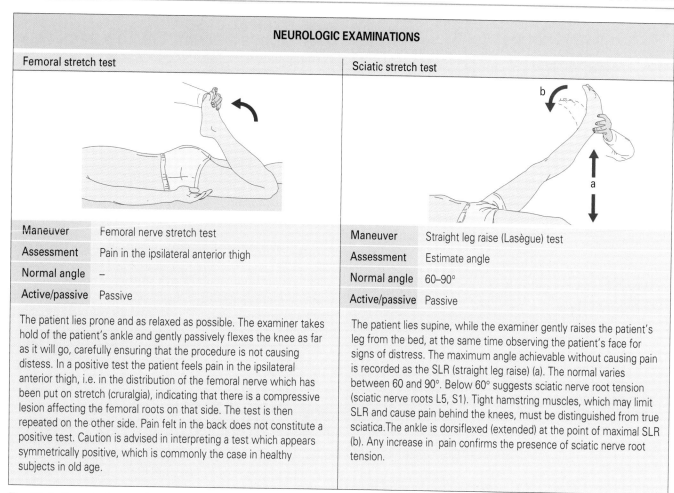

NEUROLOGIC EXAMINATIONS

Femoral stretch test

Maneuver	Femoral nerve stretch test
Assessment	Pain in the ipsilateral anterior thigh
Normal angle	–
Active/passive	Passive

The patient lies prone and as relaxed as possible. The examiner takes hold of the patient's ankle and gently passively flexes the knee as far as it will go, carefully ensuring that the procedure is not causing distress. In a positive test the patient feels pain in the ipsilateral anterior thigh, i.e. in the distribution of the femoral nerve which has been put on stretch (cruralgia), indicating that there is a compressive lesion affecting the femoral roots on that side. The test is then repeated on the other side. Pain felt in the back does not constitute a positive test. Caution is advised in interpreting a test which appears symmetrically positive, which is commonly the case in healthy subjects in old age.

Sciatic stretch test

Maneuver	Straight leg raise (Lasègue) test
Assessment	Estimate angle
Normal angle	60–90°
Active/passive	Passive

The patient lies supine, while the examiner gently raises the patient's leg from the bed, at the same time observing the patient's face for signs of distress. The maximum angle achievable without causing pain is recorded as the SLR (straight leg raise) (a). The normal varies between 60 and 90°. Below 60° suggests sciatic nerve root tension (sciatic nerve roots L5, S1). Tight hamstring muscles, which may limit SLR and cause pain behind the knees, must be distinguished from true sciatica. The ankle is dorsiflexed (extended) at the point of maximal SLR (b). Any increase in pain confirms the presence of sciatic nerve root tension.

Fig. 24.5 Neurologic examinations.

MOTOR INNERVATION OF LOWER EXTREMITIES

Region	Backward	Forward
Hip	L4, 5 extension	Flexion L2, 3
Knee	L5, S1 flexion	Extension L3, 4
Ankle	S1, 2 plantar flexion	Inversion L4 Dorsiflexion L4, 5 Eversion L5, S1

Fig. 24.6 Motor innervation of the lower extremities.

RADIOGRAPHS IN LOW BACK PAIN

Radiographs should ONLY be considered in one of the following circumstances:

Older age (onset of severe pain in people >50 years of age

Recent significant trauma

History of prolonged corticosteroid usage

Known cancer

Fevers or weight loss

Pain on lying flat with knees flexed

Drug abuse

Fig. 24.7 Indications for radiographs in low back pain.

SPINAL DISORDERS

FEATURES OF ACUTE MECHANICAL LOW BACK PAIN

- Sudden onset in association with some physical activity.
- Pain made worse by back movement and certain positions.
- Examination often reveals muscle spasm and localized tenderness may occur.
- Flexion and/or extension of the back exacerbates the pain.
- A heterogeneous condition of many causes (most cases probably result from minor tears of muscles or ligaments) – a precise anatomic cause can hardly ever be ascertained.
- Investigations are contraindicated.
- Prolonged bed rest is contraindicated.
- Should be managed with reassurance, analgesics, early mobilization, and a quick return to normal activities.
- Over 50% of cases resolve within 2 weeks, and 90% within 8 weeks. Persistence beyond 6–8 weeks should raise suspicion.
- Recurrences can occur, and all patients should be instructed on back care after resolution of an attack (see self-help for low back pain).

FEATURES OF SCIATICA

- Acute shooting pain with or without paresthesia, which affects a dermatome, usually L5 or S1, sometimes L4.
- Caused by protrusion of the nucleus pulposus of the intervertebral disc, which results in pressure on a nerve root.
- Often preceded by some episode or a period of low back pain (sometimes a clear mechanical event has ruptured the annulus fibrosus of the disc, which allows herniation of the nucleus).
- Usually accompanied by muscle spasm, a scoliosis may be present, and the sciatic stretch test is usually positive.
- Investigations and any specific interventions are contraindicated unless progressive deterioration occurs or neurologic signs of motor involvement (weakness or loss of reflexes) develop, in which case patients should be referred for consideration of surgery.
- Most cases can be managed with a short period of rest (often most comfortable with the spine flexed and/or the knees bent up) with analgesics and muscle relaxants, followed by early mobilization and a quick return to normal activities.

 TYPICAL CASE: ACUTE MECHANICAL LOW BACK PAIN

Brian is a 38-year-old bank clerk who has always been fit, active, and healthy. He has just moved house, and was lifting a heavy box of books on the weekend when he felt his back 'go', and was struck by acute low back pain that made it difficult for him to move. The pain radiates into one buttock, but no further, and is not exacerbated by coughing or sneezing. On examination you find obvious muscle spasm, and a marked reduction in flexion and extension, which clearly causes pain.

You reassure Brian and his wife Laura that nothing terrible has happened and that it is likely his pain will resolve within 2 weeks, and you tell them that prolonged bed rest is bad. You suggest regular acetaminophen (paracetamol) and early mobilization, and counsel Brian to go to work on Monday, even if his back still hurts. You provide Brian with a Self-Help Leaflet about back care (see page 344) for use after the attack subsides.

The pain resolves fairly quickly, and Brian is quite well 2 weeks later.

 TYPICAL CASE: SCIATICA

Bill is a 37-year-old car mechanic, with a history of several previous episodes of mild, resolving, mechanical low back pain. A week ago he again experienced the onset of low back pain when he was bending over a car engine to clean the carburetor. He assumed it would resolve as before. However, 2 days later he noticed the gradual onset of pains shooting down to his right foot when he moved about or coughed, which has worsened over the past few days. He is now experiencing severe back pain and lancing, shooting pains that radiate down the outside of his calf into the foot, made worse by various movements as well as by coughing or sneezing. He has noticed some tingling on the side of his right foot. Bill is worried about himself, for the first time in his life. The neighbors tell him that he has a 'slipped disc', which should be 'put back' or operated on.

On examination you find marked muscle spasm of the back, a mild scoliosis, and a positive sciatic stretch test are found, but no abnormal neurologic signs.

You reassure Bill and explain that discs do not slip in and out, and tell him that the jelly that is pressing on his nerve will slowly be absorbed by the body. You advise 3 days of bed rest, with a pillow under the knees to relieve pressure on the sciatic nerve, and with analgesics and muscle relaxants. After that some improvement occurs and you encourage Bill to start moving about and go back to work the next week. He does this, and things gradually improve. After 6 weeks Bill is back to normal.

3 TYPICAL CASE: CHRONIC LOW BACK PAIN

Sherri is 48-year-old housewife who experienced several episodes of back pain when in her 30s. She had another of her attacks about a year ago, shortly after Fred, her husband, had an affair with his secretary, Sarah. This time the pain did not go away, and she has had worsening trouble with her back over the past 9 months. She describes severe low back pain, which radiates into both buttocks, is made worse by any movement, and is present most of the time. She says that it keeps her awake, and stops her having any sort of social life. She tells you that she has tried all sorts of treatments, but nothing helps. She appears mildly depressed.

On examination you find a thin, miserable woman, who complains of tenderness on palpation of several areas around the spine. She is reluctant to move the back much, and walks carefully. There are no other specific findings.

You prescribe antidepressants, and encourage Sherri to pick up her life again, but to no avail. Secretly she blames Sarah, who is now living with her husband.

SOME OTHER TYPES/CAUSES OF LOW BACK PAIN

SPONDYLOSIS AND SPONDYLOLISTHESIS

A defect in the pars interarticularis can lead to the slip of one vertebra onto another (Fig. 24.8). It is often developmental, but may follow trauma. Patients who are symptomatic may complain of pain in the back that is made worse by extension. The defect may be palpable. Flexion exercises and reassurance, with or without a back support, are all that is usually required.

LEG LENGTH INEQUALITIES

Inequalities of leg length are a common cause of mechanical low back pain, and may respond well to a heel raise to correct the inequality.

COMPRESSION FRACTURES

Compression fractures are a common cause of acute pain in people with osteoporosis, including older women and those on corticosteroid therapy. The pain is often localized, and local bony tenderness may be present. Radiographs show the osteoporosis and compression fracture (Fig. 24.9; see also Chapter 34).

FEATURES OF CHRONIC LOW BACK PAIN

- Defined as low back pain of >6 months' duration.
- Characterized by descriptions of severe low back pain, which may radiate into the buttocks, and usually has a marked affect on lifestyle.
- Often preceded by attacks of self-limiting back pain.
- Often associated with mild depression and/or psychosocial problems.
- May be associated with occupational factors of etiological significance.
- Often unresponsive to any therapy, although treatment of associated depression may help, and pain clinics or back schools can successfully improve outcomes.
- Investigations are usually unhelpful, although a high level of suspicion of a serious disorder is required to find the occasional case of a sinister nature.

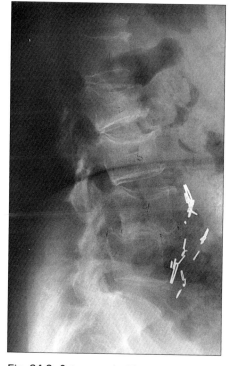

Fig. 24.9 Osteoporosis. Plain radiograph, lateral view, that demonstrates diffuse osteopenia and multiple compression fractures.

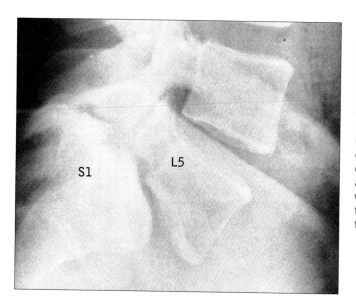

S1   L5

Fig. 24.8 A developmental spondylolisthesis at the L5–S1 level. Note the forward displacement of L5 on S1, caused by a developmental defect in the pars articularis, which controls the stability of the segment.

SPINAL INFECTIONS

Various uncommon forms of infection can affect the spine, including staphylococcal infections of the disc space, and tuberculosis. Presentations vary, but any fevers or weight loss should raise suspicion. Radiographs help in late stages only (Fig. 24.9), and referral for further investigation and treatment is necessary if there is a reasonable index of suspicion or in high-risk cases (such as intravenous drug abusers). Blood abnormalities such as raised ESR are likely to be present.

SPINAL TUMORS

The vertebrae can be affected by metastases (breast, prostate, and others), primary bone tumors (especially multiple myeloma), and by a variety of benign or malignant bone or spinal cord tumors. Presentations vary, but typically the insidious onset of back pain becomes severe and unremitting, and unresponsive to supine rest. Severe local tenderness is often present, and the ESR is generally raised.

WORK-RELATED LOW BACK PAIN

Work injuries that lead to low back pain are a common complaint. Although back pain is clearly related to some occupations that involve a lot of lifting, in many cases litigation is a major factor, and symptoms may not resolve until legal proceedings have been completed.

 MANAGEMENT

In the majority of cases no precise anatomic or pathologic cause for either acute or chronic mechanical low back pain can be found, and so the objective of therapy is simply to relieve symptoms quickly and efficiently with minimal risk of treatment toxicity.

Guidelines for the treatment of low back pain include bedrest, pain relief, spinal manipulation, and exercises.

PATIENT EDUCATION AND SELF-HELP

The importance of patient education and self-help cannot be overemphasized in the management of low back pain, and some evidence indicates that the doctor–patient relationship is of the greatest importance to outcome. Simple explanations of what is likely to be occurring may be facilitated by a back model. Reassurance and a positive attitude to outcome are important. All patients should be given instruction about back care and self-help (see Self-Help Leaflet, page 344).

PHYSICAL THERAPY

Patients with acute episodes of back pain tend to rest, but it is clear that bed rest for more than 2–3 days is harmful. Early ambulation is recommended in all cases other than those that involve a serious systemic disorder, such as infection or tumor. Local heat (or occasionally cold) packs may help to ease pain. Physical therapy can help some patients with acute or chronic mechanical low back pain, and physical therapists can play an important role in teaching patients about back care and in facilitating education, empowerment, and self-help. Manipulations can be of value in the early stages of acute episodes of low back pain, provided there is no neurologic involvement (Fig. 24.10).

GENERAL MANAGEMENT/DRUG THERAPY

The general approach to back pain should be an expectant one, beginning with general reassurance and advice about rest and activities. This may need to be combined with the use of simple non-narcotic analgesics such as acetaminophen in a dose of around 500–650mg every 4–6 hours. Nonsteroidal anti-inflammatory drugs can also assist pain relief and may be preferred for some patients, for example for those who have already tried acetominophen and failed to obtain relief, provided that they have no contraindications to NSAID use, such as peptic ulceration. In those patients in whom pain does not quickly subside other measures might be considered, including spinal manipulation and other pain-relieving drugs. The place of muscle relaxants is unclear, but they may be of value in some people, particularly those in whom there is clinical evidence of a lot of muscle spasm around the spine. Diazepam is ineffective and most benzodiazepines are contraindicated. In those with more chronic pain other pharmaceutical measures, such as low dose amitryptilline, might be considered, although this can result in drowsiness and an increased risk of falls particularly in the elderly.

Other measures, including investigations or referral, should be reserved for those in whom these simple measures have failed, and for those in whom there is good grounds for suspicion of a sinister cause, or neurological complications.

NEW ACHPR GUIDELINES ON THE TREATMENT OF LOW BACK PAIN

Bed rest for longer than 4 days is unhelpful and may debilitate the patient.

Encourage patients to ambulate as soon as this can be tolerated.

Pain relief can be achieved most safely with nonprescription analgesics (e.g. acetaminophen) or nonsteroidal anti-inflammatory drugs.

Spinal manipulation can help within the first 4 weeks of acute back pain in the absence of any neurologic component.

Low-stress aerobic exercises can safely be started within 2 weeks of any acute episode.

Patients should be encourage to return to normal work and recreational activities as soon as possible.

Fig 24.10 ACHPR guidelines on the treatment of low back pain.

INJECTION THERAPY

Local injections may be of value in some patients but should only be carried out by specialists. Severe local trigger spots can be treated with a local injection of lidocaine (lignocaine) 1% combined with a depot corticosteroid, and this can block peripheral pain input and result in some lasting benefit.

Epidural injections are sometimes used for nerve root compression, and apophyseal joint injections can be carried out under fluoroscopic control, but both techniques are controversial, with varying reports of effectiveness and side effects in the literature.

SURGERY

Less than 1% of patients with low back pain need surgery. In cases with severe or deteriorating signs and symptoms of nerve compression, surgical decompression may be required. Other operations, such as spinal fusion, have little or no place.

DIET, AND COMPLEMENTARY AND OTHER TECHNIQUES

That the medical profession cannot offer a precise diagnosis of most cases of back pain and that the management of many chronic cases is unsatisfactory have helped the development of a huge alternative therapy market in the back pain area. No useful dietary benefits have been established, other than weight loss in the obese. The most important and popular forms of complementary medicine revolve around physical means of treatment, such as osteopathy and chiropractic. Some evidence suggests that manipulation can help in the early stages of acute attacks, and many people seem to find that manipulation of some sort can cure their attacks of back pain.

Other valuable forms of therapy include transcutaneous electrical nerve stimulation and acupuncture for pain relief; the development of back classes and back schools helps chronic sufferers.

RECOMMENDATIONS FOR REFERRAL

Most people with back pain can and should be treated at home by their primary care physician.

RECOMMENDATIONS FOR REFERRAL IN PATIENTS WITH LOW BACK PAIN

Specialist referral

- Progressive neurological deficits require URGENT referral (any features of cauda equina compression, such as urinary retention, incontinence or saddle anaesthesia are particularly worrying and require very urgent intervention).
- Surgical referrals should also be considered for any person in whom you suspect a sinister cause such as an expanding abdominal aneurysm, infection or tumor, and anyone with acute vertebral collapse.
- Patients who still complain of severe pain after 4–6 weeks of conservative management should also be considered for referral to a rheumatologic or orthopaedic service.

Other services

- Spinal manipulation may be of value in the early period after an acute attack, and physiotherapy to loosen up the spine and improve mobility is of value to many patients who experience difficulty with chronic pain and disability related to back pain.

SPINAL DISORDERS

25

NECK PAIN

Pain in the neck is extremely common. Younger adults may suffer from acute attacks, but the most frequent problem is chronic pain or recurring attacks in older people. The relationship between age and neck pain is very strong (Fig. 25.1).

COMMON CAUSES OF NECK PAIN

Neck pain presents as acute attacks or as a chronic problem (often with superimposed intermittent exacerbations or acute attacks).

Cervical spine pain can be classified in much the same way as low back pain – the majority of cases are mechanical in type, a minority being either neurogenic, inflammatory, sinister, or psychogenic; as in the case of low back pain, the primary care physician's responsibilities include picking out the small minority with a serious cause from the majority with mechanical pain (see Chapter 24). The vast majority of cases are related to trauma or to spondylosis and have the features of mechanical pain – that is, pain related to movement and activities and relieved by rest.

The common causes of neck pain can also be classified in a more etiologic framework (Fig. 25.2).

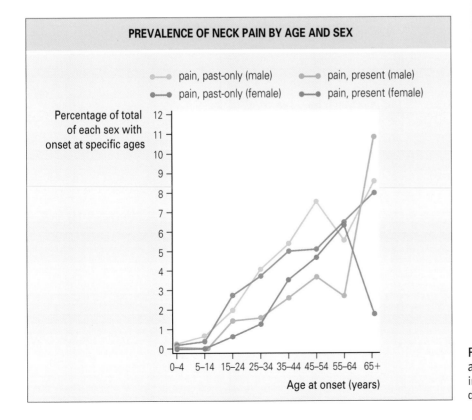

PREVALENCE OF NECK PAIN BY AGE AND SEX

- pain, past-only (male)
- pain, past-only (female)
- pain, present (male)
- pain, present (female)

Percentage of total of each sex with onset at specific ages

Age at onset (years)

KEY POINTS

- Neck pain is extremely common, particularly in older adults.
- Most forms of neck pain are mechanical in nature and related to trauma (including whiplash injury) or age-related changes in the cervical spine. The commonest patterns are acute nonspecific neck pain, chronic mechanical neck pain, cervical root irritation and whiplash injury.
- Investigations are not normally necessary. Plain radiographs can be misleading, but imaging of the cervical spine needs to be considered in the uncommon cases in which neurological signs develop, where trauma is the cause, and where there is good reason to suspect a sinister cause such as infection or tumor.
- Management involves simple ways of relieving symptoms as safely as possible while preserving the best possible range of motion of the neck.

Fig. 25.1 Prevalence of neck pain by age and sex. The prevalence is high and increases with increasing age, but no difference is found between men and women.

CAUSES AND TYPES OF NECK PAIN	
Etiology	Types of disorder that can occur
Trauma-related	Acute attacks in young adults Occupational forms Whiplash injury
Spondylosis	The main pathology associated with chronic or acute or chronic neck pains in older people Can result in root pressure (from osteophytes or disc herniation) and occasionally in cervical myelopathy
Inflammatory joint diseases	Rheumatoid arthritis can cause serious neck problems Ankylosing spondylitis and other spondyloarthropathies frequently affect the neck
Infection	Discs or bones of the neck are occasionally affected by acute or chronic infections such as tuberculosis
Tumor	Metastases from tumors of the lung, thyroid, prostate, breast, or kidney may affect the neck Myeloma can occur Occasional primary spinal tumors
Referred pain	Ischemic heart disease may cause pain in the neck

Fig. 25.2 Causes and types of neck pain.

THE HISTORY

The history helps to determine the type of pain and differentiate the likely cause. Clearly, a history of recent trauma or of any occupational factors that affect pain should be sought. Mechanical pain is characteristically worse on movement and relieved by rest, but it frequently radiates into the shoulder blades or to the top of the arm without any nerve root or spinal cord involvement. True neurologic pain is of a shooting or lancing nature and radiates in a root distribution (Fig. 25.3).

Inflammatory pain is associated with morning stiffness. Serious causes such as infections or tumor often result in pain of relatively insidious onset, which then becomes severe and constant, and is unrelieved by rest. It may be accompanied by obvious signs of systemic disease such as fevers or weight loss.

EXAMINATION

- *Look.* Inspect the whole of the cervical region, which includes the shoulders and the top of the dorsal spine, and note any swellings or deformity and the posture of the patient.
- *Feel.* Patients should be reassured by the doctor as he or she feels the neck. Local tenderness may be present, and severe tenderness localized to a bone may occasionally signify a serious disorder, but little information is gained from palpation.
- *Move.* The range of motion of the neck can be ascertained by the maneuvers shown in Figure 25.4. However, neck movements normally decrease with age. If root involvement occurs, lateral flexion away from the side affected may exacerbate the radiating pain as the affected root is stretched.

Fig. 25.3 Sensory and motor distribution of the cervical roots.

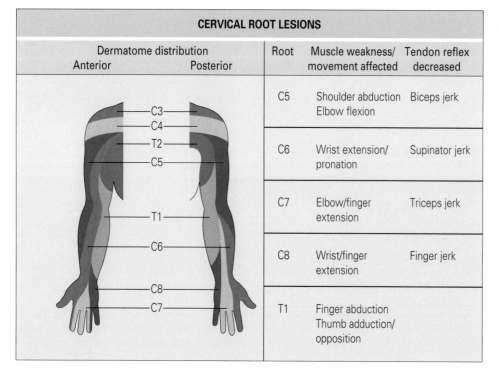

CERVICAL ROOT LESIONS				
Dermatome distribution Anterior	Posterior	Root	Muscle weakness/ movement affected	Tendon reflex decreased
C3 C4 T2 C5 T1 C6 C8 C7		C5	Shoulder abduction Elbow flexion	Biceps jerk
		C6	Wrist extension/ pronation	Supinator jerk
		C7	Elbow/finger extension	Triceps jerk
		C8	Wrist/finger extension	Finger jerk
		T1	Finger abduction Thumb adduction/ opposition	

- *Neurologic*. Any suspicion of a neurologic component requires that the arms be examined to detect any root problems (see Fig. 25.3); in cervical myelopathy the legs may also be affected (see Chapter 27).

EXAMINATION OF THE NECK

Cervical spine

Right rotation		Left rotation		Flexion	
Maneuver	Turn head to right	Maneuver	Turn head to left	Maneuver	Flex neck forward
Assessment	Estimate angle	Assessment	Estimate angle	Assessment	Estimate angle
Normal angle	60–90° diminishing with age	Normal angle	60–90° diminishing with age	Normal angle	60–90° diminishing with age
Active/passive	Active	Active/passive	Active	Active/passive	Active
The patient sits comfortably on the edge of the examining table with the legs hanging free, facing the examiner. The patient is asked to turn his/her head to the right as far as possible. The examiner gently guides the patient's jaw to ensure that the maximum range is achieved, and then estimates the angle.		The patient sits comfortably on the edge of the examining table with the legs hanging free, facing the examiner. The patient is asked to turn his/her head to the left as far as possible. The examiner gently guides the patient's jaw to ensure that maximum range is achieved, and then estimates the angle.		The patient sits comfortably on the edge of the examining table with the legs hanging free, facing the examiner. The patient is asked to bend his/her head forward as far as possible. The examiner gently guides the patient's head to ensure that the maximum range is achieved, and then estimates the angle.	

Extension		Right lateral flexion		Left lateral flexion	
Maneuver	--	Maneuver	Flex neck to right	Maneuver	Flex neck to left
Assessment	Estimate angle	Assessment	Estimate angle	Assessment	Estimate angle
Normal angle	60–90° diminishing with age	Normal angle	30–60° diminishing with age	Normal angle	30–60° diminishing with age
Active/passive	Active	Active/passive	Active	Active/passive	Active
The patient sits comfortably on the edge of the examining table with the legs hanging free, facing the examiner. The patient is asked to look up as far as he/she can. The examiner gently guides the patient's jaw to ensure that the maximum range is achieved, and then estimates the angle.		The patient sits comfortably on the edge of the examining table with the legs hanging free, facing the examiner. The patient is asked to angle his/her head to the right to try to touch his/her ear with his/her shoulder. The examiner gently guides the patient's head to ensure that the maximum range is achieved, and then estimates the angle.		The patient sits comfortably on the edge of the examining table with the legs hanging free, facing the examiner. The patient is asked to angle his/her head to the left to try to touch his/her ear with his/her shoulder. The examiner gently guides the patient's head to ensure that the maximum range is achieved, and then estimates the angle.	

Fig. 25.4 Examination of the neck.

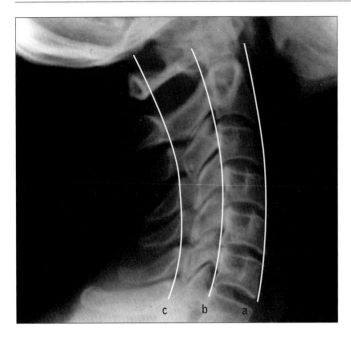

Fig. 25.5 Plain lateral radiograph of a normal cervical spine. Lines joining the anterior part of the vertebral body (a), the posterior aspect of the vertebral body (b), and the anterior border of the laminae (c), should describe a smooth arc.

INVESTIGATIONS

Investigations are not normally necessary, and can be misleading. Routine radiographs of the neck should not be taken for patients with neck pain.

- *Imaging* – The relationship between radiographic evidence of cervical spondylosis and the incidence or severity of neck pain is very poor. In common mechanical neck pain, radiographs have nothing to offer to help either diagnosis or treatment. If a neurologic problem exists, radiographs and other imaging techniques such as magnetic resonance imaging are indicated to resolve the anatomy of the lesion. Radiographs should be taken if a serious disorder is suspected, or if there is a history of significant trauma. The lateral view is the most helpful (Fig. 25.5).
- *Other tests* – Blood tests (particularly the erythrocyte sedimentation rate) may be indicated if a serious disorder, such as tumor or infection, or an inflammatory arthritis is suspected. In secondary care a number of other investigations can be carried out to define the anatomic source of the pain, such as targeted injections of anesthetic to various structures.

FEATURES OF ACUTE ATTACKS OF NONSPECIFIC NECK PAIN

- Common, especially in young adults under some stress.
- Etiology unknown, but often related to minor trauma or to occupational factors.
- Muscle spasm seems to be a major component in most cases.
- Pain is often predominantly on one side of the neck, but may be bilateral, and it often radiates to the top of the shoulder and periscapular region.
- Tender points or trigger spots may be found.
- Associated widespread trigger points may be indicative of fibromyalgia.
- Attacks normally resolve spontaneously within 2 weeks, but may recur.
- Investigations are not indicated, unless recent severe trauma has occurred.
- Treatment involves reassurance, simple analgesics, gentle voluntary mobilization of the neck with the help of local heat, and possibly some stretching of the neck.

1 | TYPICAL CASE: AN ACUTE ATTACK OF NONSPECIFIC NECK PAIN

Sylvia is a 34-year-old secretary who has been under much pressure at work recently. In the past she has noticed occasional discomfort in her neck after a long day at the keyboard. Yesterday, toward the end of the working day, she felt a sudden severe pain on the left side of her neck as she looked up from the keyboard to see who was coming in to see her boss. Her neck became 'stuck' and she went home early from work.

On examination you find a very anxious young woman complaining of severe left-sided neck pain (which radiated to the scapula and top of the shoulder) who is holding her neck rigidly still. Muscle spasm is still obvious around the neck, with some tenderness of the muscles. No neurologic signs are found.

You reassure Sylvia, advise her to gently loosen up the neck with the help of a hot bath or shower and a simple analgesic, and recommend she return to work as soon as possible. When she visits you a week later her neck is causing no problems, but you find that she is under a lot of stress, which you help to offset with counseling.

TYPICAL CASE:
CHRONIC MECHANICAL NECK PAIN

Anne is a 73-year-old woman with a long history of neck problems. She first had an attack of neck pain when she was 64 years old, and since then has suffered numerous acute attacks of severe neck pain, which usually resolve within 1 week. Now she also has an aching neck between attacks and she has noticed that it is very difficult to turn her head round to see oncoming cars when she tries to cross the road. Radiography of her neck was carried out a few years ago, as a result of which she was told that advanced degenerative changes were present.

She comes to see you in the middle of another nasty attack. You find an otherwise fit woman who is obviously in much pain, with some muscle spasm and tenderness of her neck and marked restriction of her neck movements, particularly rotation.

She says that she is very worried about the deteriorating condition of her neck and asks for further radiographs to be taken. You reassure her that nothing terrible will happen, and explain that there is no relationship between radiographic findings and the pain or prognosis of treatment. You provide her with a soft collar to use during acute attacks and a prescription for a nonsteroidal anti-inflammatory drug (NSAID), as she tells you that acetaminophen (paracetamol) does not help her pain. You advise her about the use of heat to relieve pain and muscle spasm, and provide her with a Self-Help Leaflet (see page 345).

FEATURES OF CHRONIC MECHANICAL NECK PAIN

- Very common in older people.
- Thought to be based on cervical spondylosis, but no relationship has been found between radiographic features and pain, prognosis, or treatment responses.
- Usually characterized by acute on chronic pain, with intermittent acute attacks that last a few days on the background of chronic discomfort. The pain often radiates to the scapula region and to the top of the arms.
- Neck movements are markedly reduced in most cases.
- Some tenderness around the neck may be present.
- It can be complicated by cervical root irritation or cervical myelopathy.
- Investigations are not warranted.
- Treatment should be conservative.
- Collars may help in acute attacks.
- Simple analgesics, nonsteroidal anti-inflammatory drugs, and muscle relaxants may help.
- Physical therapy may help.
- The natural history varies, but most cases persist.

3 **TYPICAL CASE:**
CERVICAL ROOT IRRITATION

Helen is a 68-year-old woman with a 5-year history of neck problems that date back to a fall she had when gardening. Ever since then she has had recurrent attacks of self-limiting neck pain, as well as some chronic discomfort and reduced neck movements.

She presents with a 4-day history of a quite different pain – a severe lancing pain that shoots down the outside of her right arm associated with some tingling.

On examination she has a rigid neck with muscle spasm, some reduced sensation in the C5 distribution, and a reduced biceps reflex on the right. Pain in the right arm is exacerbated by lateral neck flexion to the left and by vertical pressure on the head (Spurling's maneuver). You arrange for a lateral radiograph to rule out a subluxation or other serious disorder; it shows simple cervical spondylosis with disk-space narrowing at the C5/6 level, where you suspect root pressure (Fig. 25.6).

You reassure her, provide her with a collar, advise her to use local heat on the neck to relieve pain, and provide her with acetaminophen for pain relief. As she is still in pain a few days later, you refer her for physical therapy, and she receives daily light traction on the neck. The pain slowly subsides.

FEATURES OF CERVICAL ROOT IRRITATION

- A common complication of cervical spondylosis, with pressure that usually occurs on the C5, 6, or 7 nerve roots, either as a result of osteophyte pressure or from a disc herniation.
- Usually presents with sudden onset of typical nerve root pain, which may be followed by the development of sensory and motor complications.
- Root pain is often exacerbated by lateral flexion of the neck to the other side and by Spurling's maneuver (vertical pressure on the head).
- A lateral plain radiograph should be taken to exclude cervical subluxation or a major bony abnormality. No other investigations are indicated.
- Treatment should be conservative with local heat, analgesics, a collar in the acute stage, and consideration of neck traction.
- Most cases settle down within a few weeks with conservative management.
- Referral and surgery are rarely necessary and should only be considered if progressive neurologic signs or severe pain that is unremitting over a period of months occur.

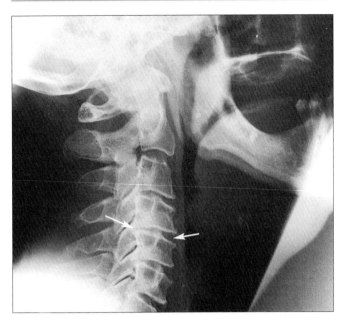

Fig. 25.6 Lateral cervical spine radiograph illustrating features of cervical spondylosis. There is loss of posterior disc height with irregularity of the disc margins at C4–C5 and C5–C6, with some subchondral sclerosis and osteophyte formation anteriorly and posteriorly at these levels.

FEATURES OF WHIPLASH INJURY

- A whiplash injury is a rapid flexion/hyperextension injury of the neck; it usually results from rear-end or side-impact car accidents.
- Typically, these injuries result in the onset of acute neck pain and stiffness within hours.
- Over 50% of cases resolve after a few weeks with the help of the conservative measures recommended for acute attacks of nonspecific neck pain.
- In about 30% of cases pain persists for many months or years.
- Neck pain may be accompanied by other symptoms, including anxiety, sleep loss, dizziness, paresthesia, or root pain.
- Radiographs should always be obtained to rule out subluxation, fractures, or other major injuries.
- In most cases of chronic whiplash the radiographs are normal, and pain may be severe but with no evidence of damage provided by any imaging modality.
- As a result of a whiplash injury a number of lesions can occur that do not show up on images (Fig. 25.7).
- Local injections of anesthetic can help reveal which of these anatomic causes is the problem in a particular patient (most commonly a zygapophyseal joint), but the pain rarely responds permanently to local injection therapy.
- Chronic cases should be fully investigated as a surgically correctable lesion is occasionally found.
- Treatment of chronic whiplash is extremely difficult, but a multidisciplinary approach to pain management should be undertaken.
- Many cases are complicated by litigation issues

4 TYPICAL CASE: WHIPLASH INJURY

Bill is a 53-year-old steel worker. About 3 years ago his car had been struck unexpectedly from behind while stationary at a red light. Over the next hour he became aware of severe neck pain. He was taken to hospital and a number of radiographs of the neck were taken – no abnormality was found. He was given a collar and analgesics, but the pain persisted and proved refractory to physical therapy, NSAIDs, and antidepressants. Repeat radiographs and CT scans show no abnormality. Injection of the zygapophyseal joint at C5/6 with local anesthetic provided temporary relief, which indicated that this was the site of the pain.

His pain is persisting and he is seeking legal compensation from the driver of the car that bumped into him.

OTHER CAUSES OF NECK PAIN

TORTICOLLIS
Torticollis describes an abnormal position of the cervical spine, and may be congenital (and painless) or acquired (and usually painful). Acute torticollis can result from a mechanical disorder or injury, or complicate a sore throat or other inflammatory disorder. Spasmodic torticollis is produced by a sudden contracture of neck muscles, which results in a rotation and tilting of the head – it can occur as a result of a movement disorder, be postencephalitic, or psychogenic.

RHEUMATOID ARTHRITIS
Rheumatoid arthritis can result in destabilization of the neck and subluxation at the atlantoaxial level or in the midcervical spine (Figs 25.8 and 25.9). This can cause devastating neurologic complications, and a high degree of awareness of possible neck problems is required in patients with chronic rheumatoid arthritis who come to surgery or are involved in accidents.

MORE COMMON WHIPLASH INJURY LESIONS AFFECTING THE CERVICAL SPINE

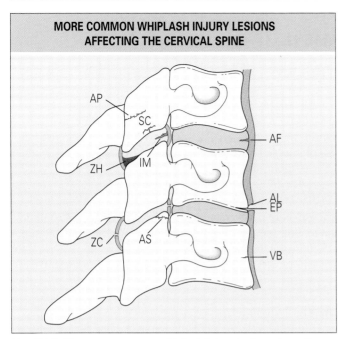

Fig. 25.7 The more common whiplash injury lesions that affect the cervical spine. AP: articular pillar fracture; SC: fracture of the subchondral plate; AF: tear of the annulus fibrosus of the intervertebral disc; ZH: hemarthrosis of the zygapophyseal joint; IM: contusion of the intra-articular meniscus of the zygapophyseal joint; AL: tear of the anterior longitudinal ligament; EP: end-plate avulsion and/or fracture; ZC: rupture of tear of the zygapophyseal joint capsule; AS: fracture involving the articular surface; VB: vertebral body fracture. (Adapted with permission from Spine, State of the Art Reviews, 1993:7.)

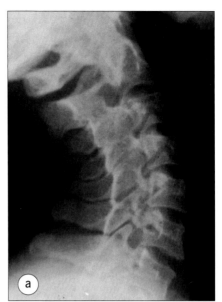

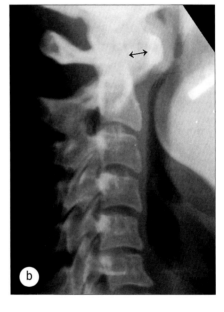

Fig. 25.8 Lateral views of the upper cervical spine in rheumatoid arthritis. (a) A film obtained in neutral position showed no significant abnormality. (b) Another film taken in the flexed position showed increased distance between the atlas and odontoid (arrows). This demonstrates laxity of the transverse ligament.

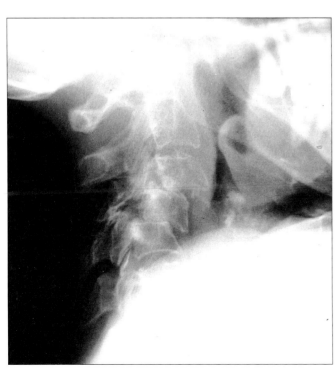

Fig. 25.9 Lateral view of the cervical spine in advanced rheumatoid arthritis. Severe osteoporosis and subaxial subluxations with loss of disc spaces are seen. (Reproduced with permission from Kantor S, Brower AC. In: Rothermich N, Whistler R, eds. Rheumatoid arthritis. Orlando: Grune & Stratton; 1985.)

INDICATIONS FOR REFERRAL

Specialist referral

- Patients with significant weakness in one arm and those with long-standing intractable pain should be considered for referral to a rheumatologic or orthopaedic service.
- Any patient with cord compression, long tract signs or severe root symptoms should be considered for referral for an orthopaedic or neurosurgic opinion.
- Some patients with long-standing or recurrent cervical pain may be considered for referral for a specialist opinion to aid reassurance.

Other services

- Any patient with severe restriction of neck movements might be considered for referral to a physiotherapist for mobilizing exercises, provided that there is no risk of instability of the cervical spine (as in rheumatoid arthritis).
- Traction of the neck can be useful in acute attacks and in those with root irritation, provided there is no risk of instability.

 MANAGEMENT

The management of neck pain aims to relieve symptoms as safely as possible, and to maintain a good range of neck motion. As in the case of low back pain, management of the acute attack is expectant, with simple measures and time alone leading to the resolution of most cases. In people in whom severe pain persists for more than a few weeks, further investigation may be considered (beginning with a lateral plain radiograph of the cervical spine) as well as other interventions and possible referral.

PATIENT EDUCATION AND SELF-HELP

Patient education and self-help is of great importance. Patients need to understand the problem and to look for any postural or occupational factors that might exacerbate the pain. Simple measures such as heat applications can relieve pain and simple exercises can be taught to keep the neck mobile (see Self-Help Leaflet, page 345).

PHYSICAL THERAPY

Physical therapists have a major role to play in patient education and empowerment. Local applications (particularly of heat) may relieve pain, and exercises such as mobilizations may help, although no good evidence for the efficacy of physical therapy is available.

Traction can be helpful for the acute event and for root irritation.

DRUGS

As in low back pain, simple analgesics are recommended, with use of muscle relaxants and NSAIDs considered in acute syndromes and antidepressants in chronic situations. Creams or gels to rub onto the painful neck often aid pain relief.

Injections into local tender spots should not generally be carried out, although in secondary care, injection therapy to specific anatomic sites can be used to help determine the cause of the pain.

COMPLEMENTARY AND OTHER TECHNIQUES

Manipulative treatments from osteopaths and chiropractors are popular, but there is little evidence available on which to base their use or reason to recommend them.

Other approaches to pain relief, such as transcutaneous electrical nerve stimulation and acupuncture, may be of value in some patients with chronic and acute problems.

SURGERY

Surgery is rarely necessary, the main indications being neurologic.

SPINAL DISORDERS

26

ANKYLOSING SPONDYLITIS

Ankylosing spondylitis (AS) is a common disease of young men, with a prevalence of 0.5–1% in Caucasians and a male-to-female ratio of about 5:1. It is the most common inflammatory disorder to present with back pain, and the most common of the group of disorders known as 'seronegative spondyloarthropathies'.

Usually AS presents with back pain and stiffness in young adults; early diagnosis is not easy, but the disease is generally identified within a few years of onset. However, it is heterogeneous in expression and can cause the gradual development of stiffness and deformity of the spine with few symptoms, and cases occasionally present late.

1 TYPICAL CASE: PRESENTATION/ EARLY ANKYLOSING SPONDYLITIS

John is a 27-year-old bank clerk who is keen on sports. He first noticed some discomfort in his spine about 4 years ago, but it came and went without troubling him much, and always eased off with exercise, so it didn't interfere with his jogging or tennis, and he didn't do anything about it.

Recently the pain has become more severe, particularly in his buttocks, and he has noticed that it is worse after periods of inactivity. It has woken him at night on two occasions and he has also noticed stiffness of his spine first thing in the morning. However, the features that made him decide to seek medical help were the spread of buttock pain down the back of his right leg, which made him think a 'slipped disc' might be the problem, and the onset of pains around his chest, which made him very worried about his heart.

On further questioning, you discover that his father has psoriasis and some back problems.

On examination, both you and John are surprised to find that he cannot touch his toes because of spinal stiffness (John feels sure that he could reach them a few years ago); you also find that very deep breathing causes pain, and that he is tender over the sacroiliac joints and the costosternal junctions. A radiograph shows mild but symmetric sacroiliitis (Fig. 26.1), which confirms your clinical diagnosis of AS.

His symptoms respond well to an exercise regime combined with regular nonsteroidal anti-inflammatory drugs (NSAIDs).

KEY POINTS

- A chronic, systemic, inflammatory rheumatic disorder with a predilection for axial skeletal involvement.
- Sacroiliitis is its hallmark.
- Strong genetic predisposition associated with HLA-B27.

Clinical features
- Chronic inflammatory low back pain.
- Characteristic radiographic findings.
- Limitation of spinal mobility.
- Acute anterior uveitis as an extra-articular manifestation.
- Association with psoriasis, chronic inflammatory bowel disease, and reactive arthritis in some patients.
- Good symptomatic response to nonsteroidal anti-inflammatory drugs.

FEATURES OF EARLY ANKYLOSING SPONDYLITIS

- Usually begins insidiously in men in their second decade.
- Chronic low back (buttock) pain and stiffness are the main symptoms.
- Symptoms are made worse by inactivity and relieved by mild exercise.
- Enthesitis around the ankles, feet, pelvis, or chest wall is common.
- Mild constitutional symptoms are common early on.
- Pain may radiate in a 'root' distribution, which mimics disc herniation.
- Loss of mobility of the lumbar spine and tenderness of the sacroiliac joints are common.
- The characteristic radiologic sign is symmetric sacroiliitis, but this only appears after a few years of disease.

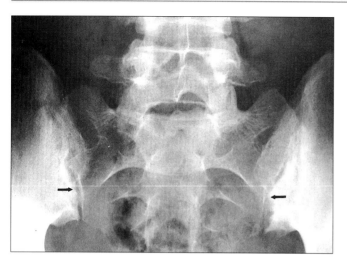

Fig. 26.1 Radiograph of the pelvis showing erosive changes of the sacroiliac joints caused by ankylosing spondylitis. These changes are more apparent on the left side than on the right. The joint areas inferior to the arrows are imaged well by this special Ferguson view (the sacroiliac joints are difficult to image and a number of radiographic positions are used). Reproduced with permission from Brower AC. The radiographic features of psoriatic arthritis. In: Gerber L, Espinoza L, eds. Psoriatic arthritis. Orlando: Grune and Stratton; 1985;125–7.

FEATURES OF ADVANCED ANKYLOSING SPONDYLITIS

- Pain has usually been present, and a history of some extra-articular features is common, in those who develop advanced ankylosing spondylitis, but occasionally the condition presents very late.
- Rigid fixation of the spine and chest wall is caused by ankylosis, with a kyphotic deformity of the spine compensated for by hip flexion and a wide-based gait.
- Lack of movement of the neck can cause great difficulties in everyday tasks such as driving or crossing the road.
- Pulmonary complications can develop as a result of the fixed chest.
- Patients can develop fractures through rigid segments of the spine.
- Neurologic complications can occur from both neck and lumbar spine disease.
- Patients occasionally become so stooped that they cannot see ahead to walk without prismatic glasses.

2 TYPICAL CASE: ADVANCED/LATE ANKYLOSING SPONDYLITIS

Jack is a 53-year-old desk clerk who prides himself on not having taken a day of sick leave from work all his life. He lives a sedentary life and has always had little interest in sports or physical activity. He had noticed that he was stooping forward more in recent years, but it did not trouble him, so he didn't seek help. Over recent months he has noticed increasing shortness of breath on activity, which is the reason for his consulting you.

On examination you notice the typical kyphotic deformity of a man with advanced AS (Fig. 26.2). He has hardly any movement of any part of his spine, and his chest wall is also rigid. Radiographs confirm the diagnosis of advanced AS with ankylosis of the sacroiliac joints and spine (Figs 26.3 and 26.4). The chest radiograph is normal.

You refer him to the physical therapist who is able to help his chest and decrease his dyspnea, but who can do nothing for his spinal movements.

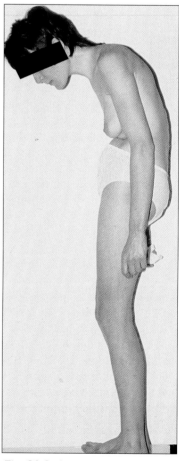

Fig. 26.2 A patient with severe ankylosing spondylitis. Characteristic features of his posture include flattened lumbar lordosis, severe dorsal kyphosis, prominent abdominal folds, and flexed knees.

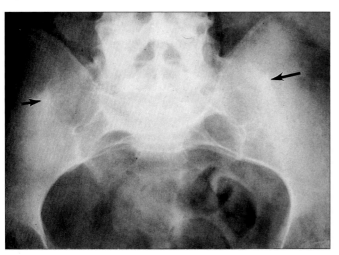

Fig. 26.3 An anteroposterior view of the sacroiliac (SI) joints in long-standing ankylosing spondylitis shows total ankylosis. Ossification of the ligaments that connect the posterosuperior aspect of the SI joints is evident (arrows).

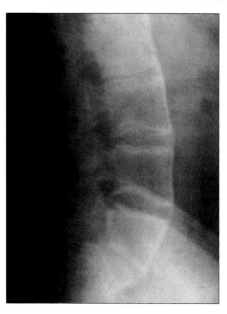

Fig. 26.4 Lateral view of the lumbosacral spine. Shown are syndesmophytes of ankylosing spondylitis, which give a bamboo appearance.

NATURAL HISTORY AND OTHER CLINICAL FEATURES

The natural history of AS is variable, with exacerbations and remissions of symptoms occurring, particularly in early disease. The condition has a tendency to start in the sacroiliac joints and lumbar spine, and subsequently spread up to the thoracic and cervical spine, although it occasionally starts in the neck. Only a minority of patients develop extraspinal involvement, usually in the form of hip disease. Most patients do well, as the condition is relatively mild in the majority, and the activity of the condition tends to subside as the patient grows older.

Extra-articular features, early severe disease, or early and/or severe involvement of the cervical spine or hips are prognostically poor, and suggest that the patient may go on to become disabled by the condition.

The extraskeletal manifestations include:
- Anterior uveitis (iritis) – this occurs at some time in about 25% of AS patients, is usually unilateral, and tends to be recurrent; it presents as a painful red eye (Fig. 26.5).
- Rarely, patients develop aortitis, which can result in aortic insufficiency, conduction abnormalities, or myocardial dysfunction.
- Stiffness of the chest wall reduces inspiration, although most patients can compensate fully with diaphragmatic breathing. In a few, progressive fibrosis of the upper lobes of the lungs develops, which can be complicated by aspergillosis.

Fractures can occur through ankylosed segments of the spine.

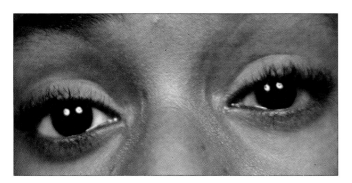

Fig. 26.5 Acute anterior uveitis in a patient with ankylosing spondylitis. The left eye has marked circumcorneal congestion.

211

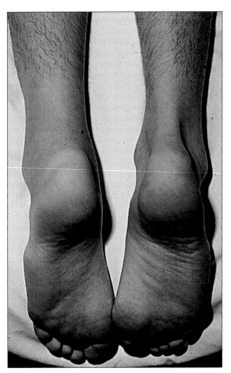

Fig. 26.6 Inflammation of the insertion of the Achilles' tendon into the calcaneum.
This is a common example of an 'enthesopathy' (lesion of a tendon or ligament insertion into bone) seen in patients with ankylosing spondylitis. It may cause visible swelling in association with marked pain, as on the left heel of this patient.

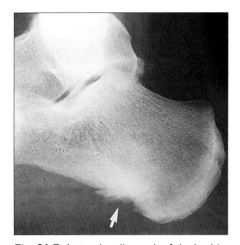

Fig. 26.7 Lateral radiograph of the heel in a patient with ankylosing spondylitis.
Shown is erosion of bone and proliferation of the plantar aponeurosis (arrow).

! POINTS TO LOOK OUT FOR

- *Hip involvement.* It is easy to compensate for stiffness of the lumbar spine so long as the hips are not involved. It is hip disease in general, and flexion deformities in particular, that lead to late kyphotic deformities and disability.
- *Untreated acute iritis.* Iritis should always be treated promptly to avoid eye damage.
- *Severe neck stiffness* – this can result in difficulties with driving or even in crossing the road, as well as a predisposition to fracture dislocation or atlantoaxial subluxation.
- *Gastrointestinal disease.* Some cases are associated with Crohn's disease or ulcerative colitis. Even if this is not the case, low-grade mucosal inflammation may occur in the gut.
- *Insidious development of disabilities.* AS is a disease with a very slow time course that results in gradual loss of spinal movement, and it is difficult to assess the disease activity. Some people adapt to the insidious development of severe disease by allowing themselves to become increasingly and unnecessarily disabled.
- *Women and AS.* Although uncommon, AS is not rare in woman. Since AS tends to evolve more slowly in women than in men, its early diagnosis is particularly difficult.
- *Presentation in children.* The onset of AS in childhood or adolescence can occur, and in these cases peripheral arthropathies and enthesopathies tend to be particularly common and severe (see Section 7).
- *Severe enthesopathies.* Some patients develop severe enthesopathies, particularly around the heels, which can be resistant to therapy and occasionally require local radiotherapy (Fig. 26.6).
- Fractures through ankylosed segments in advanced AS, and the rare complication of fracture dislocation in the cervical spine, leading to quadriplegia or cauda equina syndrome.

INVESTIGATIONS

- *Radiographs* – The main diagnostic investigation is radiography. Views of the sacroiliac joints and lateral views of the thoracolumbar spine are most likely to show changes. In addition to characteristic symmetric sacroiliitis, a number of features in the spine may be found, including syndesmophytes, squaring of vertebrae, and fusion, as well as erosive enthesopathies associated with new bone formation (Fig. 26.7).
- *Blood tests* – Many patients have mild elevation of the erythrocyte sedimentation rate or C-reactive proteins, but these are not good guides to the activity of the disease. A mild anemia and modest elevations of alkaline phosphatase are also common.
- *Tissue typing* – AS is strongly associated with HLA B-27, but as this is common in the general population, varying in different racial groups, tissue typing should not be used as a diagnostic test for AS.

DIFFERENTIAL DIAGNOSIS

In early AS, the main differential diagnosis is with other causes of low back pain in young adults such as mechanical low back pain or a prolapsed intervertebral disc (see Chapter 24). Some patients with AS also have ulcerative colitis or Crohn's disease.

Overlap occurs between AS and other members of the seronegative spondyloarthropathies (principally reactive arthritis and psoriatic arthropathy), which can cause a very similar axial arthropathy.

In late disease with spinal fusion, confusion may arise between AS and diffuse idiopathic skeletal hyperostosis (see Chapter 27).

 MANAGEMENT

OBJECTIVES OF THERAPY

The objectives of treatment in AS are to:
- Reduce pain and stiffness.
- Restore any loss of movement of the spine, hips, and chest wall.
- Maintain good posture.
- Minimize the development of disability.
- Prevent or adequately treat any complications.

PATIENT EDUCATION AND SELF-HELP

Patient education is vital in AS. Much of the onus in maintaining mobility of the chest and spine, and to prevent the development of stiffness, deformities, and disability depends on the patient regularly carrying out appropriate exercises at home.

Patients can also help themselves in a number of simple ways (see Self-Help Leaflet, page 346).

PHYSICAL THERAPY

Physical therapy is the cornerstone of AS patient treatment. All patients diagnosed with AS should be referred to a physical therapist for assessment. They should be taught a course of regular exercises to maintain good posture and full mobility of the spine and hips, which should be continued throughout life.

DRUG THERAPY

An important role in the management of AS is played by NSAIDs, as the symptoms of back pain and stiffness in AS respond well to these drugs, unlike most other forms of back pain. Regular, full-dose NSAID therapy should be used when symptoms are present and if there are no contraindications to their usage (see Chapter 9).

Corticosteroids and other drugs have little part to play in the management of AS, although in those patients with severe disease an anti-arthritic agent may be indicated ,particularly if peripheral joints are involved. Sulfasalazine is probably the most effective and appropriate drug to be used in these circumstances (see Chapter 9).

SURGERY AND OTHER TREATMENT MODALITIES

Bad hip disease can cause severe disabilities as well as pain, and may necessitate hip replacement surgery. In the occasional case of advanced AS, back deformities are so severe that spinal surgery to correct kyphosis is warranted.

Other forms of therapy are rarely required. Radiotherapy of the spine is now not used because of the increased risk of deformity and leukemia, but occasional radiotherapy for local resistant enthesopathies is warranted.

DIET AND COMPLEMENTARY TECHNIQUES

No good evidence has been established for the efficacy of any specific dietary or complementary therapeutic approach in AS. Diets high in fish oils rather than other fats, combined with NSAIDs, may provide some benefit as in other inflammatory arthropathies. Techniques such as relaxation may relieve spinal pain and help patients develop the habit of taking regular exercise.

DIFFERENTIAL DIAGNOSIS OF ANKYLOSING SPONDYLITIS

- Noninflammatory causes of low back pain.
- Ankylosing spondylitis with inflammatory bowel disease.
- Other seronegative spondyloarthropathies (reactive arthritis or psoriatic arthropathy).
- Diffuse idiopathic skeletal hyperostosis.

SUMMARY OF MANAGEMENT

- Early diagnosis, patient education, and physical therapy are essential to the successful management of ankylosing spondylitis.
- The goal of physical therapy is to restore and maintain posture and movement to as near normal as possible.
- Self-management of the disease with exercises must be continued on a life-long basis.
- Nonsteroidal anti-inflammatory drugs relieve pain and stiffness, and facilitate physical therapy.
- Other drugs, treatments, or surgery are occasionally indicated.

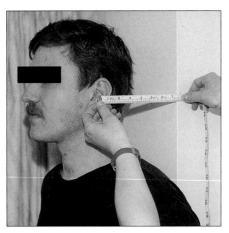

Fig. 26.8 Measurement of the wall-to-tragus distance. This is one way to assess change in spinal mobility during follow-up of patients with ankylosing spondylitis.

TREATMENT OF COMPLICATIONS

Iritis is the only common complication that requires treatment; it should always be treated quickly with topical corticosteroids and mydriatics. Protection from light may also be necessary.

In the rare cases in which severe cardiac or pulmonary complications develop, referral for specialist treatment is indicated.

MONITORING PROGRESSION AND OUTCOME

The ease with which quite severe deformities and loss of movement can develop means it is important to monitor patients carefully by simple measures of spinal movement, such as toe-to-floor distance, or tragus-to-wall distance (Fig. 26.8). Chest expansion can also be measured. Review to check on such movements should be carried out annually.

If a patient shows signs of increasing stiffness or deformity, further input from the physical therapist is indicated.

INDICATIONS FOR REFERRAL

Specialist referral
- Patients with iritis should be considered for referral to an ophthalmologic service.
- Patients with troublesome pain, stiffness, deformity or disability despite simple conventional therapy should be referred to a rheumatologist.
- Any patient with AS and severe hip disease or other peripheral joint problems should be referred to a rheumatologist, and may need to be considered for surgery.
- Patients with severe or resistant enthesopathies, and those with systemic complications such as cardiopulmonary problems should be referred to a rheumatologist.
- Patients with significant gastrointestinal problems should be referred to a rheumatologic or gastroenterologic service.
- Anyone with sudden severe worsening of back pain should be referred, as they may have suffered a fracture or dislocation of the spine.
- Anyone with significant neurologic complications should be referred urgently to a rheumatologic, orthopaedic or neurosurgical service.

Physiotherapy
- All patients with ankylosing spondylitis should be referred to physiotherapists to be taught a daily regime of exercises.
- Any patient in whom there is evidence of increasing spinal stiffness or deformity should be referred for a course of mobilizing exercises.

SPINAL DISORDERS

27

OTHER SPINAL DISORDERS

CERVICAL MYELOPATHY

IN WHAT CIRCUMSTANCES SHOULD YOU SUSPECT CERVICAL MYELOPATHY?

Any older patient with a history of cervical spondylosis or rheumatoid arthritis who has an injury to the cervical spine is vulnerable to cervical myelopathy. In addition, cervical myelopathy can gradually develop in patients with long-standing neck pain and radicular symptoms.

In any of these circumstances a careful history to elicit any symptoms, such as weakness or numbness in the legs or sphincter problems, should be taken, and a neurologic examination carried out to elicit signs of a sensory level or of upper motor neuron changes, such as a Babinski response in the lower limbs.

 MANAGEMENT

Cervical myelopathy is a medical emergency. Patients should be referred urgently for investigation and treatment. Most need urgent decompression of the cervical cord to prevent progression and subsequent paralysis.

KEY POINTS

Definition

- Compression of the spinal cord or of the spinal arteries in the cervical region.
- Can result from several different pathologies, including cervical spondylosis, disc protrusion, rheumatoid arthritis of the cervical spine, traumatic subluxation, or (less commonly) tumors or infections in the neck.

Main clinical features

- Often presents with a combination of lower motor neuron features at the site of the lesion (commonly C6/7) and upper motor neuron lesions below this.
- A clear sensory level may be present.
- Other features can include vertebrobasilar insufficiency vertigo and drop attacks, and sphincter abnormalities.

Diagnosis

- Requires urgent referral for imaging by magnetic resonance or computed tomography with contrast medium, to define the cause and anatomy of the lesion that is compressing the cord (see Figs 27.1 & 27.2).

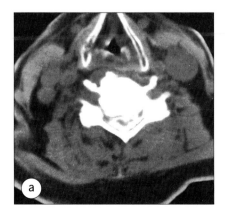
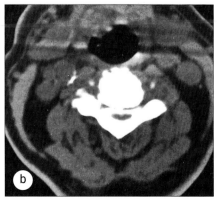

Fig. 27.1 Imaging cord compression.
(a) Computed tomography scan taken after injection of a contrast medium, which is seen forming a sleeve around the slightly flattened spinal cord. (b) In the vertebral body, obstruction of the flow of contrast by osteophytes shows they are compressing the cord.

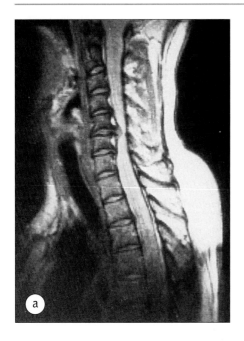

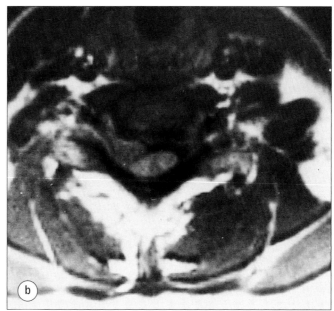

Fig. 27.2 Magnetic resonance imaging offers one of the best ways to discriminate between different types of soft tissue and imaging cord compression. (a) A large lateral disc protrusion at the C5/6 level, which is compressing the dural mater. (b) The axial scan shows the posterior disc bulge.

ENTEROPATHIC ARTHROPATHIES

KEY POINTS

Definition
- Arthropathies associated with intestinal diseases.

Main clinical features
- Various patterns occur (see text).
- Most commonly a disorder very similar to ankylosing spondylitis that occurs in patients with inflammatory bowel disease (ulcerative colitis or Crohn's disease).

Diagnosis
- Special gastrointestinal investigations, which include biopsy, may be necessary to diagnosis the intestinal disease.
- The arthropathy can usually be diagnosed clinically, but radiographs may be needed for confirmation.

IN WHAT CIRCUMSTANCES SHOULD YOU SUSPECT ENTEROPATHIC ARTHROPATHY?

Any arthritis with bowel symptoms, and any undiagnosed arthritis with a spinal component (the bowel disease is not always obvious – it may be subclinical).

PATTERNS AND TYPES OF DISEASE

The main patterns and types of enteropathic arthropathy are discussed below:
- A spinal arthritis indistinguishable from ankylosing spondylitis occurs in about 10% of patients with inflammatory bowel disease (Fig. 27.3). The activity of the spondylitis is unrelated to the activity of the bowel disease.
- A lower limb peripheral arthritis occurs in patients with inflammatory bowel disease, which does vary in activity in line with the progression of the bowel problem. Most commonly an asymmetric synovitis of knees, ankles, and metatarsophalangeal joints, tendinitis, and enthesitis can also occur (Fig. 27.4).
- Enteropathic reactive arthritis occurs as a result of a bowel infection by microorganisms such as *Salmonella*, *Shigella*, or *Yersinia* (see reactive arthritis, Chapter 22).
- A spondyloarthropathy accompanied by a subclinical bowel infection can occur, only diagnosable from histologic findings in the gut.
- A polyarthritis or arthritis that affects the spine can occur in patients with Whipple's disease or celiac disease, or in people who have had an intestinal bypass operation for obesity.

Rx MANAGEMENT

The management involves appropriate standard therapy for the bowel condition, and the same measures as used for a spondyloarthropathy or peripheral arthropathy in the absence of bowel involvement. Referral to rheumatology services for the arthropathies and to gastroenterologists for the bowel disease may be necessary.

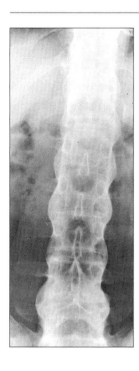

Fig. 27.3 Bamboo spine in a woman with severe Crohn's disease.

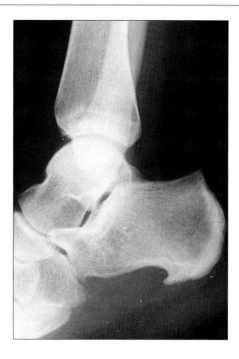

Fig. 27.4 Spur formation at the insertion of the Achilles' tendon and plantar fascia. This is a case of lower limb arthritis and enthesopathy associated with enteropathic arthritis.

DIFFUSE IDIOPATHIC SKELETAL HYPEROSTOSIS

IN WHAT CIRCUMSTANCES SHOULD YOU SUSPECT DIFFUSE IDIOPATHIC SKELETAL HYPEROSTOSIS?

Diffuse idiopathic skeletal hyperostosis (DISH) is associated with age, obesity, diabetes, gout, and hypertension, and is twice as common in men than in women. Hence, any older, overweight man, particularly if he also has one of the other associations, is quite likely to have DISH.

The presence of symptoms from the condition is unusual, but loss of significant spinal movement can cause problems, and the occasional case of spinal complications, such as cord pressure, arises.

The main importance of DISH lies in the confusion it causes on radiographs, and the chance of it being misdiagnosed as ankylosing spondylitis.

 MANAGEMENT

No treatment is needed. If spinal or peripheral joint stiffness is significant, physical therapy may help.

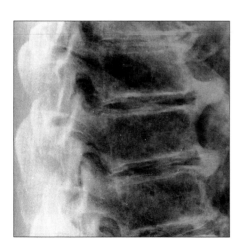

Fig. 27.5 Thoracic spine radiograph in diffuse idiopathic skeletal hyperostosis. Demonstrated are large osteophytes that fuse the disc spaces anteriorly. Disc space height is preserved.

KEY POINTS

Definition
- A common, age-related condition characterized by new bone formation at entheses (ligament–bone junctions), particularly in the spine, which results in ankylosis (Fig. 27.5).

Main clinical features
- Usually asymptomatic.
- Can cause marked stiffening of the spine, particularly in the thoracic region.
- Occasionally causes pressure problems in the spine and can result in dysphagia, cervical myelopathy, or spinal stenosis.
- Peripheral joints may become stiff, but do not ankylose.

Diagnosis
- Diagnosis depends on the typical radiographic features.
- Often a chance finding on chest or other radiographs.

SYSTEMIC DISORDERS

AN INTRODUCTION TO SYSTEMIC DISORDERS

The systemic rheumatic diseases are an important group of disorders that present a number of problems in primary care medicine. The symptoms of these disorders are typically vague and only rarely offer immediate clues to the diagnosis. The malar rash of systemic lupus or the skin thickening of scleroderma might be examples of clinical findings that are readily recognized and easily diagnosed. More often, however, patients present with vague musculoskeletal complaints, such as diffuse joint aches and pains or weakness, constitutional symptoms like fever, anorexia, or malaise, or perhaps most commonly fatigue or lack of energy. The immediate concern of deciding whether these are caused by self-limited processes, ordinary life stresses in healthy individuals, another medical condition, or a rheumatic disease is difficult and delay in diagnosis is frequent. On rare occasions, systemic rheumatic diseases are life threatening and demand prompt referral and treatment. In general, such patients are easily recognized by their high spiking fevers, rapid weight loss, and obvious signs of major organ dysfunction; infection or malignancy are often considered in the differential diagnosis. The large majority of patients with systemic rheumatic diseases, however, have chronic illnesses that are diagnosed and managed principally in a primary care setting.

These diseases are remarkably heterogeneous and have little in common in the way of presentations, clinical course, pathogenesis, or treatment. A diagnostic algorithm for the systemic rheumatic diseases is shown overleaf. It begins with the identification of patients who have fibromyalgia, unquestionably the most common of the systemic rheumatic disorders. These patients present a characteristic syndrome of profound fatigue and generalized musculoskeletal symptoms, with little in the way of objective findings on the physical examination save for tenderness in soft-tissue areas, called 'tender points'. In the remaining patients, most of whom have clear abnormalities detected by the physical examination, the antinuclear antibody (ANA) is used to separate patients into ANA positive and ANA negative groups. Although this is a reasonably convenient scheme, it is important to remember that the ANA is occasionally negative in the ANA-positive group and vice versa. The connective tissue diseases are the most potentially serious of the ANA-positive group. The remaining patients who are ANA positive, having the so-called ANA spectrum disorders, have a very broad differential diagnosis and often cause real problems in diagnosis. Most of the ANA-negative systemic disorders are vascular diseases of one sort or another, with the exception of Still's disease and hypermobility syndrome.

DIAGNOSTIC ALGORITHM FOR SYSTEMIC RHEUMATIC DISORDERS

Suspect a systemic rheumatic disease if any of the following are present: constitutional signs/symptoms, arthralg
arthritis, mucocutaneous lesions, neurologic symptoms, thrombophlebitis, muscle weakness, Raynaud's phenome

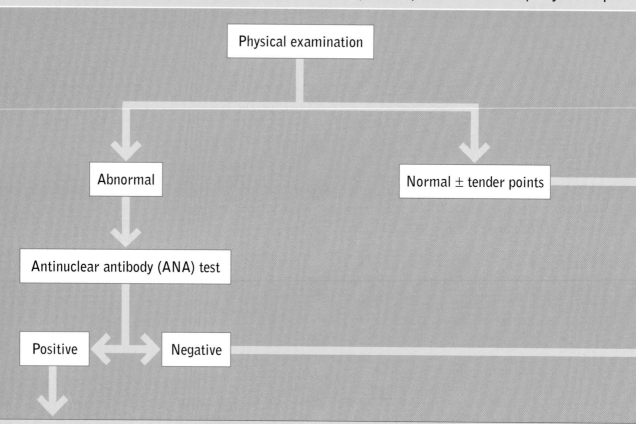

Physical examination

Abnormal

Normal ± tender points

Antinuclear antibody (ANA) test

Positive

Negative

Positive

Connective tissue diseases

- SLE (rash, arthritis, pleurisy, nephritis, etc.; Ch. 29)

- Sjögren's syndrome (dry eyes, dry mouth; Ch. 30)

- Inflammatory myopathy (muscle weakness, rashes; Ch. 33)

- Scleroderma (Raynaud's phenomenon, skin thickening, pulmonary disease; Ch. 31)

- ANA spectrum disorders (Ch. 32)

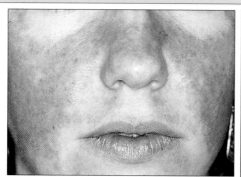

Fig. 2 A malar rash in a patient with SLE.

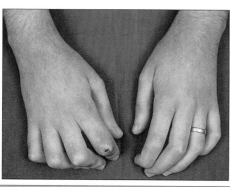

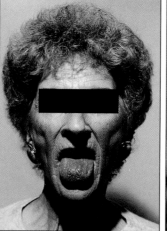

Fig. 3 Sicca syndrome in scleroderma. The tongue is parched and hypopapillated.

Fig. 4 A patient with severe proximal muscle wasting due to myositis.

Fig. 5 Contractures and ulceration in scleroderma. Note the loss of hair from the dorsum of the fingers.

Fibromyalgia (Ch. 28)
(Profound fatigue, generalized subjective musculoskeletal symptoms)

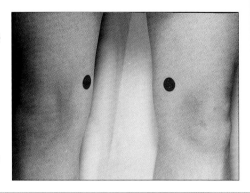

Fig. 1 Location of the knee tender points for diagnostic classification of fibromyalgia.

Negative

- Primary Raynaud's phenomenon (episodic vasospasm of extremities; Ch. 31)

- Adult's Still's disease (fevers, arthritis, rash; Ch. 33)

- Vasculitis syndromes [constitutional signs, major organ (lung, kidney, central nervous system, etc.) disease; Ch. 33]

- Behçet's syndrome (mucosal ulcers, uveitis, thrombophlebitis; Ch. 33)

- Antiphospholipid syndrome (recurrent venous/arterial thromboses, spontaneous abortion, thrombocytopenia; Ch. 33)

- Hypermobility syndrome (joint and skin laxity, noninflammatory arthropathy; Ch. 33)

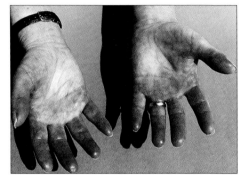

Fig. 6 Raynaud's phenonomen. Sharply demarcated cyanosis of the fingers with proximal venular congestion in a woman with scleroderma.

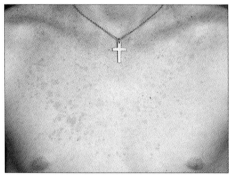

Fig. 7 The faint salmon-colored rash of Still's disease. Although the rash is most common on the trunk and upper extremities, it may also be seen on the face.

Fig. 9 Livideo reticularis. With permission from Conn DL. Polyarteritis. In: Rheumatic Disease Clinics of North America, Ch 7 Conn DL, ed. Philadelphia: WB Saunders; 1990:341–62.

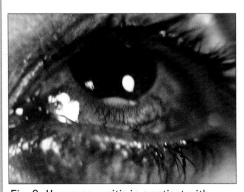

Fig. 8 Hypopyon uveitis in a patient with Behçet's syndrome.

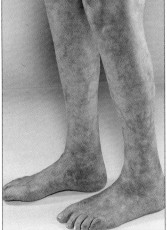

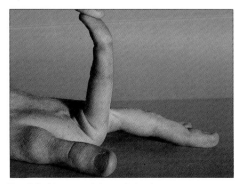

Fig. 10 Hypermobility of the finger in hypermobility syndrome.

SYSTEMIC DISORDERS

28

FIBROMYALGIA

Fibromyalgia is a common, chronic, generalized pain syndrome typically accompanied by profound fatigue and subjective musculoskeletal symptoms. The majority of patients are women between the ages of 30 and 50 years. Physical and laboratory abnormalities are notably absent except for tenderness at discrete anatomic sites called tender points. Fibromyalgia occurs commonly in patients with other rheumatic diseases, particularly rheumatoid arthritis (RA) and lupus. Fibromyalgia has a number of similarities to other 'affective' disorders, which include chronic fatigue syndrome, irritable bowel syndrome, and myofascial pain syndrome.

 TYPICAL CASE: FIBROMYALGIA

Helen is a 48-year-old, divorced copyeditor with a 10-month history of profound fatigue and 'hurting all over'. She sleeps poorly at night, waking up three or four times, and finds it difficult to get back to sleep. She feels miserable most of the time and by the end of the day is so exhausted that she collapses on the couch.

On physical examination, she is 10lb (4.5kg) overweight and looks depressed. There is no evidence of synovitis and muscle strength testing and neurologic examinations are normal. Laboratory studies reveal a normal complete blood count (CBC), an erythrocyte sedimentation rate (ESR) of 10mm/h, and normal thyroid function tests.

NATURAL HISTORY AND OTHER CLINICAL FEATURES

Patients with fibromyalgia often identify a flu-like illness or physical or emotional stress as a potential cause of their symptoms (Fig. 28.2). Diagnosis is often delayed when physicians reassure patients that nothing is wrong or alternatively refer them to specialists (infectious disease, neurology, gastroenterology, etc.) for evaluation of specific symptoms. The syndrome is generally easily and promptly recognized once it receives proper consideration (Fig. 28.3).

Although most patients have some improvement with appropriate treatment, the vast majority develop a chronic pain syndrome and true remissions are distinctly unusual. Fibromyalgia is an important cause of medical disability, and studies show that up to 50% of patients develop functional impairments that have a substantial impact on employment.

KEY POINTS

Definition
- A chronic musculoskeletal syndrome characterized by diffuse pain and tender points.
- No evidence that synovitis or myositis are causes.
- Occurs in the context of unrevealing physical, laboratory, and radiologic examinations.
- Women account for 80–90% of patients, and the peak age is 30–50 years.

Clinical features
- Generalized chronic musculoskeletal pain.
- Diffuse tenderness at discrete anatomic locations termed tender points.
- Other features, of diagnostic utility but not essential for classification of fibromyalgia, may include fatigue, sleep disturbances, headaches, irritable bowel syndrome, paresthesias, Raynaud's-like symptoms, depression, and anxiety.

FEATURES OF FIBROMYALGIA

- Chronic, poorly localized, diffuse pain; often begins in the neck and shoulders and becomes generalized.
- Profound fatigue, evident when first awakening in the morning and worsens during midafternoon.
- 'Light' sleep; awakened often during the night, with difficulty getting back to sleep.
- Tension or migraine headaches.
- Depression and anxiety.
- Subjective complaints of joint or soft-tissue swelling or muscle weakness with normal rheumatologic examination.
- Characteristic 'tender points' (Fig. 28.1).
- Normal laboratory studies.

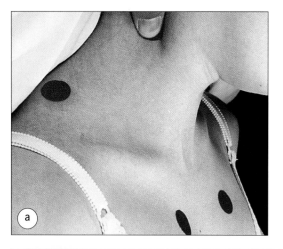

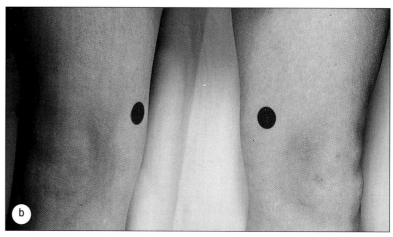

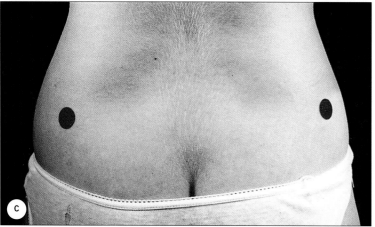

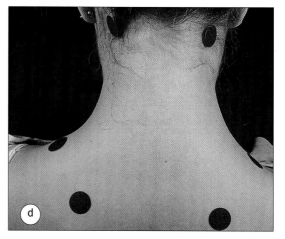

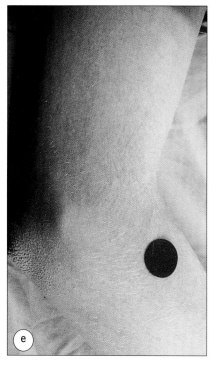

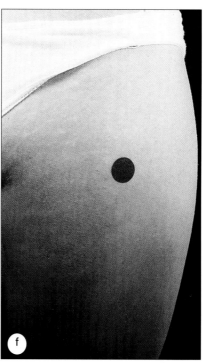

Fig. 28.1 Locations of the nine pairs of tender points for diagnostic classification of fibromyalgia.
See (g) for details.

TENDER POINTS IN FIBROMYALGIA

Pain on digital palpation must be present in at least 11 of the following 18 tender point sites:

Occiput: bilateral, at the suboccipital muscle insertions (d)

Low cervical: bilateral, at the anterior aspects of the intertransverse spaces at C5–C7 (a)

Trapezius: bilateral, at the midpoint of the upper border (d)

Supraspinatus: bilateral, at origins, above the scapula spine near the medial border (d)

Second rib: bilateral, at the second costochondral junctions, just lateral to the junctions on upper surfaces (a)

Lateral epicondyle: bilateral, 2cm distal to the epicondyles (e)

Gluteal: bilateral, in upper outer quadrants of buttocks in anterior fold of muscle (c)

Greater trochanter: bilateral, posterior to the trochanteric prominence (f)

Knee: bilateral, at the medial fat pad proximal to the joint line (b)

(g)

MOST COMMON PRECIPITATING FACTORS IN FIBROMYALGIA

Flu-like viral illness

Rheumatic disorders

HIV infection

Lyme disease

Physical trauma

Emotional trauma

Medications,
especially corticosteroid withdrawal

Fig. 28.2 Most common precipitating factors in fibromyalgia.

CLUES TO THE POSSIBILITY OF FIBROMYALGIA SYNDROME

- Past/present prolonged localized pain complaint – important tests negative

- Often prior nonspecific label – 'lumbago', 'chronic fatigue' syndrome, 'restless legs' syndrome, 'whiplash', 'growing pains'

- Past/present tension headache, irritable bowel, fluid retention or similar syndromes

- Widespread joint/muscle pain

- Poor-quality sleep

- Background stress factors (may be subtle)

Fig. 28.3 Clues to the possibility of fibromyalgia syndrome.

! POINTS TO LOOK OUT FOR

- Other rheumatic diseases – traditional inflammatory rheumatic diseases (RA, systemic lupus erythematosus, etc.) may present with (or be accompanied by) fibromyalgia symptoms. Careful review of systems, physical examination, and directed laboratory investigation are important.
- Thyroid disease – both hypo- and hyperthyroidism may produce diffuse musculoskeletal pain.
- Polymyalgia rheumatica – presents with shoulder and hip girdle pain that resembles fibromyalgia (see Chapter 42). Older patients (>50 years) and high ESR are helpful clues to diagnosis.
- Sleep apnea – may be confused with fibromyalgia – daytime napping, loud snoring, or witnessed long respiratory pauses suggest the diagnosis.

INVESTIGATIONS

Fibromyalgia is a clinical diagnosis that requires minimal screening laboratory studies to exclude other medical conditions. Imaging studies, biopsies, or other testing are not necessary and should only be directed by findings from the history or physical examination.

LABORATORY TESTS

Initial routine laboratory studies include a CBC, standard blood chemistries, ESR, and thyroid function studies in all patients. These studies are normal in fibromyalgia. Other laboratory studies are obtained only if there is clear suspicion from the history or physical examination of another disease. In particular, antinuclear antibodies or Lyme antibody studies should not be routinely ordered. There is a modest rate of low titer 'false positive' results with these studies in normal individuals (see Chapter 5), which often leads to unnecessary medical evaluations and delay in treatment of patients with fibromyalgia.

LESS COMMON FEATURES INCLUDE

- Raynaud's-like sensitivity to cold.
- Abdominal pain, bloating, alternating diarrhea/constipation (irritable bowel syndrome).
- Numbness and tingling of the extremities.
- Dry eyes and dry mouth.
- Palpitations.

DIFFERENTIAL DIAGNOSIS AND SYSTEMIC ILLNESSES THAT ARE ASSOCIATED WITH FIBROMYALGIA (FM)		
Condition	Helpful differential features	% with FM
Rheumatoid arthritis	Synovitis, serologic tests, elevated erythrocyte sedimentation rate (ESR)	12
Systemic lupus erythematosus	Dermatitis, systemic vasculitis (renal, central nervous system, etc.)	22
Sjögren's syndrome	Lymphadenopathy, biopsy of salivary glands	11
Polymyalgia rheumatica	Elevated ESR, elderly, response to corticosteroids	?
Myositis	Increased muscle enzymes, weakness more than pain	?
Hypothyroidism	Abnormal thyroid function tests	?
Neuropathies	Clinical and electrophysiologic evidence of neuropathy	?

Fig. 28.4 Differential diagnosis and systemic illnesses that are associated with fibromyalgia.

SYNDROMES THAT OVERLAP WITH FIBROMYALGIA	
Syndrome	Relationship with fibromyalgia
Depression	Present in 25–60% of fibromyalgia cases
Irritable bowel	Present in 50–80% of fibromyalgia cases
Migraine	Present in 50% of fibromyalgia cases
Chronic fatigue (CFS)	70% of CFS cases meet criteria for fibromyalgia
Myofascial pain	May be a localized form of fibromyalgia

Fig. 28.5 Syndromes that overlap with fibromyalgia.

CLASSIFICATION SCHEMA FOR CHRONIC FATIGUE SYNDROME (CFS)
Classify as CFS or idiopathic chronic fatigue if:
Fatigue persists or relapses for ≥6 months
History, physical examination, and appropriate laboratory tests exclude any other cause for the chronic fatigue
Classify as CFS if, along with the fatigue, four or more of the following are present for >6 months:
Impaired memory or concentration, sore throat, tender cervical or axillary lymph nodes, muscle pain, multijoint pain, new headaches, unrefreshing sleep, postexertion malaise

Fig. 28.6 Classification schema for chronic fatigue syndrome. (Modified from Fukuda K, Straus S E, Hickie I, Sharpe MC, Dobbins JG, Komaroff A. The chronic fatigue syndrome: A comprehensive approach to its definition and study. Ann Intern Med. 1994;121:953–9.)

COMPARISON OF FIBROMYALGIA AND MYOFASCIAL PAIN SYNDROMES		
Variable	Fibromyalgia	Myofascial pain
Examination	Tender points	Trigger points
Location	Generalized	Regional
Response to local therapy	Not sustained	'Curative'
Sex	Females:males, 10:1	(?) Equal
Systemic features	Characteristic	(?)

Fig. 28.7 Comparison of fibromyalgia and myofascial pain syndromes.

DIFFERENTIAL DIAGNOSIS

The somewhat vague and nebulous symptoms of chronic, generalized pain and fatigue are present in many rheumatic and nonrheumatic conditions (Fig. 28.4). These are typically readily excluded by a careful history and physical examination. Hypothyroidism may cause symptoms that mimic fibromyalgia and thyroid function studies should be carried out in all patients. Peripheral neuropathies, entrapment syndromes (such as carpal tunnel syndrome), and neurologic disorders (such as multiple sclerosis or myasthenia gravis) are sometimes considered in the differential diagnosis.

The most confusing conditions in the differential diagnosis are a group of similar, poorly understood, affective disorders (Fig. 28.5). The considerable overlap among these conditions is generally accepted. The two disorders that are most difficult to distinguish from fibromyalgia are chronic fatigue syndrome (Fig. 28.6) and myofascial pain syndromes (Fig. 28.7).

 ## MANAGEMENT

The goals of management of fibromyalgia are symptomatic relief and improvement of function. Self-help is the key to successful treatment (see Self-Help Leaflet, page 347 and Fig. 28.8).

PATIENT EDUCATION AND SELF-HELP

Education is critical to successful management of fibromyalgia. Patients must be reassured that the illness is real, and not imagined. They should be told that fibromyalgia is not a deforming or deteriorating condition and that it is never a life-threatening or cosmetic problem. It is often helpful to provide patients with self-help instructions or other educational material that discusses various aspects of the disease.

PHYSICAL THERAPY

Patients must be strongly encouraged to begin an aerobic exercise program and to carry out stretch and strength exercises for the abdominal and paraspinal musculature daily. Most patients derive some benefit from simple low-level aerobic training, such as a daily walking program. In addition, instructing patients in stress management tactics, such as relaxation, meditation, yoga, or similar activities, is often helpful for pain management.

DRUG THERAPY

Low doses of tricyclic antidepressant drugs given at bedtime are the mainstay of drug treatment of fibromyalgia. Patients are generally begun on 5–10mg of amitriptyline (or desipramine) 1–2 hours before bedtime. The dose may be gradually increased after 2 weeks. The final dose should be set by the patient (typically 25–50mg) based on improvement in symptoms and side effects. Even with low-dose tricyclics, side effects such as dry mouth, constipation, fluid retention, weight gain, and difficulty with concentration are common. Other tricyclic compounds and different classes of antidepressant central nervous system medications, particularly serotonin-reuptake inhibitors such as fluoxetine (Prozac™), sertraline (Zoloft™), paroxetine (Paxil™), and flovoxamine (Luvox™) may be used in patients who remain symptomatic despite maximum doses of amitriptyline.

Acetaminophen or tramadol may be useful adjuncts for pain management. Nonsteroidal anti-inflammatory drugs or corticosteroids have no effect on the disorder.

RECOMMENDATIONS FOR REFERRAL

Subspecialty
- Subspecialty referral is occasionally warranted in patients with symptoms suggesting the fibromyalgia may be secondary to another disease process. Examples include patients with arthritis or suspected connective tissue disease (rheumatology), peripheral or central nervous system signs of symptoms (neurology), or bowel disturbances (gastroenterology).

Physical therapy/rehabilitation
- Referral to physical therapy/rehabilitation may be indicated in patients lacking the motivation to begin or carry out an exercise program.

Other
- Referral to a psychologist or psychiatrist may be indicated in patients with difficulty coping with stress or with a poor self-image.

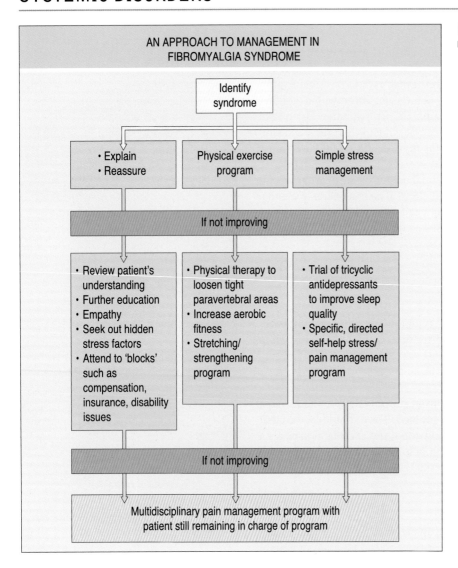

Fig. 28.8 An approach to the management of fibromyalgia.

OTHER TREATMENT MODALITIES AND COMPLEMENTARY TECHNIQUES

A variety of therapies have been advocated for fibromyalgia, but with no convincing evidence of efficacy. Although studies have suggested some benefit from acupuncture, hypnotherapy, and electromyography–biofeedback, these techniques have not gained wide acceptance. Tender points are frequently injected locally with lidocaine (lignocaine) with or without corticosteroids, but with no evidence that the procedure has any real impact on the disorder. A large percentage of patients resort to over-the-counter alternative drugs, which include nutritional supplements, herbs, vitamins, and other remedies. The role of these therapies and their cost-effectiveness remain unknown.

MONITORING PROGRESSION AND OUTCOME

Patients need to be followed at regular intervals until they have achieved improvement and stability of their symptoms. A multidisciplinary team that consists of nurse educators, psychiatrists or other mental health workers, physiatrists, and physical therapists may be needed for the more difficult patients.

RECOMMENDATIONS FOR REFERRAL

Most patients with fibromyalgia can be successfully diagnosed and managed entirely in a primary care setting.

SYSTEMIC LUPUS ERYTHEMATOSUS

Systemic lupus erythematosus (SLE) is the most common of the autoimmune, connective tissue disorders. It occurs mostly in young women (20–30 years old), African–Americans and Asians being at increased risk. Presentations of the disease are variable – most patients begin with the insidious onset of constitutional signs, with rashes and arthritis.

1 THE TYPICAL CASE: SYSTEMIC LUPUS ERYTHEMATOSUS

Mary is 20-year-old college senior. Over the past month she has been extremely tired and unable to keep up with her coursework. She falls asleep in classes and has found some difficulty with concentration. Recently, she has felt feverish, but has not bothered to take her temperature. She comments that her hair seems to be falling out after brushing or washing her hair. In addition, she has started to notice occasional swelling and stiffness in her hands and wrists.

On examination, a raised, warm rash is evident on her cheeks and small ulcerations are found on the hard palate (Fig. 29.1). Mild, tender synovitis is found in both wrists as well as in the second and third metacarpointerphalangeal joints of both hands. A small effusion is present in the left knee.

NATURAL HISTORY AND OTHER CLINICAL FEATURES

Clinical manifestations are usually most intense during the early stages of the disease. The disease course generally involves relapses ('flares') and remissions. Lupus may affect vital organs, and this may be clinically silent. It is important to recognize major organ involvement early:

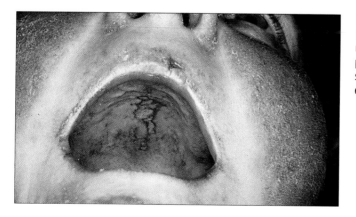

Fig. 29.1 Malar rash and mouth ulcers in a patient with systemic lupus erythematosus.

FEATURES OF SYSTEMIC LUPUS ERYTHEMATOSUS

- Young women are most commonly affected.
- Constitutional signs – fatigue, fever, and weight loss.
- Migratory polyarthritis affects the hands, wrists, and knees.
- Photosensitive rashes – acute malar erythema ('butterfly rash'; Fig. 29.2) and chronic, scarring discoid lesions (Fig. 29.3) are most common.
- Serositis – pleurisy, pericarditis, and peritonitis.
- Alopecia – may be diffuse or spotty.
- Mucosal ulcers – painless, shallow ulcerations of buccal mucosa.
- Renal disease – proteinuria, active urine sediment, and impaired renal function.
- Neurologic (headaches, seizures, etc.) and psychologic difficulties such as depression.
- Mild anemia and leukopenia evident in most patients.
- Positive antinuclear antibody in all patients.

- Renal disease – clinical evidence of nephritis occurs in about 50% of patients; peripheral edema is infrequent, but when present is a sign of nephrotic syndrome; most often renal involvement is detected on screening urinalysis or blood tests.
- Neurologic or psychiatric disease – broad spectrum of neurologic manifestations includes seizures, acute strokes, movement disorders, and transverse myelopathy; most serious psychiatric features are organic brain syndromes and neurocognitive dysfunction.

! POINTS TO LOOK OUT FOR

- Infection – lupus patients are highly prone to infections and the development of persistent or high-spiking fevers requires careful evaluation of the patient.
- Hypertension – typically a sign of active renal disease.
- Renal failure – may occur insidiously in otherwise well patients such that urinalysis and blood urea nitrogen (BUN) need to be monitored periodically.
- Dyspnea – may indicate lupus pneumonitis, pulmonary hypertension, or shrinking lung syndrome.
- Thrombophlebitis – this occurs with pulmonary emboli in a subset of lupus patients with the so-called antiphospholipid syndrome.
- Chronic hip or knee pain – osteonecrosis (Fig. 29.4) is common in patients treated with corticosteroids (see Chapter 9).
- Chest pain – typically from pleurisy/pericarditis, but need to consider angina pectoris.

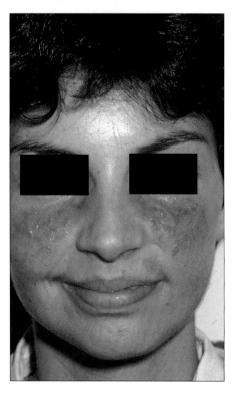

Fig. 29.2 Erythematous rash of systemic lupus erythematosus. Note that the rash does not cross the nasolabial fold.

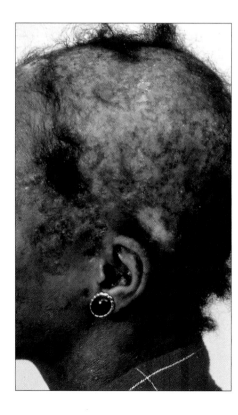

Fig. 29.3 Scarring discoid lupus of the scalp with permanent alopecia.

INVESTIGATIONS

LABORATORY TESTS

Positive antinuclear antibody (ANA) is typically found in high titer. Other immunologic tests include antibodies to DNA, depressed complement levels (particularly in patients with nephritis), and false-positive tests for syphilis, mild anemia, and leukopenia. Analyses for renal function (BUN and creatinine tests) and albumin are carried out, as is urinalysis for proteinuria cells and/or casts in urine sediment.

DIFFERENTIAL DIAGNOSIS

The differential diagnosis includes:

- drug-induced lupus; drugs (Fig. 29.5) may produce positive antinuclear antibodies and a syndrome that resembles lupus; findings are reversible on stopping the drug;
- other ANA-positive rheumatic syndromes with arthritis, in particular rheumatoid arthritis, Sjögren's syndrome, and dermatomyositis (see Chapter 32);
- chronic infections that may be associated with fever, arthritis, and positive ANA (e.g. subacute bacterial endocarditis, syphilis).

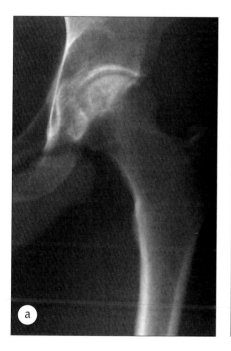 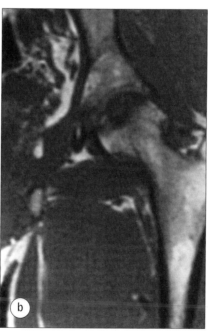

Fig. 29.4 Imaging appearance of osteonecrosis of the hip in systemic lupus erythematosus. (a) Radiograph of the hip shows typical sclerotic features of osteonecrosis in the femoral head. (b) The corresponding coronal T1-weighted MRI shows a pathognomonic pattern of subchondral marrow replacement with wavy margins. Early collapse of the articular surface of the central femoral head can be seen.

Fig. 29.5 Drugs implicated in drug-induced lupus.

DRUGS IMPLICATED IN DRUG-INDUCED LUPUS		
Carbamazepine	Hydralazine	Procainamide
Chlorpromazine	Isoniazid	Quinidine
Diphenylhydantoin	Methyldopa	Sulfasalazine
Ethosuximide	Penicillamine	

Subspecialty

- Patients in whom diagnosis is questionable or those with evidence of severe or major organ lupus should be referred to a rheumatologist who typically coordinates evaluation and treatment. Other subspecialty referrals, most commonly nephrology, neurology, or psychiatry, are dictated by the organs affected .

Orthopedic surgery

- Patients with osteonecrosis, a common complication in SLE patients, should be referred to orthopedic surgery for consideration of joint replacement.

Other

- Pregnant lupus patients are at risk of losing the pregnancy and should be under the care of obstetricians trained in high-risk pregnancies.

 MANAGEMENT

Lupus management is guided by the concept of 'lupus activity', with therapy dictated by the degree and severity of clinical manifestations:

- Nonsteroidal anti-inflammatory drugs (NSAIDs) are important for the treatment of musculoskeletal symptoms, mild serositis, and constitutional signs.
- Antimalarial drugs are highly effective for acute and chronic lupus rashes.
- Most clinical manifestations of SLE respond promptly to corticosteroids, but corticosteroid toxicities account for substantial morbidity.
- Immunosuppressive drugs, particularly intravenous cyclophosphamide, are useful in patients with major organ involvement, such as lupus nephritis.

OBJECTIVES OF THERAPY

The objectives of treatment of SLE are to:

- relieve pain associated with local inflammation (arthritis, serositis, etc.);
- aggressively treat involvement of major organs to prevent damage and loss of organ function.

PATIENT EDUCATION AND SELF-HELP

Education is important in SLE, for which pamphlets and books are helpful. Since most patients are photosensitive, they need to be advised against intense sun exposure and to liberally use sun screens.

DRUG THERAPY

Low-dose corticosteroids, NSAIDs, and antimalarial drugs such as hydroxy-chloroquine play an important role in the management of mild lupus. Brief courses of high-dose corticosteroids and/or cytotoxic drugs (e.g. cyclophosphamide) are used for patients with serious or progressive major organ involvement.

MONITORING PROGRESSION AND OUTCOME

Clinical signs and symptoms are generally a good monitor of lupus activity; however, routine urinalysis, blood chemistries, and blood counts are important to detect silent involvement of vital organs. In most patients, lupus manifestations can be fully brought under control and patients need to be followed regularly to slowly withdraw drugs (particularly corticosteroids) with close monitoring of blood studies and urinalysis.

RECOMMENDATIONS FOR REFERRAL

Patients with mild lupus not affecting major organs (i.e. kidneys, central nervous system, cardiopulmonary system, and so on) can typically be diagnosed and managed in a primary care setting.

SYSTEMIC DISORDERS

30

SJÖGREN'S SYNDROME

Sjögren's syndrome is a chronic, progressive immunologic disorder that primarily affects the exocrine glands. The classic signs and symptoms include enlargement of the parotid and lacrimal glands, with mucosal dryness manifested by dry mouth (xerostomia) and dry eyes (xerophthalmia). It is commonly found in patients with other autoimmune disorders, which include rheumatoid arthritis, systemic lupus, and scleroderma (so-called secondary Sjögren's syndrome; Fig. 30.1), but it may also occur as a primary, idiopathic disease. Sjögren's syndrome is the most common form of autoimmunity disorder and is seen mostly in women (female:male ratio 9:1) in the fourth and fifth decades of life.

TYPICAL CASE OF SJÖGREN'S SYNDROME

Sophia is a 60-year-old seamstress with a 3-month history of fatigue, arthralgias, and troublesome dryness of her eyes and mouth. She awakens 4–5 times during the night to drink water, and it has been extremely difficult for her to chew dry foods like bread or biscuits. Over the past year she has had a problem with severe dental caries that required a number of tooth extractions.

Physical examination reveals a prominent enlargement of the parotid glands (Fig. 30.2). Laboratory studies reveal mild anemia with a hematocrit of 32%, a positive rheumatoid factor (RF) and antinuclear antibody (ANA), and an erythrocyte sedimentation rate (ESR) of 60mm/h (Westergren). A Schirmer's test is abnormal, with 3mm wetting in 5 minutes, and a biopsy of minor salivary glands shows prominent lymphocytic infiltration.

ASSOCIATION OF SJÖGREN'S SYNDROME WITH OTHER AUTOIMMUNE RHEUMATIC DISEASES (SECONDARY SJÖGREN'S SYNDROME)

Rheumatoid arthritis

Systemic lupus erythematosus

Scleroderma

Mixed connective tissue disease

Primary biliary cirrhosis

Myositis

Vasculitis

Thyroiditis

Chronic active hepatitis

Mixed cryoglobulinemia

Fig. 30.1 Association of Sjögren's syndrome with other autoimmune rheumatic diseases (secondary Sjögren's syndrome).

KEY POINTS

Definition
- A slowly progressive, inflammatory, autoimmune disease that affects primarily the exocrine glands.
- Lymphocytic infiltrates replace functional epithelium, which results in decreased exocrine secretions (exocrinopathy).
- Characteristic autoantibodies, anti-Ro(SS-A) and anti-La(SS-B), are produced.

Clinical features
- Mucosal dryness manifested in keratoconjunctivitis sicca, xerostomia, xerotrachea, and vaginal dryness.
- Major salivary gland enlargement and atrophic gastritis.
- Nonerosive polyarthritis; Raynaud's phenomenon without telangiectasia or digital ulceration.
- Extraglandular disease that affects lungs, kidneys, liver, and blood vessels.
- Association with other autoimmune diseases (rheumatoid arthritis, systemic lupus erythematosus, systemic sclerosis, polymyositis).
- Increased risk of lymphoid malignancy.

SYSTEMIC DISORDERS

FEATURES OF SJÖGREN'S SYNDROME

- Mucosal dryness – eyes, mouth, trachea, vagina.
- Enlargement of parotid or lacrimal glands.
- Arthritis or arthralgia, most commonly of the hands and wrists.
- Raynaud's phenomenon.

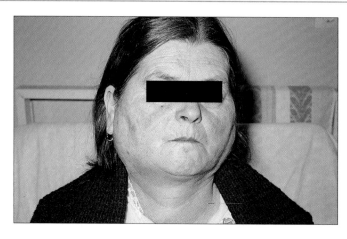

Fig. 30.2 Patient with primary Sjögren's syndrome. Parotid gland enlargement.

INITIAL MANIFESTATIONS OF PRIMARY SJÖGREN'S SYNDROME

	Percent
Subjective xerophthalmia	47
Subjective xerostomia	42.5
Parotid gland enlargement	24
Dyspareunia	5
Fever/fatigue	10
Arthralgias/arthritis	28
Raynaud's phenomenon	21
Lung involvement	1.5
Kidney involvement	1.5

Fig. 30.3 Initial manifestations of primary Sjögren's syndrome.

SJÖGREN'S SYNDROME – SYSTEMIC FEATURES INDICATIVE OF LYMPHOMA

Fever	Pulmonary infiltrates
Night sweats	Renal insufficiency
Increasing malaise	Worsening of anemia
Lymphadenopathy	Falling serum immunoglobulin M
Hepatosplenomegaly	Monoclonal gammopathy
Parotid enlargement	

Fig. 30.4 Findings that alert the physician to possible lymphoma in a patient with Sjögren's syndrome.

NATURAL HISTORY AND OTHER CLINICAL FEATURES

In most patients, Sjögren's syndrome runs a rather slow and benign course. Initial manifestations (Fig. 30.3) can be non-specific and typically 8–10 years elapse from the initial symptoms to the full-blown development of the syndrome.

! POINTS TO LOOK OUT FOR

- Occlusion of parotid duct with bacterial parotitis (typically acute and unilateral with painful swelling and erythema).
- Acute or chronic pancreatitis.
- Lymphoma (Fig. 30.4).

INVESTIGATIONS

LABORATORY TESTS

Routine laboratory studies should include a complete blood count, ESR, RF, and ANA. Mild anemia, elevated ESR, and positive RF and ANA are found in most patients. Auto-antibodies to the cellular ribonuclear antigens SS-A(Ro) and SS-B(La) are found in the majority of patients. Hyper-gammaglobulinemia is common.

FUNCTIONAL STUDIES OF EXOCRINE SECRETION

Functional studies of exocrine secretion include:
- Schirmer's tear test, which measures tear secretion by the lacrimal glands (Fig. 30.5);
- Rose bengal staining and slit-lamp examination of the eye to detect devitalized or damaged epithelium of the conjunctiva and cornea from reduced lacrimal secretions, termed keratoconjunctivitis sicca (Fig. 30.6);
- sialometry, sialography, and scintigraphy to measure salivary gland flow rates, architecture, and inflammation of salivary glands.

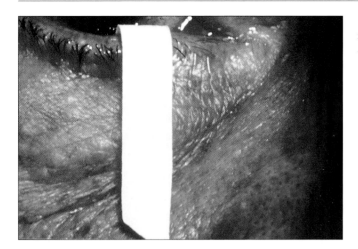

Fig. 30.5 Schirmer's test in a patient with Sjögren's syndrome. Wetting of <5mm/5min of the filter paper strip is abnormal and indicates reduced lacrimal secretions.

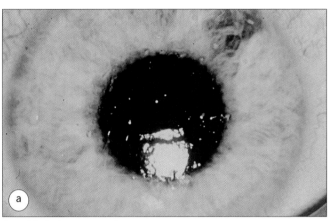
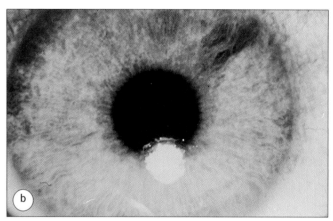

Fig. 30.6 Rose bengal staining. (a) In a normal volunteer and (b) in a patient with Sjögren's syndrome; retention of the stain in the cornea is apparent.

MINOR SALIVARY BIOPSY

Minor salivary gland biopsy is the cornerstone of diagnosis. Typical pathologic findings include focal aggregates of lymphocytes, plasma cells, and macrophages.

DIFFERENTIAL DIAGNOSIS

A number of infectious and infiltrative diseases can affect the parotid glands to produce parotid enlargement or disrupt secretions and lead to oral dryness (Fig. 30.7). In particular, human immunodeficiency virus infection (see Chapter 21), sarcoidosis (see Chapter 23), and hepatitis B and C (see Chapter 21) must be considered. A number of rare, infiltrative processes affect the lacrimal and salivary glands, including sarcoidosis, hemochromatosis, lymphoma, and amyloidosis. In addition, glandular swelling can result from the deposition of fat in the glands in diabetes mellitus, alcoholism, pancreatitis, cirrhosis, and hypertriglyceridemia. Drugs with anticholinergic side effects that cause dry mouth must be excluded; common examples include antidepressants (amitriptyline, doxepin), antihypertensives (clonidine, prazosin), and decongestants (ephedrine, pseudoephedrine).

DIFFERENTIAL DIAGNOSIS OF PAROTID GLAND ENLARGEMENT
Bilateral
Viral infection (mumps, influenza, Epstein–Barr, coxsackie A, cytomegalovirus, HIV)
Sjögren's syndrome
Sarcoidosis
Miscellaneous (diabetes mellitus, hyperlipoproteinemia, hepatic cirrhosis, chronic pancreatitis, acromegaly, gonadal hypofunction)
Recurrent parotitis of childhood
Unilateral
Salivary gland neoplasm
Bacterial infection
Chronic sialadenitis

Fig. 30.7 Differential diagnosis of parotid gland enlargement.

RECOMMENDATIONS FOR REFERRAL

Subspecialty
- Patients with a suspected secondary cause typically require a more thorough evaluation, which is generally carried out by a rheumatologist.

Other
- Patients with Sjögren's syndrome are prone to periodontal disease and dental caries, and require close follow-up by a dentist.
- Patients with severe sicca may require referral to an ophthalmologist or dentist.

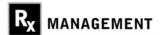

MANAGEMENT

The treatment of patients with Sjögren's syndrome is mainly symptomatic – the goal is to keep mucosal surfaces moist.

PATIENT EDUCATION AND SELF-HELP
The instruction of patients in daily self-management routines is the key to treatment. Regular use of artificial tears is essential to minimize the occurrence of dry eyes and prevent keratoconjunctivitis sicca. A variety of preparations are available that differ primarily in viscosity and preservative. Patients usually need to try several different preparations to determine which is most suitable for their own individual requirements. Soft contact lenses may help to protect the cornea, but the lenses themselves require wetting, and patients must be followed carefully because of the risk of infection. Home humidifiers and the avoidance of windy and low-humidity environments are helpful. Cigarette smoking is discouraged and drugs with anticholinergic side effects are avoided.

Treatment of dry mouth is difficult. Most patients learn to carry water with them at all times and keep water at the bedside. Stimulation of salivary flow by sucking sugar-free, flavored lozenges such as lemon drops, or chewing gum, generally helps, and dry foods are avoided. Careful attention to oral hygiene after meals is essential to prevent dental disease. Topical treatment with stannous fluoride enhances dental mineralization and retards damage to tooth surfaces.

Vaginal dryness is treated with lubricant jellies and dry skin with moisturizing lotions.

DRUG THERAPY
Drugs have a very limited role in the management of Sjögren's syndrome. Nonsteroidal anti-inflammatory drugs and antimalarial drugs are often beneficial in patients with persistent musculoskeletal complaints. Systemic corticosteroids and immunosuppressive drugs such as cyclophosphamide are used for severe extraglandular diseases, which include diffuse interstitial pneumonitis, glomerulonephritis, vasculitis, and neurologic involvement.

SURGERY AND OTHER TREATMENT MODALITIES
Surgical occlusion of the puncta at the medial aspect of the lower lids by electrocautery is occasionally helpful in patients with severe, progressive dry eyes.

MONITORING PROGRESSION AND OUTCOME

In the vast majority of patients with Sjögren's syndrome, regular monitoring of the disease is not necessary. Patients need to be reminded of the importance of seeking medical attention if they develop local (dental caries, bacterial parotitis, etc.) or systemic, extraglandular complications.

RECOMMENDATIONS FOR REFERRAL
The majority of patients with Sjögren's syndrome present with mild symptoms which can easily be managed entirely in a primary care setting.

SYSTEMIC DISORDERS

31

RAYNAUD'S PHENOMENON

Raynaud's phenomenon is the occurrence of episodic attacks of digital ischemia provoked by exposure to the cold or to emotional stress. It is common (found in 20% of the general population) and occurs most often in females (female:male ratio 4:1). Symptoms typically first develop in the teenage years. Raynaud's phenomenon is generally divided into primary (idiopathic) and secondary forms, based on whether an underlying cause or disease associated with peripheral vasospasm can be identified.

1 TYPICAL CASE OF RAYNAUD'S PHENOMENON

Ginny is a 34-year-old secretary with a long history of her fingers turning blue in the winter. The problem has become much worse recently, such that her fingers are blue most of the time, and, in addition, the fingers have become painful with numbness and tingling. She indicates that her health otherwise seems good. She hasn't noted any rashes or changes in her skin, weight loss, or joint complaints. She smokes a pack of cigarettes a day and her only medication is birth control pills that she has taken for more than 10 years.

All the fingers on both hands are strikingly cold and appear markedly cyanotic (Fig. 31.1). The remainder of the physical examination is unremarkable. Laboratory studies show a normal complete blood count (CBC), an erythrocyte sedimentation rate (ESR) of 15mm/h, and positive antinuclear antibody (ANA, speckled) at a titer of 1:80.

NATURAL HISTORY AND OTHER CLINICAL FEATURES

A careful history is essential to establish the diagnosis of Raynaud's phenomenon and to screen for evidence of signs and symptoms suggestive of a secondary cause. Patients complain of episodic attacks of well-demarcated, white or blue

---

KEY POINTS

- Periodic, vasospastic disorder of the extremities.
- Most commonly affects the fingers, with attacks of digital ischemia provoked by exposure to the cold or to emotional stress.
- Digits have a triphasic color change of pallor, cyanosis, and hyperemia.
- The vast majority of patients have a benign, chronic course (primary Raynaud's phenomenon).
- Conditions associated with secondary Raynaud's phenomenon include systemic rheumatic syndromes, occupational (vibration) injury, and drug or chemical exposure.

FEATURES OF RAYNAUD'S PHENOMENON

- Episodic attacks of color changes (white, blue, or red) of the fingers induced by exposure to cold (or stress).
- Attacks typically last for minutes to hours.
- On rewarming, the digits may become bright red with throbbing pain.
- Occasionally the toes, tip of the nose, ear lobes, or nipples may be involved.

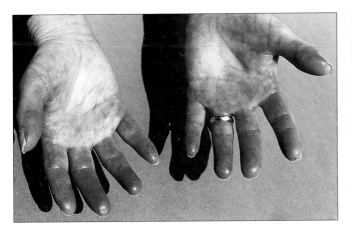

Fig. 31.1 Raynaud's phenomenon. Sharply demarcated cyanosis of the fingers with proximal venular congestion (livedo reticularis) is seen.

digits on exposure to the cold and that are sometimes induced by emotional stimuli. Often only a portion of the digit is affected and typically the thumbs are spared. The classic tricolor change (white to blue to red) described in most textbooks is rarely volunteered by patients, most of whom describe only blanching of the digits accompanied by numbness. During the attacks, one or more of the fingers or toes may be numb and may be described as 'dead'. On rewarming, the digits may become bright red and throbbing pain may occur. When pain is a prominent symptom in the ischemic phase, a secondary cause is likely. Attacks may last for minutes to hours. Patients may experience one or more attacks per cold season or multiple attacks throughout the year. Although the fingers and toes are most commonly involved, the attacks may involve the nose, ear lobes, or nipples.

A careful review of systems is important to screen for symptoms of connective tissue disease (arthralgias, arthritis, dysphagia, heartburn, rash, photosensitivity, skin changes, muscle weakness, or sicca), a drug-related etiology, an obstructive arterial disease (intermittent claudication), continuous finger trauma, and exposure to vibratory tools.

! POINTS TO LOOK OUT FOR

- Trophic changes of the digit (loss of pulp, ulcers, pits, gangrene) indicates severe ischemia.
- Tightness or thickening of the skin suggests scleroderma (see Chapter 33).
- Dysphagia, esophageal reflux, or dyspnea suggests scleroderma (see Chapter 33).

INVESTIGATIONS

LABORATORY TESTS

A CBC, ESR, and ANA are obtained for all patients to screen for connective tissue diseases. Laboratory studies are normal in patients with primary Raynaud's phenomenon. A high ESR or high titers of ANA suggest a connective tissue disease.

NAILFOLD CAPILLARY MICROSCOPY

Nailfold capillary microscopy is a useful procedure to distinguish primary from secondary Raynaud's phenomenon. Capillary microscopy may be performed with a hand-held ophthalmoscope at powers <20D with water-soluble gels (such as K-Y jelly) as the moisturizing agent to increase transluceny of the epidermis. Whereas patients with primary Raynaud's phenomenon have capillaries of relatively normal and uniform appearance, patients with Raynaud's phenomenon secondary to connective tissue diseases typically have enlarged, deformed capillary loops surrounded by avascular areas (Fig. 31.2).

IMAGING

Digital angiography is occasionally indicated in patients for whom reconstructive vascular surgery is considered. Patients with Raynaud's phenomenon and a positive Adson's test (loss of radial pulse with neck extension and rotation of the head to the side examined) should have a chest radiograph to look for a cervical rib.

DIFFERENTIAL DIAGNOSIS

In patients with unequivocal Raynaud's phenomenon, the challenge in diagnosis is to determine whether the patient has a primary or secondary form of the disease (Fig. 31.3). The connective tissue diseases, particularly scleroderma (see Chapter 33), are the most common cause of secondary Raynaud's phenomenon.

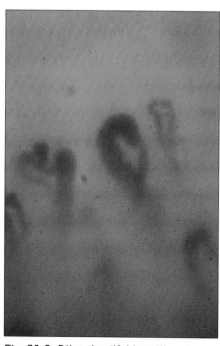

Fig. 31.2 Dilated nailfold capillary loops in Raynaud's phenomenon. Dilatation and dropout of capillaries may suggest eventual evolution to connective tissue disease.

Raynaud's phenomenon may occasionally be confused with other conditions that cause color changes or symptoms in the digits, such as cold digits, chilblain (pernio), livedo reticularis, and acrocyanosis. Many patients complain of cold, sometimes painful, digits that do not undergo color changes. This condition probably represents one extreme of the spectrum of normal sympathetic nervous system activity. Chilblain is an inflammatory condition of the skin of the extremities induced by cold. Patients develop a bluish-red discoloration and edema, which typically involves the lower limb, associated with warmth, erythema, and burning. Livedo reticularis is a bluish discoloration of the skin of the extremities with a characteristic lacy, irregular appearance. The bluish discoloration becomes more intense on exposure to cold and may disappear in a warm environment. Most patients are entirely asymptomatic, although livedo reticularis may be a feature of the antiphospholipid syndrome, in which patients are at increased risk for venous and arterial thromboses, thrombocytopenia, and pregnancy losses (see Chapter 33). In acrocyanosis, the hands and (less commonly) the feet develop a persistent, bluish discoloration. The blue color is intensified by exposure to cold, and becomes purplish or red by warming; a pallor phase is absent. The skin is cold and the palms are often wet and clammy from sweat. Trophic changes or ulcerations are rarely observed.

Rx MANAGEMENT

The management of Raynaud's phenomenon (either primary or secondary) is guided by the frequency and severity of attacks and complications from ischemia (Fig. 31.4). Secondary forms of Raynaud's phenomenon also require treatment directed at the underlying medical disorder, discontinuation of drugs implicated as the cause of the vasospasm, or occupation modifications.

PATIENT EDUCATION AND SELF-HELP

Mild Raynaud's phenomenon is generally easy to control with lifestyle changes to minimize exposure to the cold, such as dressing warmly with loosely fitted, layered clothing and keeping the thermostat a few degrees higher than normal. Limiting time spent outdoors in winter or wearing insulated gloves and using hand or foot warmers are usually helpful. Patients are taught to recognize and terminate attacks promptly by returning to a warmer environment and applying local heat to the hands (e.g. placing their hands in warm water or using a hairdryer). Patients are strongly encouraged to stop smoking and to avoid passive smoke situations, since nicotine induces cutaneous vasoconstriction. Stress modification and social support are valuable aspects of treatment to minimize vasoconstriction induced by hyperactivity of the sympathetic nervous system. Counseling, training in relaxation, or medications may be helpful. Some patients benefit from conditioning programs, such as biofeedback training.

DRUG THERAPY

Drug therapy is usually reserved for patients with prolonged or frequent attacks that fail to respond to conservative measures. The calcium channel blockers are, by far, the most widely used and effective of the drugs employed to treat Raynaud's

DIFFERENTIAL DIAGNOSIS OF RAYNAUD'S PHENOMENON
Structural vasculopathies
Large and medium arteries
Thoracic outlet syndrome
Brachiocephalic trunk disease
(atherosclerosis, Takayasu's)
Crutch pressure
Small artery and arteriolar
Systemic lupus erythematosus
Dermatomyositis
Overlap syndromes
Cold injury
Vibration disease
Arteriosclerosis (thromboangiitis obliterans)
Chemotherapy (bleomycin, vinblastine)
Polyvinyl chloride disease
Normal vessels – abnormal blood elements
Cryoglobulinemia
Cryofibrinogenemia
Paraproteinemia
Cold agglutinin disease
Polycythemias
Normal blood vessels – abnormal vasomotion
Primary (idiopathic) Raynaud's phenomenon
Drug-induced (β–blockers, ergots, methysergide)
Pheochromocytoma
Carcinoid syndrome
Other vasospastic disorders (migraine, Prinzmetal)

Fig. 31.3 Differential diagnosis of Raynaud's phenomenon.

phenomenon. Nifedipine (10–20mg t.i.d. or q.i.d) or diltiazem (60mg t.i.d. or q.i.d.) are helpful, although side effects such as fluid retention, light headedness, and heartburn often limit therapy. Both reserpine (0.1–0.5mg daily) and guanethidine (10–40mg daily) increase capillary blood flow in patients during cold exposure and have the advantage of once-a-day administration. Other sympatholytic drugs that may be used include methyldopa, phenoxybenzamine, and tolazoline. Topical nitroglycerin paste (2%) may be beneficial.

TREATMENT OF RAYNAUD'S PHENOMENON	
Mild	Complete abstinence from smoking Keep entire body warm (not just hands) Avoid cold exposure, particularly winter sports
Moderate	Nifedipine Prazosin Topical nitroglycerin

Digital ulcers	Maximal doses of calcium channel blockers
	'Occlusive' dressing:
	  soak in antiseptic liquid, air dry, apply
	  antibiotic ointment, bandage

Acute ischemia	Sympathetic blocks Prostaglandin E$_1$ or prostacyclin (where available) Microvascular surgery Digital sympathectomy
Gangrenous, infected ulcers	Antibiotics Adequate pain control Surgical debridement Amputation (last resort)

Fig. 31.4 Treatment of Raynaud's phenomenon.

SURGERY AND OTHER TREATMENT MODALITIES

Sympathectomy (thoracic, lumbar, or digital) may be a consideration for the management of patients with refractory disabling attacks or with an acutely ischemic digit that is unresponsive to other measures. Surgical debridement or amputation may be required in patients with digital gangrene (Fig. 31.5).

DIET AND COMPLEMENTARY TECHNIQUES

Dietary therapy with fish-oil supplements that contain omega-3 fatty acids may be beneficial in patients with primary, but not secondary, Raynaud's phenomenon.

MONITORING PROGRESSION AND OUTCOME

The vast majority of patients with primary Raynaud's phenomenon have a chronic, stable course with periodic attacks of self-limited digital ischemia and do not require any medical monitoring. Progression to a secondary form, most commonly a connective tissue disease such as scleroderma, occurs in approximately 15% of patients over the first 10 years following the onset. Variables predictive of a transition to a secondary form include nailfold capillary abnormalities, hand swelling, positive Allen's test and ANAs. Patients with secondary Raynaud's phenomenon are much more likely to develop ischemic complications as a result of fixed vasculature damage.

Fig. 31.5 Digital gangrene. Sharply demarcated gangrene of several weeks' duration affecting multiple fingertips in a woman with a recent onset of systemic sclerosis. Ultimately, the disease was managed using surgical debridement.

RECOMMENDATIONS FOR REFERRAL

Subspecialty
- Patients with Raynaud's phenomenon, a positive antinuclear antibody in high titer, and/or symptoms suggestive of a systemic rheumatic disease, should be referred to a rheumatologist for evaluation.

Other
- Patients with severe, acute ischemia ('dead white finger') or evidence of gangrene should be referred to a vascular surgery specialist for management.

SYSTEMIC DISORDERS

32

ANTINUCLEAR ANTIBODY SPECTRUM DISORDERS

Antinuclear antibody (ANA) tests are frequently carried out in patients with signs or symptoms that suggest a rheumatic disease, most commonly as a screening test for systemic lupus erythematosus (SLE). However, positive ANAs can be present in many other diseases, and also in healthy people (Fig. 32.1). Patients with no clear diagnosis who are found to have a positive ANA in the course of evaluation are commonly encountered in clinical practice.

1 TYPICAL CASE IN SPECTRUM OF ANTINUCLEAR ANTIBODY DISORDERS

Margo is a 32-year-old aerobics dance instructor who has presented with fatigue, fevers, and pain in her knees for the past several months. Her older sister, who has similar symptoms, was recently diagnosed as having lupus.

KEY POINTS

- Positive antinuclear antibody test.
- Constitutional, musculoskeletal, or organ-specific signs or symptoms.
- Most common causes include rheumatic diseases, drugs, and normal findings.
- Evaluation requires careful history and physical examination, and chest radiograph, liver enzyme tests, and cultures as appropriate.

Fig. 32.1 Conditions associated with antinuclear antibodies.

CONDITIONS ASSOCIATED WITH ANTINUCLEAR ANTIBODIES	
1. Rheumatic diseases	**5. Pulmonary diseases**
Systemic lupus erythematosus Polymyositis Sjögren's syndrome Scleroderma Vasculitis Rheumatoid arthritis	Idiopathic pulmonary fibrosis Asbestos-induced fibrosis Primary pulmonary hypertension
	6. Chronic infections
	7. Malignancies
2. Normal, healthy individuals	Lymphoma Leukemia Melanoma Solid tumors (ovary, breast, lung, kidney)
Females > males, prevalence increases with age Relatives of patients with rheumatic diseases ? Pregnant females	
	8. Hematologic disorders
	Idiopathic thrombocytopenic purpura Autoimmune hemolytic anemia
3. Drug-induced	
4. Hepatic diseases	**9. Miscellaneous**
Chronic active hepatitis Primary biliary cirrhosis Alcoholic liver disease	Endocrine disorders (type I diabetes mellitus, Graves' disease) Neurologic diseases (multiple sclerosis) End-stage renal failure After organ transplantation

SYSTEMIC DISORDERS

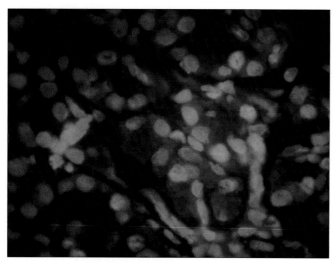

Fig. 32.2 Homogeneous antinuclear antibody immunofluorescence pattern. (Courtesy of Dr N Rothfield.)

Margo is worried that she too might be developing lupus. Physical examination is essentially normal except for a faint blush over the malar regions of her cheeks. No evidence of arthritis, other skin rashes, oral ulcers, or hair loss is found. Laboratory studies reveal normal complete blood count, blood chemistries, and erythrocyte sedimentation rate, and a positive (1:80) ANA in a homogeneous pattern (Fig. 32.2).

! POINTS TO LOOK OUT FOR WITH A POSITIVE ANA TEST

- Fever – suggests a rheumatic disease or infection.
- Weight loss – suggests rheumatic disease, hyperthyroidism, or malignancy.
- Dyspnea – suggests rheumatic disease (particularly scleroderma), pulmonary fibrosis, or primary pulmonary hypertension.

DIFFERENTIAL DIAGNOSIS

There is a broad differential diagnosis for a positive ANA test.

HEALTHY PEOPLE
Normal, healthy people can develop a positive ANA test. In general, the antibody titer is low (<1:80) and of a homogeneous or diffuse pattern. The frequency increases with age (25% by age 60 years), with a higher prevalence in females and in relatives of patients with a rheumatic disease.

RHEUMATIC DISEASES
Virtually all of the systemic, immune-mediated rheumatic disorders are associated with ANAs, including SLE, scleroderma, inflammatory myopathies, Sjögren's syndrome, systemic vasculitis, and rheumatoid arthritis. In general, patients with classic rheumatic diseases have clinical signs and symptoms such that a diagnosis is evident before the results of the ANA test are available. On occasion, testing for disease-specific autoantibodies to nuclear or cytoplasmic antibodies may help to clarify the diagnosis (Fig. 32.3). In some patients, the symptoms and positive ANA test occur as part of an early, undifferentiated rheumatic disease in which patience and time are needed before a diagnosis is possible.

INFECTION
Although ANAs are most commonly associated with chronic infections, almost any acute bacterial or viral disease can cause a transient increase in ANA titers. Acute infectious mononucleosis can be easily confused with SLE and must be considered in the differential diagnosis in young patients who present with a lupus-like syndrome. Up to one-third of patients with Gram-negative urinary tract infections, such as *Klebsiella* spp. and *Escherichia coli* have ANA positivity. Parasitic infections, particularly malaria, have an extraordinarily high prevalence of ANA positivity.

AUTOANTIBODIES HELPFUL IN THE DIAGNOSIS OF SPECIFIC RHEUMATIC DISEASES	
Disease suspected	Autoantibody
Systemic lupus erythematosus	Anti-dsDNA Anti-Sm Anti-Ku
Drug-induced lupus	Antihistones
Mixed connective tissue disease	Anti-RNP
Polymyositis/ dermatomyositis	Anti-Jo-I (histidyl tRNA synthetase)
Scleroderma	Anti-Scl-70 (topoisomerase 1) Anticentromere
Sjögren's syndrome	Anti-Ro(SS-A) Anti-La(SS-B)
Wegener's granulomatosis	Antineutrophil cytoplasmic antibody

Fig. 32.3 Autoantibodies helpful in the diagnosis of specific rheumatic diseases.

LIVER DISEASE

Positive ANA titers have been associated with various forms of chronic liver disease, which include chronic active hepatitis, primary biliary cirrhosis, and even alcoholic liver disease. In viral hepatitis positive for hepatitis B surface antigen, ANAs typically resolve despite persistence of viral markers. Antibodies to centromere proteins develop in patients with primary biliary cirrhosis, and presumably such patients have a forme fruste of limited scleroderma (see Chapter 33).

LUNG DISEASE

Positive ANA titers have been found in a wide range of chronic pulmonary disorders, which include idiopathic pulmonary fibrosis, fibrotic lung disease following asbestos exposure, and primary pulmonary hypertension. The frequency of positive ANA tests is higher in females and correlates with the duration of pulmonary findings, the presence of Raynaud's phenomenon, and digital vasculitis.

DRUGS

Many drugs have been associated with a positive ANA test (Fig. 32.4). Procainamide and hydralazine are, by far, the most frequent offenders, and

DRUGS ASSOCIATED WITH A POSITIVE ANTINUCLEAR ANTIBODY TEST		
Drugs with good evidence of association		
Carbamazepine	Hydralazine	Procainamide
Chlorpromazine	Isoniazid	Quinidine
Diphenylhydantoin	Methyldopa	Sulfasalazine
Ethosuximide	Penicillamine	
Case reports		
Acebutolol	Interferon (α,γ)	Phenylethylacetylurea
Allopurinol	Labetalol	Pindolol
Aminoglutethimide	Leuprolide acetate	Practolol
Amoproxan	Levodopa	Prazosin
Anthiomaline	Levomepromazine	Primidone
Atenolol	Lithium carbonate	Promethazine
Benoxaprofen	Lovastatin	Propranolol
Canavanine (L-)	Mephenytoin	Propylthiouracil
Captopril	Methimazole	Psoralens
Chlorprothixene	Methysergide	Pyrathiazine
Chlorthalidone	Metoprolol	Pyrithoxine
Cimetidine	Minoxidil	Reserpine
Cinnarizine	Nalidixic acid	Spironolactone
Clonidine	Nitrofurantoin	Streptomycin
Danazol	Nomifensine	Sulindac
Dapsone	Oral contraceptives	Sulfadimethoxine
Debrisoquin	Oxprenolol	Sulfamethoxypyridazine
Diclofenac	Oxyphenisatin	Sulfonamides
1,2-Dimethyl-3-hydroxypyride-41 (L1)	Para-aminosalicylic acid	Tetracyclines
	Penicillin	Tetrazine
Disopyramide	Perazine	Thionamide
Ethylphenacemide	Perphenazine	Thioridazine
Gold salts	Phenelzine	Timolol
Griseofulvin	Phenopyrazone	Tolazamide
Hydrazines	Phenylbutazone	Tolmetin
Ibuprofen		Trimethadione

Fig. 32.4 Drugs associated with a positive antinuclear antibody test.

RECOMMENDATIONS FOR REFERRAL

Subspecialty

- Patients with an unexplained positive ANA and clear signs of major internal organ or musculoskeletal involvement should be referred to a rheumatologist for diagnosis.

roughly three-fourths of patients treated with these drugs develop a positive ANA. The vast majority of patients with drug-induced ANAs are entirely asymptomatic and there is no need to discontinue or change drug treatment. A small percentage of patients develop a lupus-like syndrome characterized by fever, and musculoskeletal and pleuropulmonary symptoms (Fig. 32.5). The development of drug-induced lupus requires stopping the drug thought to be responsible for the positive ANA and most symptoms completely resolve within several months.

MALIGNANCY

Various malignancies have been reported to be associated with a positive ANA, including malignant melanoma, leukemias and lymphoma, and solid tumors. In large, granular lymphocytic leukemia – a chronic leukemia of T-cell origin that occurs in a subset of Felty's syndrome – approximately one-half the patients are ANA positive. Disappearance of the antibody has been documented in patients in whom a remission is induced by chemotherapy or following resection of a solid tumor.

RECOMMENDATIONS FOR REFERRAL

In most patients the ANA helps to confirm a clinical diagnosis (i.e. SLE) and referral is generally not indicated. The finding of a positive ANA in healthy people does not require further evaluation.

CLINICAL FEATURES OF PROCAINAMIDE- AND HYDRALAZINE-INDUCED LUPUS		
Clinical features	Procainamide-induced lupus (%)	Hydralazine-induced lupus (%)
Arthralgia	77	85
Myalgia	44	57
Fever	41	38
Skin rash	9	27
Adenopathy	8	14
Hepatomegaly	25	24
Splenomegaly	12	14
Pleuropulmonary conditions	75	30
Pericarditis	16	5
Neuropsychiatric conditions	1	4
Renal	<1	13

Fig. 32.5 Clinical features of procainamide- and hydralazine-induced lupus. (Data from Yung RL, Richardson BC. Drug-induced lupus. Rheum Dis Clin North Am. 1994;20:61–86.)

OTHER SYSTEMIC DISORDERS

INFLAMMATORY MYOPATHIES (MYOSITIS)

IN WHAT CIRCUMSTANCES ARE INFLAMMATORY MYOPATHIES SUSPECTED?

Patients typically present with complaints of proximal muscle weakness, such as falling or finding it difficult to get out of a chair or bathtub, to climb stairs, or to raise their arms above shoulder height. The differential diagnosis of proximal muscle weakness is extensive (Fig. 33.1) – primary neurologic disorders, connective tissue diseases, and cancer are the most common.

DIFFERENTIAL DIAGNOSIS OF MUSCLE WEAKNESS
Denervating conditions: spinal muscular atrophies*, amyotrophic lateral sclerosis*
Neuromuscular junction disorders: Eaton–Lambert syndrome*, myasthenia gravis*
The genetic muscular dystophies: Duchenne's facioscapulohumeral, limb girdle*, Becker's, Emery–Dreifuss type*, distal, ocular
Myotonic diseases: dystrophia myotonica*, myotonia congenita
Congenital myopathies: nemaline, mitochondrial, centronuclear, central core
Glycogen storage diseases: adult onset acid maltase deficiency*, McArdle's disease
Lipid storage myopathies: carnitine deficiency*, carnitine palmityltransferase deficiency*
The periodic paralyses
Myositis ossificans*: generalized and local
Endocrine myopathies*: hypothyroidism, hyperthyroidism, acromegaly, Cushing's disease, Addison's disease, hyperparathyroidism, hypoparathyroidism, vitamin D deficiency myopathy, hypokalemia, hypocalcemia
Metabolic myopathies*: uremia, hepatic failure
Toxic myopathies*: acute and chronic alcoholism, drugs including penicillamine*, clofibrate*, chloroquine, emetine
Nutritional myopathies: vitamin E deficiency*, malabsorption*
Carcinomatous neuromyopathy*: carcinomatous cachexia
Acute rhabdomyolysis*
Proximal neuropathies: Guillain–Barré syndrome*, acute intermittent porphyria*, diabetic lower limb chronic plexopathies*, chronic autoimmune polyneuropathy
Microembolization by atheroma or carcinoma
Polymyalgia rheumatica*
Other collagen vascular diseases: rheumatoid arthritis, scleroderma, systemic lupus erythematosus, polyarteritis nodosa
Infections: acute viral, including influenza, mononucleosis, rickettsia, coxsackievirus, rubella and rubella vaccination, acute bacterial including typhoid
Parasites: including *Toxoplasma*, *Trichinella*, *Schistosoma*, *Cysticercus*, *Sarcosporidia*
Septic myositis: including staphylococcal, streptococcal, *Clostridium perfringens* (*welchii*) and leprosy
* Indicates the conditions that are most commonly confused with muscle weakness.

KEY POINTS

Definition
- Inflammatory myopathies are diseases characterized by acute and chronic inflammation of skeletal muscle.

Main clinical features
- Weakness typically first evident in arms and legs.
- May be accompanied by fever, characteristic rashes, polyarthritis, or dyspnea from interstitial lung disease.

Diagnosis
- Elevations of muscle enzymes (creatine kinase, aldolase, and transaminases) found in essentially all patients.
- Muscle biopsy, electromyogram, or magnetic resonance imaging usually needed to confirm diagnosis.
- Antinuclear antibody positive in the majority of patients.

Fig. 33.1 Differential diagnosis of muscle weakness.

PATTERNS OF DISEASE TYPICAL OF INFLAMMATORY MYOPATHIES	
Myopathy	Pattern
Uncomplicated polymyositis	Disease confined to proximal muscle weakness
Systemic myositis	Fevers, arthritis, and/or overlap with other connective tissue disease. Most serious complication is progressive dyspnea from interstitial lung disease (Fig. 33.3)
Dermatomyositis	Polymyositis in association with characteristic rashes including Gottron's papules (Fig. 33.4), malar rash (Fig. 33.5), and 'machinist's hands' (Fig. 33.6)
Childhood dermatomyositis	Proximal muscle weakness in young children. Disease may be complicated by heliotrope rash over eyelids, subcutaneous calcifications (Fig. 33.7), or systemic vasculitis
Inclusion body myositis	Seen in older patients, predominantly men; presents with both proximal and distal muscle weakness and only mild elevations of muscle enzymes

Fig. 33.2 Patterns of disease typical of inflammatory myopathies.

WHAT PATTERNS OF DISEASE ARE TYPICAL OF INFLAMMATORY MYOPATHIES?

Patterns of disease typical of inflammatory myopathies are outlined in Figure 33.2.

HOW ARE INFLAMMATORY MYOPATHIES MANAGED?

Patients with suspected myositis should be referred to a rheumatologist or neurologist to assist with diagnosis and planning management. High-dose corticosteroids, typically in combination with cytotoxic drugs, are needed in the majority of patients. Rehabilitation programs must be used in conjunction with medical therapies.

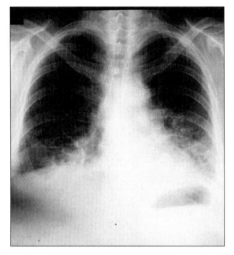

Fig. 33.3 Interstitial lung disease of polymyositis–dermatomyositis. Chest radiograph of a patient with interstitial lung disease and dermatomyositis demonstrating severe basilar fibrosis as well as mid-lung interstitial changes.

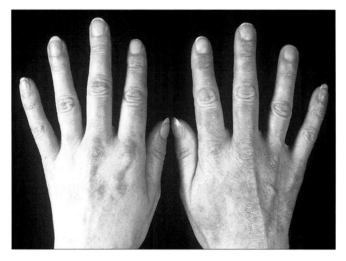

Fig. 33.4. Gottron's papules. Raised red plaques typically affect the knuckles.

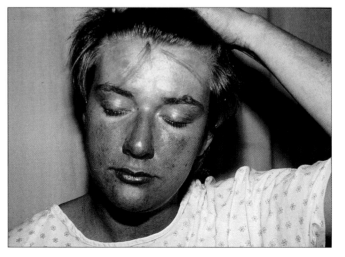

Fig. 33.5 The facial rash of dermatomyositis. Note the malar-like rash of dermatomyositis which involves the nasolabial area (an area often spared in systemic lupus erythematosus). Patchy involvement of the forehead and chin is also present in this patient.

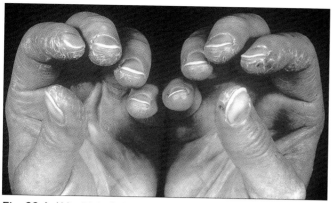

Fig. 33.6 'Machinist's hands'. Note the cracking and fissuring of the distal digital skin of the fingerpads in this patient with dermatomyositis. (Courtesy of Dr Frederick W Miller.)

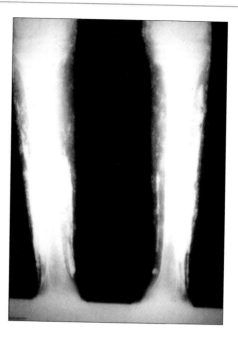

Fig. 33.7 Extensive calcinosis of the legs in a patient with dermatomyositis.

ADULT STILL'S DISEASE

IN WHAT CIRCUMSTANCES IS ADULT STILL'S DISEASE SUSPECTED?

Adult Still's disease is suspected in young patients with unexplained, persistent fevers accompanied by arthritis and other systemic signs of illness, particularly pleuritis or pericarditis or hepatosplenomegaly. The Still's rash is diagnostically helpful, although it is usually intermittent and often so subtle that it is missed by both the patient and physician alike. The clinical picture along with the marked leukocytosis ($\geq 15,000/mm^3$) and increase in neutrophils usually first suggest infection and require blood and fluid cultures, skin testing, and other serologies, which are found to be normal. Diffuse systemic diseases such as rheumatoid arthritis or systemic lupus are considered, although the absence of a rheumatoid factor or antinuclear antibody indicate the problem is not one of these disorders.

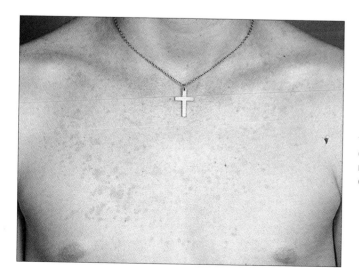

Fig. 33.8 Still's rash. The faint salmon-colored rash of Still's disease. Although the rash is most common on the trunk and upper extremities, it may also be seen on the face.

KEY POINTS

Definition
- Adult Still's disease is an acute febrile syndrome of young (16–35 years old) adults.

Main clinical features
- High-spiking, daily fevers ($\geq 39°C$), arthralgia, or arthritis, transient maculopapular rash (Fig. 33.8), sore throat, lymphadenopathy, hepatosplenomegaly, and pleuritis/pericarditis.
- Elevation of erythrocyte sedimentation rate, anemia, and leukocytosis.

Diagnosis
- In absence of characteristic Still's rash, the disease is typically diagnosed late after infectious diseases or other disorders associated with chronic, unexplained fevers (Fig. 33.9) have been excluded.
- Criteria that are helpful once the disease is considered are given in Figure 33.10.

247

DIFFERENTIAL DIAGNOSIS OF ADULT STILL'S DISEASE	
Granulomatous disorders	Sarcoidosis, idiopathic granulomatous hepatitis, Crohn's disease
Vasculitis	Serum sickness, polyarteritis nodosa, Wegener's granulomatosis, thrombotic thrombocytopenic purpura, Takayasu's arteritis
Infection	Viral infection, such as hepatitis B, rubella, parvovirus, coxsackie, Epstein–Barr virus, cytomegalovirus, or human immunodeficiency virus Subacute bacterial endocarditis, chronic meningococcemia, tuberculosis, Lyme disease, syphilis, rheumatic fever
Malignancy	Leukemia, lymphoma, angioblastic lymphadenopathy
Connective tissue disease	Systemic lupus erythematosus, mixed connective tissue disease

Fig. 33.9 Differential diagnosis of adult Still's disease.

CRITERIA FOR THE DIAGNOSIS OF ADULT STILL'S DISEASE
A diagnosis of adult Still's disease requires the presence of all of the following:
Fever ≥39°C
Arthralgia or arthritis
Rheumatoid factor <1:80
Antinuclear antibody <1:100
in addition to any two of the following:
White blood cell count ≥15,000cells/mm^3
Still's rash
Pleuritis or pericarditis
Hepatomegaly, splenomegaly, or generalized lymphadenopathy

Fig. 33.10 Criteria for the diagnosis of adult Still's disease. (Adapted from Cush JJ, Medsger Jr TA, Christy WC, Herbert DC, Cooperstein LA. Adult-onset Still's disease: clinical course and outcome. Arthritis Rheum. 1987;30:186–94.)

HOW IS ADULT'S STILL'S DISEASE MANAGED?

Patients with suspected adult Still's disease should be referred to a rheumatologist to help with the diagnosis and plan drug management. Nonsteroidal anti-inflammatory drugs (NSAIDs) or corticosteroids are useful in the early stages of the disease, and second-line antirheumatic drugs are beneficial in patients who develop a chronic course, typically with polyarthritis.

VASCULITIS SYNDROMES

KEY POINTS

Definition
- Vasculitis syndromes are serious, life-threatening, systemic rheumatic disorders caused by inflammation within and through the walls of arteries and veins leading to ischemia.

Main clinical features
- Systemic signs of illness (fever, weight loss, anorexia) in association with dysfunction of affected organs.
- Polyarthritis often accompanies the vasculitis.
- Mono- or polyneuropathy, glomerulonephritis, bowel ischemia or infarction, multifocal neurologic events, and pulmonary infiltrates or nodules are examples of organ pathology secondary to vasculitis.

Diagnosis
- Definitive diagnosis generally requires tissue biopsy with findings of vascular inflammation.
- Angiography is useful in patients with medium-sized or large-vessel disease.
- Antineutrophil cytoplasmic antibody is positive in patients with pulmonary–renal vasculitis syndromes.

IN WHAT CIRCUMSTANCES IS VASCULITIS SUSPECTED?

Most patients initially present with generalized disease characterized by anorexia, weight loss, and fever, which suggest either cancer or an infection. The presence of physical findings related to the skin, nervous system, or vital organ provides clues to vasculitis. Vasculitis is divided into syndromes based on size and type of blood vessels affected and, in particular, on distinctive clinical features (Fig. 33.11).

PATTERNS OF DISEASE TYPICAL OF VASCULITIS

There are several major disease patterns typical of vasculitis (Fig. 33.12). Characteristic clinical findings include palpable purpura (Fig. 33.13), urticarial lesions (Fig. 33.14) and necrotizing vasculitis with ulcerations (Fig. 33.15).

Fig. 33.11 Key clinical features that distinguish the major vasculitis syndromes.

KEY CLINICAL FEATURES THAT DIFFERENTIATE THE MAJOR VASCULITIC SYNDROMES			
Vasculitis syndrome	Age range (years)	Sex ratio (M:F)	Major clinical features
Takayasu's	15–25	1:9	Arm or leg claudication, decreased pulses, subclavian/aortic bruit
Giant cell arteritis	60–75	1:3	Headache, tongue or jaw claudication, hip or shoulder girdle stiffness, diplopia
Polyarteritis	40–60	2:1	Weight loss, livedo reticularis, mono/polyneuropathy, hypertension
Churg–Strauss	40–60	2:1	Asthma, atopic history, mono/polyneuropathy, pulmonary infiltrates, eosinophilia
Primary angiitis of central nervous system	30–50	1:2	Severe headache, progressive dementia, multifocal neurologic events
Wegener's granulomatosis	30–50	1:1	Sinusitis, oral ulcers, otitis media, hemoptysis, active urinary sediment
Leukocytoclastic vasculitis	30–50	1:1	Palpable purpura, maculopapular rash, medication history
Behçet's	20–35	1:1	Oral or genital ulcers, folliculitis, uveitis, thrombophlebitis
Kawasaki disease	1–5	1.5:1	Fever, conjunctivitis, cervical adenopathy, mucositis, polymorphous exanthema
Lymphomatoid granulomatosis	40–60	2:1	Pulmonary symptoms (cough, progressive dyspnea), constitutional (fever sweats, weight loss)
Henoch–Schönlein purpura	5–20	1:1	Palpable purpura, abdominal pain, bloody diarrhea

PATTERNS OF DISEASE TYPICAL OF VASCULITIS	
Vasculitis	Pattern
Cutaneous vasculitis	Palpable purpura, urticarial lesions, and nodular or ulcerative lesions most common
Mono- or polyneuropathy	Typically affects median (weakness of opposing thumb and little finger), ulnar (weakness of finger or adductors), common and deep peroneal (foot drop), and tibial (weakness of plantar flexion) nerves
Single or multiple organ system failure	Glomerulonephritis, pneumonitis, ischemia of gastrointestinal tract, focal or diffuse neurologic dysfunction

Fig. 33.12 Patterns of disease typical of vasculitis.

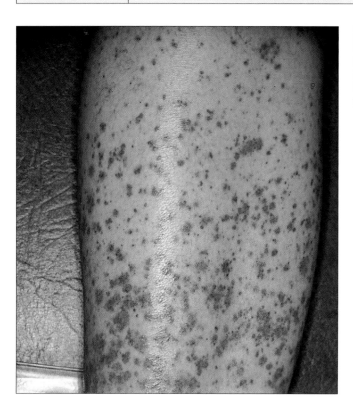

Fig. 33.13 Palpable purpura representing a leukocytoclastic vasculitis.

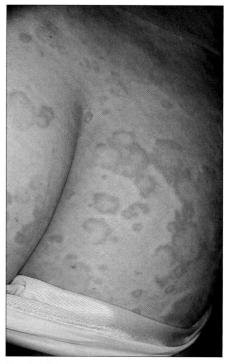

Fig. 33.14 Urticarial vasculitis.

Fig. 33.15 Severe ulcers of the lower leg caused by necrotizing vasculitis in rheumatoid arthritis.

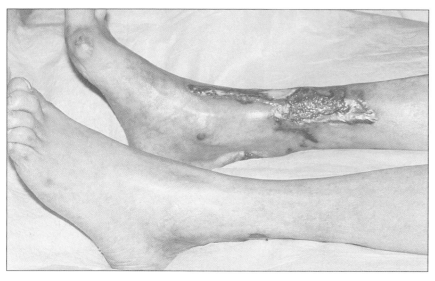

HOW ARE VASCULITIS SYNDROMES MANAGED?

Prompt referral of patients with suspected vasculitis to a rheumatologist is critical. Vasculitis syndromes are potentially life-threatening and early diagnosis and aggressive treatment are key to successful management. Vascular imaging studies (Fig. 33.16) and/or biopsy of affected organs (Fig. 33.17) help to confirm the diagnosis. Drug management differs among the various vasculitis syndromes; in general, courses of high-dose corticosteroids combined with cytotoxic drugs are important in patients with serious vasculitis.

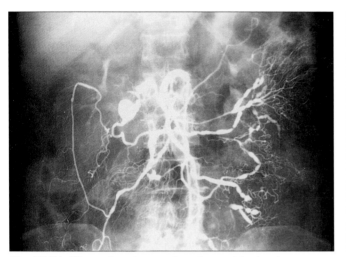

Fig. 33.16 Visceral angiogram in polyarteritis showing areas of segmental narrowing and aneurysms. (With permission from Conn DL. Polyarteritis. In: Conn DL, ed. Rheumatic Disease Clinics of North America, Ch. 7. Philadelphia: WB Saunders; 1990:341–62.)

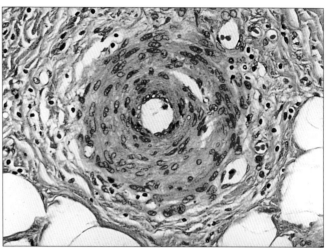

Fig. 33.17 Chronic polyarteritis with intimal proliferation and chronic fibrotic changes. (With permission from Conn DL. Polyarteritis. In: Conn DL, ed. Rheumatic Disease Clinics of North America, Ch. 7. Philadelphia: WB Saunders; 1990:341–62.)

BEHÇET'S SYNDROME

IN WHAT CIRCUMSTANCES IS BEHÇET'S SYNDROME SUSPECTED?

Severe, recurrent, aphthous ulcers are seen in virtually all patients with Behçet's syndrome and provide the initial clue to the diagnosis. Other often helpful clinical features include the presence of follicular or pustular lesions (Fig. 33.18) and chronic, relapsing bilateral uveitis, which may produce an exudate of white cells that settles in the anterior chamber of the eye (Fig. 33.19). Behçet's syndrome is one the few vasculitis syndromes to affect large veins and must be considered in patients with a diffuse systemic disorder associated with thrombophlebitis or occlusion of the more central veins (Fig. 33.20).

HOW IS BEHÇET'S SYNDROME MANAGED?

Colchicine, topical corticosteroids to oral and genital ulcers, and NSAIDs for arthritis have a general role in the management of most patients. Patients with uveitis require prompt referral to an ophthalmologist – mydriatic agents are used in the initial stages of the disease to prevent synechiae formation and cyclosporine is important in patients with severe, progressive disease. High-dose corticosteroids combined with cytotoxics are used in patients with central nervous system involvement. The role of anticoagulation in patients with thrombophlebitis is less clear.

KEY POINTS

Definition
- Behçet's syndrome is a form of systemic vasculitis that affects arteries and veins of all sizes.
- Most commonly seen in patients from Eastern Mediterranean countries (Turkey, Iran, and North Africa) and Japan.

Main clinical features
- Oral and genital ulcers, skin lesions that resemble erythema nodosum or acne, bilateral uveitis, thrombophlebitis, arthritis, and neurologic abnormalities.

Diagnosis
- Clinical diagnosis based on characteristic syndrome complex.
- So-called 'pathergy' reaction with the formation of a papule or pustule after minor trauma to the skin may help in the diagnosis.

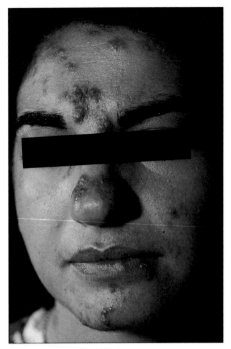

Fig. 33.18 Follicular and pustular lesions. These are not usually distinguishable from severe acne.

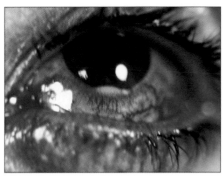

Fig. 33.19 Hypopyon uveitis. A precipitate of white cells is formed in the anterior chamber of the eye.

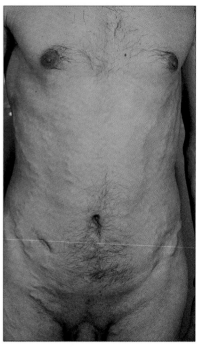

Fig. 33.20 Vena caval obstruction leading to collaterals.

ANTIPHOSPHOLIPID SYNDROME

KEY POINTS

Definition
- Antiphospholipid syndrome involves recurrent venous or arterial thromboses, pregnancy loss, and thrombocytopenia associated with elevated levels of antiphospholipid antibodies.

Main clinical features
- Recurrent deep and superficial venous thromboses, strokes, or transient ischemic attacks, and spontaneous abortions.
- Rare findings include thrombocytopenia, vegetations on cardiac valve leaflets that lead to valvular insufficiency, and migraine headaches.

Diagnosis
- Medium-to-high titer of immunoglobulin G anticardiolipin antibodies (enzyme-linked immunosorbent assay) or a positive lupus anticoagulant test is required for diagnosis.

IN WHAT CIRCUMSTANCES IS ANTIPHOSPHOLIPID SYNDROME SUSPECTED?

The antiphospholipid syndrome is suspected in women with multiple, failed pregnancies (spontaneous abortion or fetal wastage) or in patients with recurrent thrombotic events that involve veins or arteries. Most patients have prominent livedo reticularis of the skin (Fig. 33.21), which provides a ready clue to the diagnosis. Laboratory abnormalities suggestive of the syndrome include biologic false-positive tests for syphilis as well as unexplained elevations of the partial thromboplastin time. The antiphospholipid syndrome often coexists with systemic lupus erythematosus, and a number of other causes of recurrent venous thromboses need to be excluded (Fig. 33.22).

HOW IS ANTIPHOSPHOLIPID SYNDROME MANAGED?

For patients with the antiphospholipid syndrome who have not had thrombosis, prophylaxis with aspirin (325mg daily) is recommended. Acute management of venous or arterial thrombosis requires anticoagulation with warfarin. Typically, patients with recurrent thromboses are placed on chronic (?life-long) anticoagulant treatment. Pregnant women with

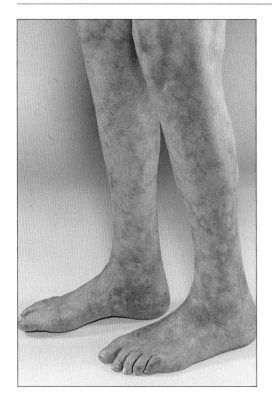

Fig. 33.21 Livedo reticularis. (With permission from Conn DL. Polyarteritis. In: Conn DL, ed. Rheumatic Disease Clinics of North America, Ch. 7. Philadelphia: WB Saunders; 1990:341–62.)

DISEASE STATES THAT SHOULD BE EXCLUDED IN PATIENTS WITH UNEXPLAINED VENOUS THROMBOSIS	
Malignancy	Protein C deficiency
Nephrotic syndrome	Protein S deficiency
Polycythemia	Factor V Leyden
Thrombocytosis	Dysfibrinogenemia
Antithrombin-III deficiency	Paroxysmal nocturnal hemoglobinuria
	Homocystinuria

Fig. 33.22 Disease states that should be excluded in patients with unexplained venous thrombosis.

the antiphospholipid syndrome are best managed by high-risk obstetric specialists who carry out regular ultrasound and Doppler studies to detect evidence of fetal distress. Warfarin cannot be used in pregnant females, and subcutaneous heparin, intravenous immunoglobulin, and prednisone have all been shown to prevent fetal loss.

HYPERMOBILITY SYNDROME

IN WHAT CIRCUMSTANCES IS HYPERMOBILITY SYNDROME SUSPECTED?

Hypermobility syndrome is considered in patients with complaints that involve multiple joints but who have no evidence of synovitis on examination. Most patients are 'double-jointed' and able to extend joints well beyond normal limits (Fig. 33.23). Hyperextensions of the fingers, elbows, knees, and wrists (Fig. 33.24) and a provisional set of diagnostic criteria (Fig. 33.25) are used in diagnosis. Skin findings (thinning, striae, scars) or mitral valve prolapse provide clues to the diagnosis. Hypermobility syndrome must be distinguished from Marfan's syndrome, Ehlers–Danlos syndrome, and osteogenesis imperfecta.

HOW IS HYPERMOBILITY SYNDROME MANAGED?

Patients should be reassured of the benign nature of the disorder. Drugs have no role in the management and a regular program of stretching exercises is often of benefit (Fig. 33.26).

KEY POINTS

Definition
- A syndrome of generalized ligamentous and skin laxity in otherwise healthy individuals.

Main clinical features.
- Joint hypermobility with the development of traumatic and overuse injuries, typically of the shoulder, patella, metacarpophalangeal or temporomandibular joints; patients may develop chronic noninflammatory arthropathy of affected joints.

Diagnosis
- The diagnosis is based on the patient's ability to perform a series of exaggerated joint movements (Beighton Scoring System).

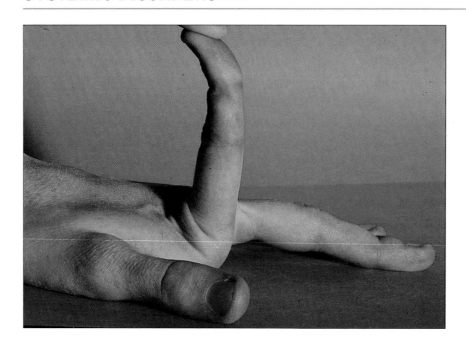

Fig. 33.23 Hypermobility of the finger in hypermobility syndrome.

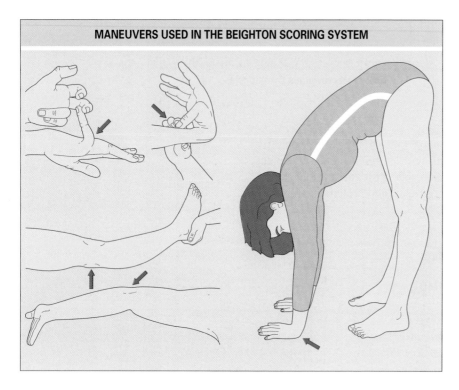

MANEUVERS USED IN THE BEIGHTON SCORING SYSTEM

Fig. 33.24 Maneuvers used in the Beighton scoring system for joint hypermobility.

PROVISIONAL SET OF DIAGNOSTIC CRITERIA FOR HYPERMOBILITY SYNDROME

Major criteria

Beighton score of 4/9 or greater (either currently or historically)

Arthralgia for longer than 3 months in four or more joints

Minor criteria

Beighton score of 1–3/9 (0–3 if over 50 years of age)

Arthralgia in 1–3 joints, back pain, spondylosis, spondylolisthesis

Dislocation in more than one joint, or in one joint or more on more than one occasion

Three or more soft tissue lesions (e.g. epicondylitis, tenosynovitis, bursitis)

Marfanoid habitus (tall, slim, span >height, upper segment:lower segment ratio ⩽0.89, arachnodactyly)

Skin striae, hyperextensibility, thin skin or abnormal scarring

Eye signs: drooping eyelids, myopia or antimongoloid slant

Varicose veins, hernia or uterine/rectal prolapse

Mitral valve prolapse (by echocardiography)

Hypermobility syndrome diagnosis requires

Two major criteria *or*

one major- two minor criteria *or*

four minor criteria *or*

two minor criteria and unequivocally affected first-degree relative

Hypermobility syndrome is excluded by presence of Marfan or Ehlers–Danlos syndromes

Fig. 33.25 Proposed diagnostic criteria for hypermobility syndrome.

EXAMPLES OF MUSCLE STRETCHING EXERCISES FOR SYMPTOMATIC JOINTS

Fig. 33.26 Examples of muscle stretching exercises. The patient can learn and perform these for whichever joints are symptomatic.

SCLERODERMA

IN WHAT CIRCUMSTANCES IS SCLERODERMA SUSPECTED?

Scleroderma is suspected in patients with Raynaud's phenomenon who develop changes of the skin or show evidence of gastrointestinal, pulmonary, or kidney disease. Skin changes are often first noticed in the hands with diffuse edema (Fig. 33.27), which may progress to tightening with contractures in advanced disease (Fig. 33.28). In generalized scleroderma, skin thickening and contractures also develop on the trunk (Fig. 33.29) and the face (Fig. 33.30). Additional skin findings that may be seen in scleroderma include telangiectasias (Fig. 33.31), subcutaneous calcifications (Figs 33.32 & 33.33) and localized skin lesions such as morphea or linear scleroderma (Fig. 33.34). Gastrointestinal (dysphagia, reflux) and pulmonary (dyspnea on exertion, nonproductive cough)

KEY POINTS

Definition
* Scleroderma is a generalized disorder of connective tissue that affects the skin and internal organs.

Main clinical features
* Raynaud's phenomenon, tightening and thickening of the skin, esophageal and small bowel dysfunction, dyspnea secondary to pulmonary fibrosis, severe hypertension and renal failure (renal crisis).

Diagnosis
* Diagnosis based on characteristic clinical findings.
* Antinuclear antibody positive in the majority of patients.

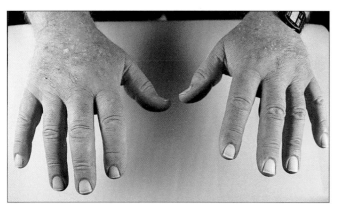

Fig. 33.27 Early puffy scleroderma. Extensive edema of the fingers and hands in a man with several months of preceding Raynaud's phenomenon. The skin was not clinically thickened, but became so on follow up.

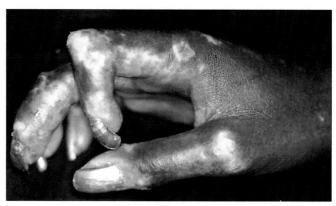

Fig. 33.28 Digital and hand scleroderma. Here, advanced changes of scleroderma have caused digital contractions and limitation of finger movement.

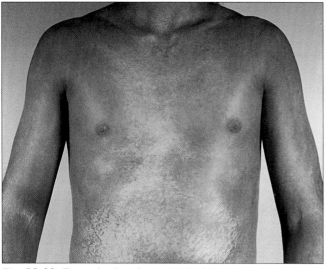

Fig. 33.29 Truncal scleroderma. Skin thickening of the chest and abdomen of a patient with diffuse scleroderma. Both hyperpigmentation and hypopigmentation are demonstrated.

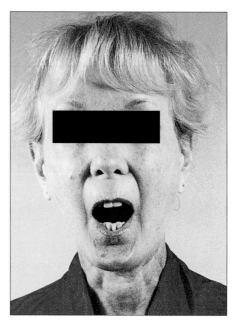

Fig. 33.30 Facial scleroderma. Taut, smooth skin over the face of a woman with long-standing disease. Her oral aperture is reduced and radial furrowing is present about the lips.

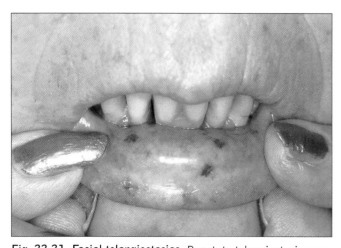

Fig. 33.31 Facial telangiectasias. Punctate telangiectasias are present on the lips and cheeks of this woman with long-standing, limited scleroderma.

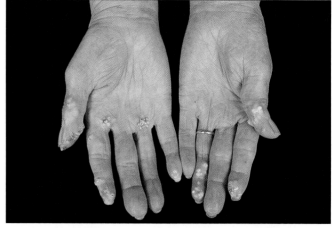

Fig. 33.32 Calcific subcutaneous deposits in the fingers. This patient has limited scleroderma (calcinosis cutis, Raynaud's phenomenon, esophageal dysfunction, sclerodactyly and telangiectasia syndrome).

are common. Approximately 10% of patients present with (or develop) accelerated hypertension with rapidly progressive renal failure (scleroderma renal crisis). Scleroderma must be differentiated from a broad range of disorders that produce skin thickening or have similar major organ involvement (Fig. 33.35).

PATTERNS OF DISEASE TYPICAL OF SCLERODERMA
Patterns of disease typical of scleroderma are given in Figure 33.36.

HOW IS SCLERODERMA MANAGED?
Patients with suspected scleroderma should be referred to a rheumatologist to assist with diagnosis and in most cases to assume primary management. Drug therapies are aimed at vascular ischemia, immune modulation, and fibrosis. Angiotensin-converting enzyme inhibitors play an important role in scleroderma renal crisis and the combination of corticosteroids and cytotoxic drugs stabilizes pulmonary function in patients with progressive pulmonary fibrosis.

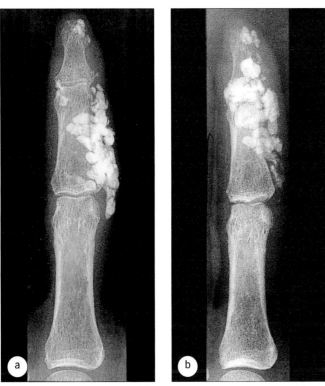

Fig. 33.33 Soft-tissue calcifications. (a) The soft tissue of the fingers in a patient with scleroderma has calcifications. (b) Following treatment with low-dose sodium warfarin for 18 months, the calcifications redistributed but with no decrease in extent.

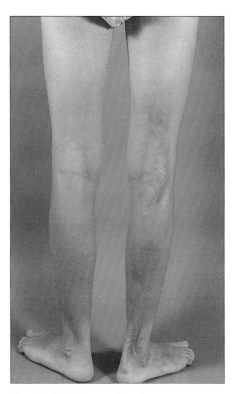

Fig. 33.34 Linear scleroderma. Present since 5 years of age in this 12-year-old girl, atrophy of the thigh and calf are apparent. As growth continues, leg length discrepancy is anticipated.

DIFFERENTIAL DIAGNOSIS OF SCLERODERMA

Disorders characterized by similar presentations	Disorders characterized by skin thickening

Systemic lupus erythematosus
Rheumatoid arthritis
Inflammatory myopathy
	Affecting the fingers
	   Diabetic digital sclerosis
	   Vinyl chloride disease
	   Vibration syndrome
	   Bleomycin-induced scleroderma
	   Chronic reflex sympathetic dystrophy
	   Amyloidosis
	   Acrodermatitis

Disorders characterized by similar visceral features	

Primary pulmonary hypertension
Primary biliary cirrhosis
Idiopathic intestinal hypomotility
Collagenous colitis
Idiopathic interstitial pulmonary fibrosis
	Sparing the fingers
	   Scleredema/scleromyxedema
	   Eosinophilic fasciitis
	   Eosinophilia–myalgia syndrome
	   Generalized subcutaneous morphea
	   Fibrosis associated with augmentative mammoplasty
	   Amyloidosis
	   Carcinoid syndrome
	   Pentazocine-induced scleroderma

Fig. 33.35 Differential diagnosis of scleroderma.

PATTERNS OF DISEASE TYPICAL OF SCLERODERMA

Scleroderma	Pattern
Diffuse scleroderma	Truncal and acral skin involvement At risk for interstitial lung disease, gastrointestinal involvement, myocardial involvement, and renal crisis Antibodies to topoisomerase-I (Scl 70) in 30% of patients
Limited scleroderma	Skin involvement restricted to extremities distal to elbows and knees and face At risk for interstitial lung disease and isolated pulmonary hypertension Also referred to as CREST syndrome (subcutaneous calcinosis, Raynaud's phenomenon, esophageal dysmotility, sclerodactyly, and telangiectasis) Anticentromere antibodies in 80% of patients Several forms of limited scleroderma are recognized, including morphea and linear scleroderma
Scleroderma sine scleroderma	Rare syndrome of major organ involvement typical of scleroderma (renal crisis, interstitial fibrosis) in absence of skin changes
Localized scleroderma	Fibrotic reaction limited to the skin without Raynaud's phenomenon or major organ involvement

Fig. 33.36 Patterns of disease typical of scleroderma.

SECTION
6

DISEASES OF THE BONE

AN INTRODUCTION TO DISEASES OF BONE

Bone diseases are an important cause of musculoskeletal symptoms, which may mimic joint diseases and other conditions.

Osteoporosis is by far the most common condition, numerically responsible for far more fractures and problems than all the rest of bone diseases put together. All other bone conditions are comparatively rare, but many are potentially serious, and include: tumors, metabolic disorders of bone, Paget's disease, and osteonecrosis (Fig. 1).

The two key manifestations of bone diseases are fractures and pain. Fractures are most likely to be osteoporotic, but it is possible for them to be secondary to tumors or metabolic bone disease. Bone pain is more likely to be caused by tumors or other forms of bone disease than by simple osteoporosis.

The most important investigation is the plain radiograph, which helps to differentiate the various conditions, as well as to diagnose the presence of fractures. Other imaging and biochemical tests can also be of value (Fig. 2). A diagnostic algorithm for bone diseases is given overleaf.

COMMON FORMS OF BONE DISEASE
• Osteoporosis (with or without fractures)
• Metastatic or primary tumors of bone
• Metabolic bone diseases such as osteomalacia and hyperparathyroidism
• Paget's disease of bone (see Section 8)
• Osteonecrosis

Fig. 1 Common forms of bone disease.

INVESTIGATION OF BONE DISEASE
• Plain radiograph
• Other imaging modalities, such as bone scans and magnetic resonance imaging
• Biochemical investigations, such as serum calcium, phosphorus, alkaline phosphatase, vitamin D, and parathyroid hormone levels

Fig. 2 Investigation of bone disease.

DIAGNOSTIC ALGORITHM FOR BONE DISEASES

1. Is there a fracture?

A recent fracture is suggested by local pain, swelling, and immobility. Old fractures may be most apparent from the history and from kyphosis of the thoracic spine, which often develops silently as a consequence of vertebral collapse in osteoporotic women. Fractures occur with minimal trauma in people with any form of bone disease.

YES

NO

If fractures are present

- The diagnosis is most likely to be osteoporosis, particularly in elderly women.

- If not in the risk category for osteoporosis, and/or if 'bone pain' or features of systemic illness are present consider the possibility of a pathologic fracture.

2. Is the condition symptomatic?

Uncomplicated osteoporosis is generally asymptomatic. Other conditions may cause either generalized aches and pains, or more severe 'bone pain'. Bone pain is characteristically unremitting severe pain that persists at night and is not relieved by rest – this suggests a possible serious cause such as tumor.

YES

NO

If pain is present

- General aches and pains are characteristic of osteomalacia and hyperparathyroidism, and fractures can occur in both.

- Local pain can occur in metabolic bone disease, Paget's disease, or osteonecrosis. Severe, unremitting pain suggests the possibility of a tumor.

3. What risk group does the patient fit into?

This, accompanied by a radiograph, is probably the most important question, as most bone disorders are associated with a clear set of risk factors, and also have characteristic radiographic features.

Condition	Risk factors
Osteoporosis (Ch. 34)	• High age • Female • White; pale skin; thin • Corticosteroid treatment • Early menopause • Low physical activity • Smoking and high alcohol intake
Osteomalacia (Ch. 35)	• Institutionalized patients • Poor diet • Low exposure to sunlight • Gastrointestinal or renal disease
Hyperparathyroidism (Ch. 35)	• Primary is most common in women in their sixth decade • Secondary is usually associated with chronic renal disease • Characterized by 'moans, groans, and stones'
Osteonecrosis (Ch. 35)	• Corticosteroid therapy • Alcoholism • Previous fracture • Hyperlipidemia • Sickle-cell disease, Gaucher's disease, and caisson disease
Metastatic tumors (Ch. 35)	• Usually come from breast, prostate, or lung • Risk factors as for these tumors
Primary tumors of bone (Ch. 35)	• Rare, found in men more than women, younger and middle aged (myeloma, osteoid osteoma and osteosarcoma)
Paget's disease (Ch. 44)	• Common age-related condition • More common in men than in women

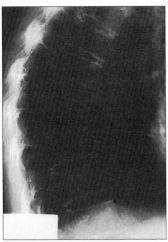

Fig. 3 Radiographic features of osteoporosis.

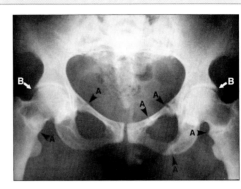

Fig. 4 Radiographic features of osteomalacia.

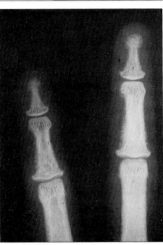

Fig. 5 Radiographic features of hyperparathyroidism.

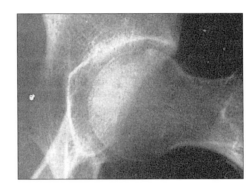

Fig. 6 Radiographic features of osteonecrosis.

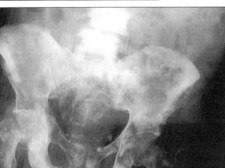

Fig. 7 Radiographic features of metastatic tumors.

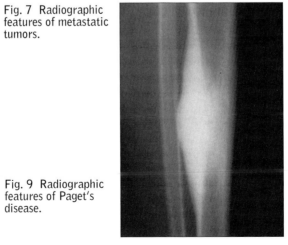

Fig. 8 Radiographic features of primary tumors.

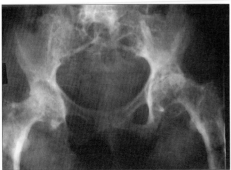

Fig. 9 Radiographic features of Paget's disease.

DISEASES OF BONE

34

OSTEOPOROSIS

Osteoporosis is the most common form of bone disorder, is very strongly age related, and much more common in women than in men. The main consequence of osteoporosis is bone fractures, which particularly affect the vertebrae, hips, and wrists, and are responsible for a huge health care and social burden in Western society.

TYPICAL CASE: VERTEBRAL OSTEOPOROSIS

Lilly is an 83-year-old Caucasian woman who for the past 15 years has noticed that she has gradually become more bent over. Her grandchildren tell her that she is much shorter than she used to be. She comes to see you because over the previous few months she has experienced discomfort in her back as well as some pains at the bottom of her rib cage.

On examination you find a thin, pale woman with an obvious Dowager's hump (Fig. 34.1a). On examination of the abdomen you find the typical folds of skin caused by loss of height and you note that the bottom ribs abut onto the top of the pelvis, and that Lilly is tender in this area.

FEATURES OF VERTEBRAL OSTEOPOROSIS

- Vertebral osteoporosis is extremely common, especially in elderly women.
- Vertebral compression fractures are the main consequence, and they occur principally between T4 and L5.
- The mean age of first fracture of the vertebrae is 70 years.
- Fractures are often asymptomatic, and many patients gradually develop a kyphosis with height loss and some restriction of activities, with little or no pain.
- As the condition advances, back pain may arise from apophyseal joint damage, and if the ribs rest on the iliac crests this can cause a lot of pain.
- Severe problems, such as spinal cord damage, are rare, although patients can develop restrictive respiratory problems.

KEY POINTS

Definition
- Osteoporosis is clinically defined as reduced bone mass (osteopenia) and increased bone fragility to an extent sufficient to result in fracture with minimal trauma.
- Osteoporosis is the most common disease that affects bone. Fractures are not usually manifest until the patient's bone mass is 30–40% below normal values.
- Osteoporosis is a multifactorial disease and not solely the inevitable consequence of aging.

Clinical features
- Osteoporotic fractures are most frequent in the spine, the hip, and wrist, but virtually any bone can be affected.
- Osteoporosis is more common in women than in men, but is an increasing public health problem in both sexes in aging populations.
- One-third of women over the age of 65 years have vertebral fractures, and the life-time risk of hip fracture in Caucasian women is 16% and in men 5%.
- Osteoporosis is associated with high morbidity and, in the case of hip fracture, increased mortality.
- Osteoporosis is of considerable socioeconomic importance because of the high prevalence of fracture and the enormous costs in health care required to deal with the consequences of these fractures.
- Osteoporosis can be prevented in patients at risk by maximizing peak bone mass and preventing major bone loss. Therapies are also available to restore bone mass in those patients with existing bone loss.

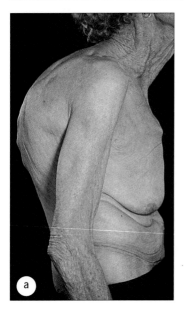
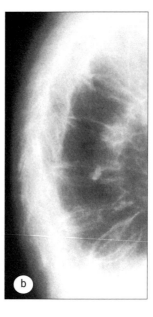

Fig. 34.1 Dowager's hump. (a) Marked thoracic kyphosis due to multiple osteoporotic fractures in an elderly woman with (b) the corresponding radiograph.

You obtain a radiograph, which confirms multiple compression fractures of the thoracic and lumbar spine (Fig. 34.1b). You advise Lilly to take calcium at night, look into possible risk factors for falls, and advise her to use hip protectors to reduce the risk of a hip fracture.

FEATURES OF VERTEBRAL FRACTURES

- Vertebral fractures are very common in elderly women, especially those who have been taking corticosteroids.
- Presentation of vertebral fractures is highly variable, but can involve sudden severe pain after bending, lifting, or coughing.
- Pain is variable in quality, but is usually localized to the site of the fracture, and occasionally radiates anteriorly to the abdomen.
- Acute pain usually subsides within 4–6 weeks, and more persistent pain may mean the diagnosis is incorrect.

2 TYPICAL CASE: SYMPTOMATIC VERTEBRAL FRACTURE

Mary is a 79-year-old woman who has taken corticosteroids for asthma for many years. She presents with a history of the sudden onset of lower thoracic back pain when bending down to pick something off the floor. She has severe localized pain, which is aggravated by movement.

On examination you note a thin, elderly woman who has thin skin and evidence of corticosteroid-related bruising, and a mild kyphosis. She moves very cautiously, keeping her back as rigid as possible. Examination of the spine shows some muscle spasm and she is tender on palpation over the spinous process of T7.

You reassure her that the pain will subside, prescribe analgesics, and advise her to keep as active as possible in spite of the pain. After 1 month she is symptom free, but a few centimeters shorter.

3 TYPICAL CASE: FRACTURE OF THE PROXIMAL FEMUR

Rose is a 77-year-old Caucasian woman who had a mild stroke 4 years ago and has been a little unsteady on her feet ever since. Earlier today she fell gently backward onto the floor of her kitchen and was unable to stand up again, in part because of pain in the groin. She was found by a neighbor, who took her to the emergency room.

On examination you find a thin, pale, frightened woman. She is anxious about any movement of the right leg, which produces groin pain; the right leg appears shorter than the left and is held in external rotation.

A radiograph is obtained (Fig. 34.2), which confirms the suspected diagnosis of a fractured neck of femur; Rose is treated surgically.

FEATURES OF FRACTURED FEMUR

- Femoral fractures are the most important consequence of osteoporosis, being associated with a high morbidity and mortality, as well as high health-care costs.
- Most hip fractures occur with minor falls, usually backward and generally from standing, with no serious trauma.
- Vulnerability to falls (immobility, history of stroke, cognitive impairment, postural hypotension, and dizziness on standing) is an important risk factor for femoral fractures.
- Osteoporosis is the other major risk factor, and the presence of vertebral fractures or a Dowager's hump is a strong risk factor for a femoral fracture.
- Femoral fractures usually cause immediate pain and immobility, although they are occasionally silent.
- Considerable blood loss from the fracture site may occur.
- The leg is usually held rigid and deformities, including shortening and external rotation, are usually present.
- Suspicion of a femoral neck fracture requires immediate hospitalization for surgical treatment.
- Rehabilitation after the fracture is often a major problem.

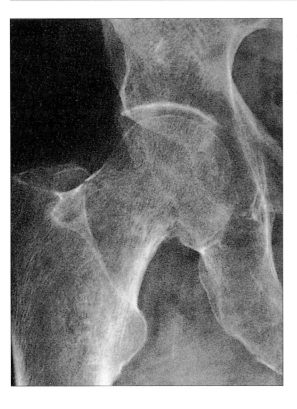

Fig. 34.2 Radiograph from an 77-year-old woman who fell in her kitchen. A typical nondisplaced, midcervical fracture of the femoral neck is seen; note the fracture line in the midcervical region.

FEATURES OF COLLES' FRACTURE

- Colles' fracture is a fracture of the distal radius with dorsal dislocation of the radial fragment.
- Colles' fracture is commonly caused by a forward fall onto the outstretched hand.
- Osteoporosis is an important risk factor, but Colles' fractures are not as strongly related to bone density as vertebral or femoral neck fractures.
- Colles' fracture always results in immediate pain, swelling, and loss of function, and requires prompt treatment.
- Reduction and splinting result in good healing in most cases.
- Mild residual dysfunction, algodystrophy, and carpal tunnel syndrome can develop subsequently, but long-term disability following a Colles' fracture is uncommon.

4 ## TYPICAL CASE: FRACTURE OF THE FOREARM (COLLES' FRACTURE)

Ellen is a 69-year-old Caucasian woman who had a hysterectomy and ovariectomy when aged 45 years, but has otherwise been well all her life. On the first snow storm of the winter, she slips when out shopping, falls forward onto her outstretched left hand, and experiences immediate pain in the wrist. She comes to your office for a consultation.

You note a thin, well-looking, but anxious woman. A deformity of the wrist is obvious, as is much pain on any attempted movement. You take a radiograph, on which a Colles' fracture is confirmed (Fig. 34.3). You refer her to the orthopedic surgeon; the wrist is reduced under anesthetic and splinted. It heals well.

Some years later Ellen develops carpal tunnel syndrome of the left wrist, which requires surgical decompression.

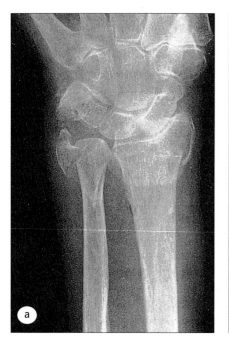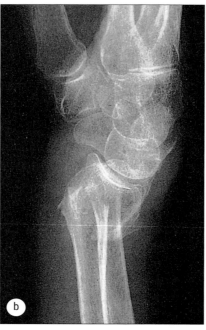

Fig. 34.3 Radiographs of the distal forearm demonstrate the features of Colles' fracture. (a) On the posteroanterior projection a decrease in the radial angle and an associated fracture of the distal ulna are evident. (b) The lateral view reveals the dorsal angulation of the distal radius, as well as a reversal of the palmar inclination. On both views the radius is foreshortened secondary to bayonet-type displacement.

RISK FACTORS FOR FRACTURES	
Risk factors for osteoporosis:	Family history positive
	Female
	White, fair, pale skinned
	Thin body habitus
	Late menarche/early menopause
	Nulliparity
	Low dietary calcium
	Sedentary lifestyle
	Smoking and excess drinking
	Drugs (corticosteroids, anticonvulsants)
Risk factors for falls:	Immobility
	History of stroke
	Cognitive impairment
	Dizziness on standing
	Postural hypotension
	Poor vision
	Environment (e.g. slippery floors)
Force of impact:	Type of fall (e.g. forward or backward)
	Protection available (e.g. hip protectors)

Fig. 34.4 Risk factors for osteoporosis and falls.

NATURAL HISTORY AND OTHER CLINICAL FEATURES

Osteoporosis is a condition characterized by a gradual decrease of bone density. By the time it presents with one fracture, the threshold below which fractures are common has obviously been reached, and the patient is at risk of sustaining further fractures.

As fractures of the hip have more severe consequences than any other type, it is important to find ways of preventing hip fractures. These include diagnosing and treating osteoporosis and countering the risk factors both for the disease and for falls (Fig. 34.4), which may require the use of hip protectors and consideration of whether bone density might be improved by treatment.

Although fractures of the vertebrae, femur, and wrist are by far the most common, fractures can occur at any other site, including the ribs and upper limbs.

Osteoporosis is often accompanied by comorbidities, which render the consequences of any fracture more devastating and the need for treatment more urgent.

 POINTS TO LOOK OUT FOR

The diagnosis of an osteoporotic fracture is generally straightforward. However, other causes of fractures occur in older people, which include osteomalacia and neoplasia, and if the patient does not have risk factors for osteoporosis (see Fig. 34.4), another cause is likely.

A pathologic fracture caused by neoplasia can be difficult to differentiate from an osteoporotic fracture, and sophisticated imaging techniques such as computed tomography (CT) or magnetic resonance imaging may be needed to confirm the diagnosis. Features that might suggest a neoplastic cause include general ill health, recent weight loss and other systemic features of neoplastic disease, and persistent bone pain, which does not subside within a few weeks of the fracture.

Osteomalacia might be suspected if patients have generalized aches and pains and/or muscle weakness, and if the bones are tender. Biochemical investigations are needed to make the diagnosis (decreased calcium and vitamin D levels, increased alkaline phosphatase).

The diagnosis of osteoporosis and osteoporotic fractures in men requires a high index of suspicion. Osteoporotic fractures are not uncommon in elderly men, the chief risk factors being age, hypogonadism, corticosteroids, and alcohol abuse, as well as falls.

INVESTIGATIONS

Over recent years the increasing awareness of osteoporosis in the population has led to increasing demands from the public for regular special investigations, particularly to assess bone density. However, the use of bone density and other investigations in osteoporosis remains a contentious issue.

When considering the investigation of osteoporosis it is particularly important to remember that no investigation can be justified if patient management will not be influenced by the result.

Investigations might be indicated to:

- detect or assess fractures
- aid the differential diagnosis
- assess bone mineral density, and
- to assess bone turnover.

The detection and assessment of fractures can be achieved by plain radiography alone, and this is clearly indicated if fracture is suspected.

The most important differential diagnoses are osteomalacia and pathological fractures related to neoplastic disease. If osteomalacia is likely, calcium, phosphorus, alkaline phosphatase and vitamin D may need to be measured (the most appropriate screening test is for elevated alkaline phosphatase, but it must be remembered that elevation of this enzyme may also occur after a fracture). If a pathological fracture due to neoplastic disease is suspected referral may be indicated, as a variety of special investigations may be needed to detect a primary fracture as well as to visualize bone deposits (such as CT or MRI, for example).

Bone mineral density can be assessed in a variety of ways. Plain radiographs are an insensitive technique, as some 20–40% of calcium must be lost before osteopenia will be detected this way. Quantified computed tomography (QTC) is an old but still widely used and effective way of measuring bone density, but involves significant exposure to X-rays. Dual energy absorptiometry is now the technique of choice in most specialist centers, providing accurate measurements in a short time and with minimal radiation exposure. More recently the simpler and cheaper technique of ultrasound assessment of calcaneal bone density has become popular, but the value of this in longitudinal studies has yet to be fully evaluated and validated.

The application of these techniques in practice is currently a disputed subject. It is widely agreed that population screening cannot be recommended on current evidence. Use for individual patients is more contentious. Single time-point measures are of limited value, partly because of the wide range of normal density measures for any given age and sex. Change over time on repeated measures, using exactly the same technique, is arguably more valuable as it allows the physician to see if bone loss is progressing faster or more slowly than might be expected, and to assess the influence of any change of therapy on the rate of bone loss.

The main indication for bone density measurement at present is for patients at high risk of fracture (Fig 34.4) in whom therapy will be considered only if a low reading is obtained, in those with a previous fracture, and in patients whose therapy can be followed over a time period of years.

Assessment of bone turnover using biochemical measures of bone formation and resorption is of little relevance in primary care, but is used in specialist centers to help decide on the best form of therapy, particularly in younger patients with osteoporosis.

 ## MANAGEMENT

Three aspects of management are considered here:
- Primary prevention.
- Prophylaxis in menopausal women.
- Treatment of established osteoporosis.

PRIMARY PREVENTION
The development of osteoporosis in later life depends on the peak bone mass achieved in early years. This can be improved by a diet with a high calcium and vitamin D intake and plenty of exercise in childhood, adolescence, and early adulthood (peak bone mass is reached at around 25–30 years of age). Maintaining a high level of physical activity, without smoking or excess alcohol, helps preserve bone mass in adulthood.

PROPHYLAXIS IN MENOPAUSAL WOMEN
Bone loss starts after about 30 years of age in both sexes, but accelerates markedly after the menopause in women (Fig. 34.5). This postmenopausal bone loss can be prevented by hormone replacement therapy (HRT), which also reduces fracture rates. To be most effective, HRT should be started immediately after the menopause and continued for many years – a minimum of 5, and up to 15 years. However, in addition to its beneficial effects on osteoporosis and cardiovascular disease, HRT increases the risk of breast cancer (especially in those with a family history) and unopposed estrogen carries a risk of endometrial tumors. Thrombosis is considered a contraindication to HRT.

As yet, the risk–benefit ratio for an individual cannot be defined, which makes it difficult to give clear recommendations and necessitates an individual approach, in which the wishes of each woman are of paramount importance. Many practitioners only recommend HRT to those women at high risk of osteoporosis who have a relatively early menopause.

TREATMENT OF ESTABLISHED OSTEOPOROSIS
The aims of treatment of established osteoporosis are to:
- Reduce pain and other symptoms or disability.
- Reduce the risk of subsequent fractures.
- Reduce further bone loss, or to increase bone density above the fracture threshold.

IMMEDIATE TREATMENT OF A PAINFUL FRACTURE
Immediate treatment of a painful fracture includes an analgesic [normally acetaminophen (paracetamol) or a codeine preparation], as well as fixation if necessary (or other surgical treatment such as a hip replacement in femoral neck fractures). Union is not delayed. A short period of rest may be necessary after a painful fracture of the vertebrae, but rest and immobilization are avoided when possible, in view of the adverse effect on bone density. Calcitonin is sometimes used if the pain is severe, as it has analgesic properties as well as effects on bone, but any severe, unremitting, or long-lasting pain indicates a pathologic fracture and a different form of bone disease.

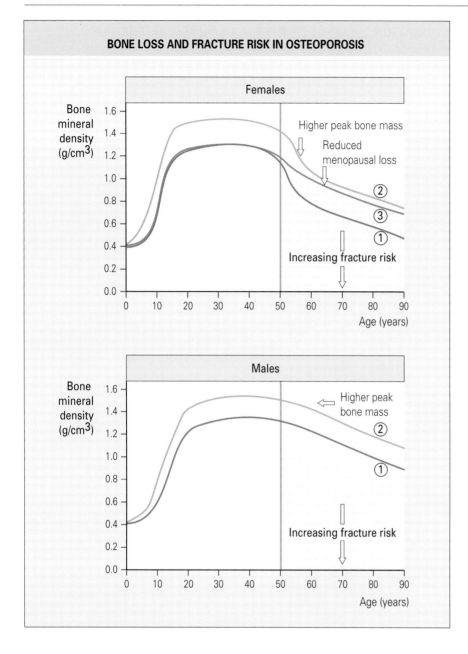

Fig. 34.5 Bone loss and fracture risk in osteoporosis. Bone density in both sexes increases from early childhood to reach a peak in early adulthood. It remains relatively stable until the late 40s or early 50s and then slowly declines in both males and females (1). In women, postmenopausal bone loss is superimposed on this age-related bone loss. Thus, bone mineral density in later life depends upon peak bone mass achieved and subsequent age and menopause-related bone loss. Fracture risk is dependent in large part upon bone mineral density in these later years. In females and males, increased peak bone mass results in higher bone density in later life (2), while prevention of postmenopausal bone loss in women is equally protective (3).

REDUCTION OF THE RISK OF SUBSEQUENT FRACTURES

Reduction of the risk of subsequent fractures involves attempts to reduce the risk of falls (see above), protecting against the consequences of falls with the use of hip protectors in those at highest risk (the institutionalized patient with osteoporosis), increasing physical activity, and treatment of the bone problem.

ATTEMPTS TO REDUCE FURTHER BONE LOSS OR INCREASE BONE DENSITY

Attempts to reduce further bone loss or increase bone density are primarily pharmacologically based. All patients are given calcium supplements and vitamin D, and estrogens are considered for postmenopausal women if no contraindications are present (those at high risk of breast or uterine cancer or thromboembolic events). Bisphosphonates are a valuable alternative to estrogen therapy, and a variety of preparations are now available, which are of proved efficacy and have low side effects. Calcitonin is another alternative.

RECOMMENDATIONS FOR REFERRAL

Subspecialty

Those at high risk of fractures (see Fig. 34.4) and anyone who has already had one osteoporotic fracture should be considered for referral to the local service that takes a special interest in osteoporosis, which may be rheumatologic or endocrinologic. In addition, patients with persistent pain should be considered for referral to a rheumatologist.

Physical therapy/rehabilitation

Elderly patients with deformity and disability due to osteoporosis (for example those with bad spinal deformity causing chest and abdominal problems) may be helped by a rehabilitation program. In addition, as exercise helps increase bone density and/or prevent any further loss of bone, referral to help educate patients about a regime of appropriate exercises to be continued on a regular basis may be considered.

Orthopedic surgery

Fractures of long bones require management by orthopedic surgeons.

EDUCATION, SELF-HELP, DIET, AND PHYSICAL THERAPY

Education, self-help, diet, and physical therapy are all important in the management of osteoporosis. A wealth of patient information on the subject is now available through publications, the internet, and other sources. Physical therapy to help maintain bone and muscle strength and increase general activity is advisable where possible, and dietary advice includes the use of calcium supplements at night for all patients (see Self-Help Leaflet, page 351).

RECOMMENDATIONS FOR REFERRAL

Referral of patients with osteoporosis, along with the investigation of bone mineral density, is a contentious issue. Policies vary widely in different countries and areas according to availability of different specialists and techniques, and because of financial/regional public health policy reasons. Furthermore, in many countries, patient pressure is one of the main factors dictating referral to specialists. This makes it difficult for us to provide clear guidance.

DISEASES OF BONE

35

OTHER BONE DISEASES

OSTEOMALACIA

IN WHAT CIRCUMSTANCES IS OSTEOMALACIA SUSPECTED?

Osteomalacia is not uncommon in the elderly. The main risk factors are a poor diet and lack of sunlight, and seen predominantly in older people who do not go out much, or who keep their skin covered. It is common in women who tend to stay indoors, avoid exposure to sunlight, and have a diet low in vitamin D; it also occurs in institutionalized people.

Other causes are gastrointestinal, because of reduced absorption of nutrients (as in gastrectomy, pancreatic insufficiency, and malabsorption syndromes), and renal disease, either hereditary renal tubule syndromes (such as renal tubule acidosis) or acquired renal disease with major tubule damage.

℞ MANAGEMENT

Osteomalacia is treated with vitamin D2 or D3 800–4000IU (0.02–0.1mg) daily for 6–12 weeks followed by 200–400IU (0.005–0.01mg) daily. Calcium is given as well for those with severe disease. A metabolic response should result, with a brisk rise in serum phosphate levels; absence of this rise suggests vitamin D resistance.

KEY POINTS

Definition
- Osteomalacia is a defect of skeletal mineralization caused by vitamin D deficiency.

Main clinical features
- Axial bone pain, which may be vague and poorly localized.
- Bone tenderness.
- Proximal myopathy with weakness, which may result in a 'waddling' gait.
- Spontaneous fractures of the femur and other sites.

Diagnosis
- Characterized by low serum calcium, phosphorus, and vitamin D levels, and a high alkaline phosphatase.
- Radiographs may show 'Looser's zones' (Fig. 35.1).
- Can be confirmed by bone biopsy (Fig. 35.2).

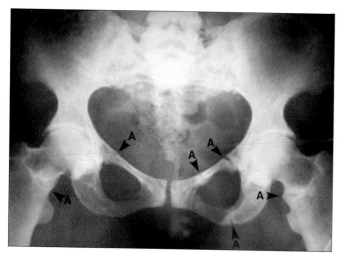

Fig. 35.1 Radiograph of the pelvis showing multiple Looser's zones (arrowhead) in a woman with severe osteomalacia.

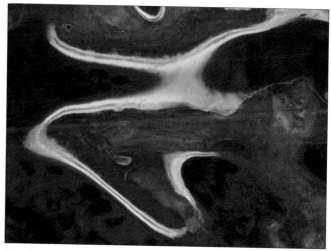

Fig. 35.2 Microscopic appearance of an iliac crest bone biopsy viewed under ultraviolet light. Apparent is the fluorescence produced by prior tetracycline labeling, which shows up the mineralization fronts; this technique can be used to measure the mineralization rate, which slows down in osteomalacia.

HYPERPARATHYROIDISM

KEY POINTS

Definition
- Primary hyperparathyroidism equates to hypercalcemia caused by overactivity of one or more parathyroid glands.
- Secondary hyperparathyroidism results from prolonged parathyroid gland stimulation from hypocalcemia, most likely caused by chronic renal disease.

Main clinical features
- Most common in women in the 6th decade of life.
- Musculoskeletal features include diffuse bone pains, arthralgias, and pathologic fractures.
- Hyperparathyroidism also causes renal stones, fatigue, emotional lability, and other neuropsychiatric features.

Diagnosis
- Serum calcium is raised in all cases.
- Radiographs may show classic changes (Figs 35.3 & 35.4).
- The diagnosis can be confirmed by raised serum parathyroid hormone levels.

IN WHAT CIRCUMSTANCES IS HYPERPARATHYROIDISM SUSPECTED?

Although most common in women in their sixth decade of life, this condition can present at any age, and in a variety of ways.

Classically, the patient has 'groans, stones, and moans' that relate to musculoskeletal pains, a tendency to renal stones, and neuropsychiatric disturbances. Diagnosis requires a high index of suspicion and screening with serum calcium assessment.

℞ MANAGEMENT

Parathyroidectomy is the only treatment for primary hyperparathyroidism, although is still unclear which patients should have surgery.

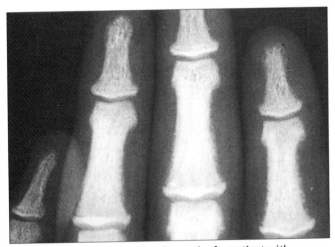

Fig. 35.3 Part of the hand radiograph of a patient with hyperparathyroidism. Shown are the characteristic subperiosteal resorption of the phalanges and lace-like trabecular pattern.

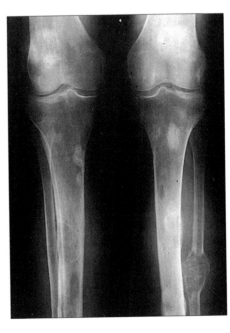

Fig. 35.4 Radiograph of the legs of a patient with severe hyperparathyroidism. The classic lytic lesions caused by 'brown tumors' are seen. (Courtesy of Professor M Kahn.)

METASTATIC BONE DISEASE

IN WHOM IS METASTATIC BONE DISEASE SUSPECTED?

Metastatic bone disease presents in two different contexts – in people with known primary tumors, in which case the development of bone pain or a fracture should raise immediate suspicion, or *de novo* in the absence of a known primary tumor, in which case the diagnosis is much more difficult. Factors that raise suspicion of this category of disease include unremitting severe bone pain and systemic features of disease, such as weight loss.

Metastatic bone deposits most commonly occur in the spine or hip, and can cause pathologic fractures. Most deposits cause osteolytic lesions, but prostatic and breast tumor deposits can be osteosclerotic.

KEY POINTS

Definition
- Metastatic bone disease is caused by metastatic deposits, most commonly related to primary tumors of the prostate, lung, or breast.

Main clinical features
- Bone pain (unrelieved by rest) is common.
- Pathologic fractures and hypercalcemia can occur.

Diagnosis
- Radiographs may show the lesions (Fig. 35.5).
- Bone scans are more sensitive than radiographs (Fig. 35.6).
- Biochemistry (raised serum calcium and alkaline phosphatase) and serum tumor markers may help.
- Biopsy may be required.

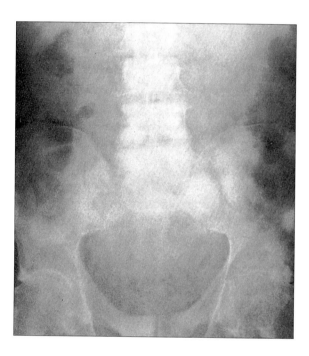

Fig. 35.5 Radiograph of the lumbar spine and pelvis in a patient who presented with back pain. The multiple sclerotic deposits are from a previously undiagnosed prostatic carcinoma.

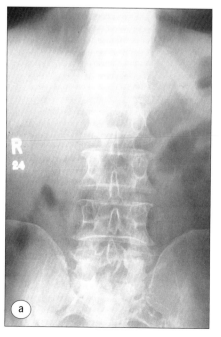
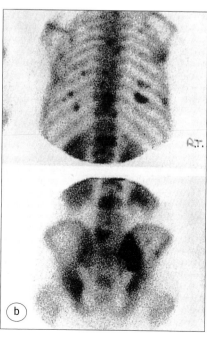

Fig. 35.6 Radiograph and bone scans in a patient who had a bronchial carcinoma and complained of back pain. (a) Normal lumbar spine radiograph. (b) The isotope bone scans reveal multiple metastases in the lumbar spine and pelvis. Note also metastases in the thoracic vertebrae and ribs.

PRIMARY TUMORS OF BONE

KEY POINTS

Definition
- Primary tumors of the bone are primary malignancies of bone.
- They can arise from bone, cartilage, vascular and other tissues, or from the marrow.
- These are rare conditions, but the most common forms are osteosarcomas in children, and osteoid osteomas and myeloma in adults.

Main clinical features
- Can present in a variety of ways.
- Bone pain (constant pain not relieved by rest) may be present.
- Pathologic fractures can occur.
- Generalized features of malignancy may be present.

Diagnosis
- Radiographs are of great value.
- In myeloma, the erythrocyte sedimentation rate is raised and serum and urinary proteins are abnormal.

IN WHOM IS A PRIMARY BONE TUMOR SUSPECTED?

Primary bone tumors are rare. Suspicion is raised for anyone with constant pain in the bones, which is unrelieved by rest and not affected by activity. Other systemic features such as weight loss, tiredness, and fevers may be present.

FEATURES OF THE MOST COMMON TUMORS
MYELOMATOSIS

Myelomatosis is the most common primary bone tumor. It occurs most often in men aged 40–50 years, and is a malignancy of the B-lymphoid cells. Bone pain is usual, vertebral fractures often occur, and systemic features such as weight loss and anemia are typically present. Radiographs may show osteolytic lesions (Figs 35.7 & 35.8), the erythrocyte sedimentation rate is raised, and protein electrophoresis in the serum usually shows a monoclonal band. Chemotherapy is required for treatment of the disease.

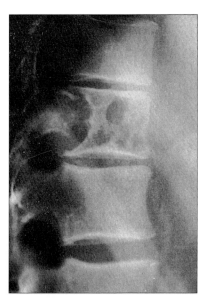

Fig. 35.7 Myeloma can cause generalized osteopenia with radiographic features that look just like osteoporosis. In addition, multiple radiolucencies may occur within the vertebrae, as shown here.

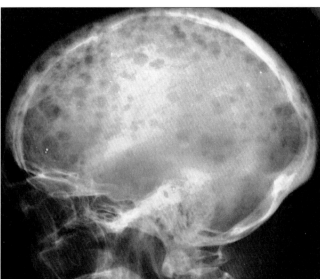

Fig. 35.8 Myeloma that affects the skull can produce the characteristic punched out lesions shown here.

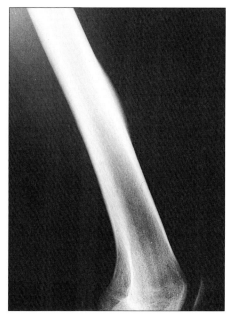

Fig. 35.9 Osteoid osteoma. Lateral radiograph of the shaft of the femur shows reactive bone sclerosis on the outer and inner surface of the anterior femur.

OSTEOID OSTEOMAS

Osteoid osteomas are benign, slow-growing, bone-forming tumors that are most commonly seen in the long bones, most often in adolescents and young adults, and they occur more commonly in men than in women (Fig. 35.9). Constant pain is the main feature, which may be exacerbated by alcoholic drinks and relieved by aspirin.

OSTEOSARCOMAS

Osteosarcomas are malignant bone tumors seen predominantly in males 10–30 years of age, and they have a predilection for the lower end of the femur and upper end of the tibia. They often present with pain, swelling, and tenderness (Fig. 35.10).

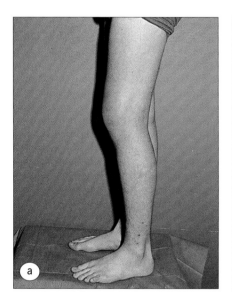
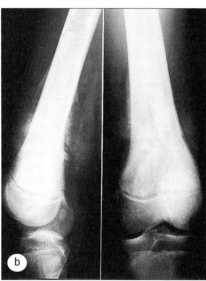

Fig. 35.10 Osteosarcoma. The patient was a 16-year-old boy. (a) He complained of a painful swelling above the left knee. (b) The radiograph showed evidence of an osteosarcoma, with a patchy increase in bone density and periosteal reaction.

DISEASES OF BONE

OSTEONECROSIS

KEY POINTS

Definition
- Osteonecrosis equates to the death of a segment of bone.

Main clinical features
- Osteonecrosis occurs most commonly in the head of the femur.
- It can occur on the convex surface of other bones, such as the medial condyle of the femur.
- Major risk factors include corticosteroid treatment, alcoholism, trauma, and hyperlipidemia (other causes include sickle cell disease, caisson disease, and Gaucher's disease).
- Variable presentation – it may be silent, or may cause a great deal of pain.
- If untreated, osteonecrosis often progresses to local bone destruction

Diagnosis
- Radiographs show characteristic changes in late stages, but they do not pick up the early stages (Figs 35.11 & 35.12).
- Early changes can be detected on bone scans and MRI.

IN WHAT CIRCUMSTANCES IS OSTEONECROSIS SUSPECTED?

Osteonecrosis (also called avascular or aseptic necrosis) is uncommon in the absence of one of the major risk factors. Corticosteroid therapy (particularly for systemic rheumatic diseases) and alcoholism are the most important risk factors, but osteonecrosis is also a complication of other conditions such as sickle cell disease and Gaucher's disease, and should be suspected in such patients. In addition, osteonecrosis is a frequent late complication of a fracture at a vulnerable site such as the neck of femur.

The presentation is variable, and osteonecrosis can present as a radiographic finding with no symptoms. In most patients, pain is present. In osteonecrosis of the femoral head, the pain is usually felt in the groin or thigh, and is worse on weight bearing. A limp may develop.

℞ MANAGEMENT

Osteonecrosis is a condition that requires a high index of suspicion, as early treatment can help prevent subsequent destruction of the head of the femur, or other bones involved. Medical treatment includes keeping the patient nonweight bearing and using analgesics such as acetaminophen (paracetamol) or nonsteroidal anti-inflammatory drugs. Surgical decompression can be of great value in selected early cases.

Late cases may require total joint replacement.

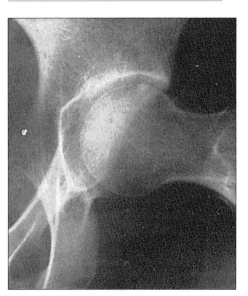

Fig. 35.11 Osteonecrosis of the femoral head. The characteristic crescent sign with flattening of the femoral head is seen.

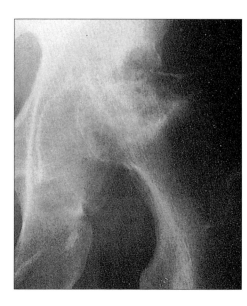

Fig. 35.12 Extensive destruction of the femoral head secondary to osteonecrosis.

CHILDHOOD RHEUMATIC DISEASES

AN INTRODUCTION TO CHILDHOOD RHEUMATIC DISORDERS

Symptoms and signs that arise from the musculoskeletal system are common in children, but serious rheumatic diseases are relatively rare.

Diagnosis can be more difficult than in adults for a number of reasons, which include the relatively uncommon complaint of pain in children (the presentation often being related to change in function rather than an overt symptom) and the attendant high levels of anxiety among many parents. Treatment is a highly specialized area of medicine, and requires a team approach. For these reasons, any child thought likely to have a significant rheumatic disease must be referred for specialist help.

The majority of symptoms are confined to a single joint area and are caused by minor deformities or growth abnormalities, and by trauma. More generalized pains are also common and usually arise from a variety of nonorganic causes, including growing pains, fibromyalgia, school phobias, and attention seeking.

Less commonly, musculoskeletal signs or symptoms in childhood may herald a major rheumatic or systemic disease. In such cases it is usual for some physical signs to be present, such as joint swelling in the case of arthritis, or fever or rashes in the case of a systemic disorder.

Disorders in childhood can thus be broken down according to the algorithm shown.

DIAGNOSTIC ALGORITHM FOR CHILDHOOD RHEUMATIC DISORDERS

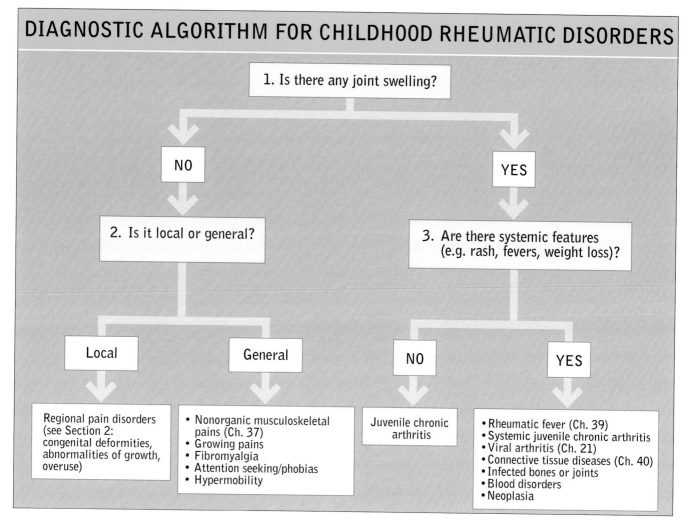

1. Is there any joint swelling?

NO

YES

2. Is it local or general?

3. Are there systemic features (e.g. rash, fevers, weight loss)?

Local

General

NO

YES

Regional pain disorders (see Section 2: congenital deformities, abnormalities of growth, overuse)

• Nonorganic musculoskeletal pains (Ch. 37)
• Growing pains
• Fibromyalgia
• Attention seeking/phobias
• Hypermobility

Juvenile chronic arthritis

• Rheumatic fever (Ch. 39)
• Systemic juvenile chronic arthritis
• Viral arthritis (Ch. 21)
• Connective tissue diseases (Ch. 40)
• Infected bones or joints
• Blood disorders
• Neoplasia

CHILDHOOD RHEUMATIC DISORDERS

36

REGIONAL MUSCULOSKELETAL DISORDERS IN CHILDREN

Most of the regional musculoskeletal disorders seen in children result from congenital or acquired deformities or growth anomalies, or from trauma, but serious conditions such as osteomyelitis also occur.

As in adults, regional musculoskeletal pain in children may be caused by articular disorders or periarticular problems, or be referred from more proximal structures (e.g. spinal disease presenting as a leg problem). Lower limb problems are much more common than upper limb disorders, and the most common presentations are:

- Parents who bring toddlers or children to see doctors because of concern about an apparent deformity.
- Limp, with or without pain.

SOME COMMON DEFORMITIES OF THE LOWER LIMBS IN CHILDREN

CLUB FOOT

The two forms of club foot that occur are:

- Positional talipes caused by intrauterine compressions, a common minor disorder that corrects easily and spontaneously.
- Talipes equinovarus, a serious complex disorder with a male preponderance, characterized by an inverted, supinated foot, which interferes with function (Fig. 36.1) – early treatment is needed, and either serial casting and/or surgical correction easily corrects it.

BOW LEGS AND KNOCK KNEES

Bow legs and knock knees are common in toddlers and young children (Fig. 36.2), are generally of no significance, and usually resolve, although occasional cases of bow legs may be caused by rickets.

> ### KEY POINTS
>
> - Most regional disorders in children result from congenital or acquired deformity, growth anomalies, or trauma.
> - Lower limb disorders are more common than upper limb disorders.
> - Common presentations include the child with a limp, and parental concerns about apparent deformity.
> - Serious disorders such as osteomyelitis occur occasionally.
> - Specific disorders described in this chapter include toxic synovitis of the hip, osteochondritis dissecans, and anterior knee pain in the adolescent.

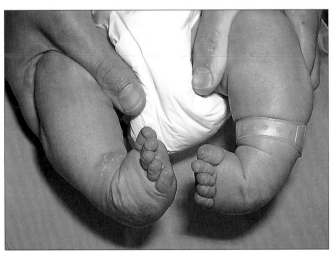

Fig. 36.1 Talipes equinovarus. (Reproduced with permission of Dr T. Lissauer, from Illustrated Textbook of Pediatrics, Tom Lissauer and Graham Clayden, Mosby, 1997.)

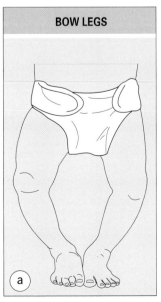

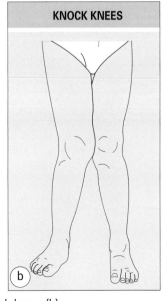

BOW LEGS

KNOCK KNEES

Fig. 36.2 Bow legs (a) and knock knees (b).

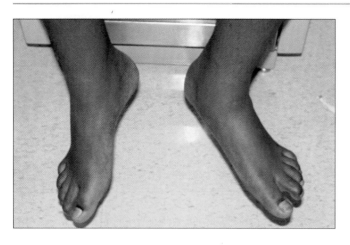

Fig. 36.3 Flat foot in a 12-year-old boy who has a peroneal spastic flat foot secondary to tarsal coalition in the left foot. The right foot is normal. (Courtesy of Kevin Murray.)

HIP DISORDERS THAT MIGHT CAUSE A LIMP IN A CHILD		
Age (years)	With pain	Without pain
1–3	Transient synovitis Trauma/osteomyelitis Septic arthritis	Congenital dislocation of the hip
3–10	Transient synovitis Juvenile chronic arthritis	Legg–Perthes disease
11–16	Acute slipped epiphysis Juvenile ankylosing spondylitis (boys) Conversion hysteria (girls)	Chronic slipped epiphysis

Fig. 36.4 Hip disorders that might cause a limp in a child.

FLAT FEET

Mobile flat feet are common and usually painless. The longitudinal arch is restored when standing on tiptoe. Pain is uncommon and is relieved by arch supports.

Painful rigid flat feet are usually caused by a tarsal coalition (Fig. 36.3).

IN-TOEING AND OUT-TOEING

In-toeing and out-toeing are mild anomalies that may be a source of concern to parents, but rarely signify an important deformity and usually resolve.

HIP DISORDERS AS A CAUSE OF LIMPING IN CHILDREN

Limping is a common presentation of hip disorders in children (Fig. 36.4). There may or may not be a history of pain.

FEATURES OF TOXIC SYNOVITIS OF THE HIP (IRRITABLE HIP)

- The most common cause of hip pain and a limp in children; boys are affected more than girls.
- A benign, self-limiting condition of unknown etiology.
- Occasionally bilateral or recurrent, but either suggests an alternative pathology.
- Presents with limping and pain, and a mild fever and raised erythrocyte sedimentation rate (ESR), which frequently makes differential diagnosis from more serious disorders, such as osteomyelitis or septic arthritis, difficult (aspiration of the hip may be needed).
- Fever greater than 38°C and an ESR >20mm/h suggest hip sepsis and the child must be referred.
- Most cases can be treated at home with bed rest and acetaminophen (paracetamol), with mobilization once the child is pain free; severe pain may require traction and nonsteroidal anti-inflammatory drugs.

1 TYPICAL CASE: TOXIC SYNOVITIS OF THE HIP

Shaun is a 4-year-old boy who presents with a 2-day history of limping and pain in the right hip. He had an upper respiratory tract infection a week ago, but is now well. There was painful restriction of hip movements.

Investigations were undertaken, and he was found to have a slightly raised erythrocyte sedimentation rate but a normal radiograph. As he was well, he was treated with acetaminophen (paracetamol) and bed rest at home with no further investigations, but the parents were told that they must return if the condition worsened or if there was any fever.

Shaun recovered fully in a week.

OTHER HIP DISORDERS OF CHILDREN

Congenital dislocation of the hip usually affects girls, particularly after breech births. Most cases are detected by neonatal screening, but some are missed or present late; if the disorder is suspected, the child is referred for treatment with splinting.

Legg–Perthes disease is an idiopathic ischemic necrosis of the femoral head, and is most common in boys of age 5–8 years. The onset is usually insidious, with a limp and little, if any, pain – any pain present may be referred to the knee. The diagnosis can be made by radiography, which also allows staging and prognostic classification (Fig. 36.5). Mild cases, particularly in younger children, can be treated conservatively, but severe cases may need traction or surgical intervention.

Slipped femoral epiphysis is most common in obese boys. Radiographs are required to confirm the diagnosis, and surgical fixation is necessary in most cases.

KNEE PAIN IN CHILDREN

Knee pain in those below the age of 10 years is uncommon, but usually significant. As in any other age group, it may be referred from the hip and can be periarticular (beware of osteomyelitis), but it is most commonly articular – disorders include meniscal tears (and a developmental discoid meniscus), septic arthritis, the onset of juvenile chronic arthritis, or the most common and specific disorder, osteochondritis dissecans.

In adolescents a number of periarticular lesions, such as Osgood–Schlatter disease and Larsen–Johansson disease can occur, in addition to the same articular diseases that may be seen in younger children. In girls in particular, anterior knee pain is a very common problem.

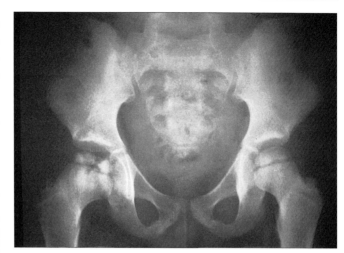

Fig. 36.5 A classic case of Legg–Perthes disease in the right hip. (Courtesy of Kevin Murray.)

2 TYPICAL CASE: OSTEOCHONDRITIS DISSECANS

Paul is a 12-year-old boy of short stature who complains of aching pain in his right knee during and after gym classes at school. He is otherwise well. He is unclear about the onset and duration, but it seems that he has gradually become more reluctant to take part in any physical activity, and his parents have noticed that he sometimes limps. He thinks he might have injured his knee some months ago, but cannot remember exactly when.

On examination, you find wasting of the right quadriceps muscle, some clicking of the joint on movement, and a small effusion.

A radiograph shows the typical features of osteochondritis dissecans (Fig. 36.6). Paul is pleased with the advice to rest his knees and the letter which lets him off gym at school, but he is less happy with being told that his mother must bully him to keep the knee moving and to do his quadriceps exercises each day.

After a few months the discomfort settles, radiographs show that the lesion is healing, and Paul is able to gradually resume normal activities.

FEATURES OF OSTEOCHONDRITIS DISSECANS

- Most common in short boys in their second decade.
- Sometimes a family history and/or a history of trauma.
- Gradual onset of activity-related discomfort in the knee.
- Quadriceps wasting, clicking, locking, and an effusion may be present.
- The lesion is separation of a subchondral bone fragment.
- Most common on one of the femoral condyles, but can affect the patella.
- Radiographic appearances are characteristic and diagnostic.
- Rest usually allows the lesion to heal.
- Surgical refixation is occasionally necessary, particularly in older children.

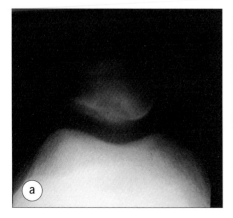
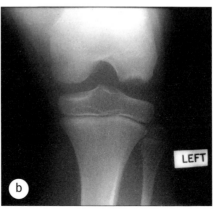

Fig. 36.6 Radiographic appearances of osteochondritic lesions. (a) Patella and (b) lateral femoral condyle.

3 TYPICAL CASE: ANTERIOR KNEE PAIN

Fiona is a 17-year-old girl who complains of pain around the patellae of both knees. She says it is difficult to sit in movie theater seats with her knees bent up, and it is difficult for her to dance at the local club. She is dressed in a short skirt, and shoes with very high heels.

On examination she appears to have rather weak quadriceps muscles, but there is no other abnormality that you can find.

She finds your reassurance that the pain will resolve difficult to believe, and does not heed your advice to not wear high-heeled shoes and to exercise daily to strengthen her quadriceps muscles.

Nevertheless, when you meet her a few years later, she cheerfully admits that the condition slowly got better, and that her knees are now quite normal.

OTHER KNEE PAIN SYNDROMES IN CHILDREN

Osgood-Schlatter disease is a traction apophysitis of the tibial tuberosity, related to overuse and most common in those aged 10–14 years. Local pain and tenderness occurs (Fig. 36.7), and radiographic findings are typical of the condition (Fig. 36.8). It usually settles with rest. Larsen–Johannson lesion is a similar disorder that occurs at the inferior pole of the patella.

SHOULDER PAIN IN CHILDREN

Shoulder pain in children or young adults can be caused by rotator cuff tendinitis (see Chapter 10), or by glenohumeral instability.

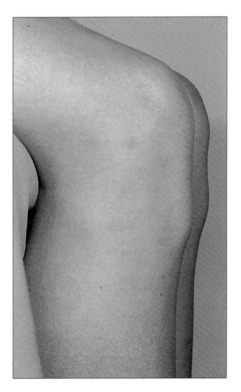

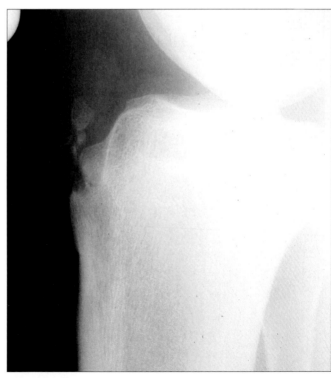

Fig. 36.7 Osgood–Schlatter disease. Enlarged tibial tuberosity.

Fig. 36.8 Osgood–Schlatter disease. Loose ossicles in the patellar tendon.

TYPICAL CASE – GLENOHUMERAL INSTABILITY

James is a 17-year-old boy who loves all sports. In the winter he plays a lot of soccer and in the summer concentrates on track and field. He presents with a painful shoulder, which makes it difficult for him to throw the javelin. The history and examination suggest rotator cuff tendinitis. However, on further questioning you elicit a history of shoulder dislocation after a football injury a few months previously, and stress tests for glenohumeral instability prove positive.

You refer him for physical therapy, and a program of muscle strengthening exercises accompanied by an improved technique for javelin throwing cures the problem.

FEATURES OF GLENOHUMERAL INSTABILITY

- The syndrome includes a wide range of disorders, in which various degrees of anatomic abnormality and directions of subluxation occur.
- Many cases experience mild subluxation, complicated by rotator cuff tendinitis, rather than frank dislocation of the shoulder.
- The diagnosis requires a high index of suspicion and careful clinical examination.
- Many cases respond to physical therapy and to alterations in activities that stress the shoulder and result in subluxation or dislocation.
- Arthroscopy can be used to confirm any anatomic abnormality and for minor repair procedures. Full surgical repair is occasionally necessary.

CHILDHOOD RHEUMATIC DISORDERS

37

NONORGANIC MUSCULOSKELETAL PAINS IN CHILDREN

INTRODUCTION

Joint aches and pains in children are common, but a serious cause or a major rheumatic illness is unlikely. Musculoskeletal pain with no apparent organic cause is reported to occur in 4–15% of children in the community, and nonorganic musculoskeletal pain is the diagnosis in about 25% of patients who attend pediatric rheumatology clinics.

The duty of the primary care physician is to differentiate those cases that might have a serious organic cause from those that do not. The major causes of nonorganic musculoskeletal pain in childhood are listed in Figure 37.1.

THE MAJOR CAUSES OF NONORGANIC MUSCULOSKELETAL PAIN IN CHILDHOOD
Diagnostic criteria
• Attention seeking
• Growing pains/recurrent limb pains
• School phobia
• Fibromyalgia and related disorders
• Conversion hysteria

Fig. 37.1 The major causes of nonorganic musculoskeletal pain in childhood.

KEY POINTS

- Commonly nonorganic.
- Causes include growing pains, school phobia, attention seeking, fibromyalgia, and conversion hysteria.
- Stress factors often contribute to the problem, whatever the cause.
- Organic causes must be excluded through a careful history (from parents as well as the child) and physical examination; simple investigations may be necessary.
- Management includes graded physical therapy and the treatment of any reversible stress factors that contribute.

1 TYPICAL CASE: 'GROWING PAINS'

John is an 11-year-old boy brought to you by his mother because of the severe pains in his legs that he has at night. Over the past few weeks he has repeatedly woken at night, crying because of pains in his calves, shins, and thighs; these pains tend to settle down when his mother rubs them. He has no pain during the day. His mother tells you that he has also complained of some headaches recently, and that she is worried that he may be being bullied at school. The examination is entirely normal.

You reassure the mother and the condition slowly resolves without treatment.

FEATURES OF GROWING PAINS OR RECURRENT LIMB PAIN IN CHILDHOOD

- Growing pains or recurrent limb pains are a common, distinct entity (affects about 4% of all children).
- Most frequently occur in the age range 6–13 years, with equal sex incidence.
- Characterized by severe pains in the calves, shins, and thighs, which wake the child at night, but respond to being rubbed.
- Attacks occur repeatedly over several months.
- In one third of cases the upper limbs or trunk are also involved.
- Recurrent abdominal pains or headaches at the same time or later are common.
- Parents often describe similar problems during their childhood.
- Stress factors, such as bullying, domestic problems or lack of friends, are common.

FEATURES OF SCHOOL PHOBIA AND ATTENTION-SEEKING BEHAVIOR IN CHILDHOOD

- Young children soon learn that the complaint of pain receives notice, and may reproduce musculoskeletal pains that occur in other family members.
- In school children, school phobia is characterized by vague aches and pains in the limbs, which usually occur the night before, or on the morning of a school day.
- The pains rarely occur at the weekends or at holiday times.
- Stress factors are commonly present.

FEATURES OF FIBROMYALGIA IN CHILDHOOD

- Most common in pubescent girls.
- The musculoskeletal pains may be generalized, or (less commonly) in one region.
- Onset often follows a minor injury or other illness.
- Headaches and abdominal pains are common.
- The child feels generally unwell.
- Pain, disability, and malaise may be incapacitating, but the child is generally cheerful.
- Skin hyperesthesia may be present.
- Signs of autonomic dysfunction may be present, as in reflex sympathetic dystrophy (see Fig. 37.2) and many children fit the classic criteria of this condition or of fibromyalgia in adults (see Chapter 28).
- Usually some abnormal family dynamics are in play, and many stress factors occur, with a very close relationship between the mother and child.

TYPICAL CASE: NONORGANIC MUSCULOSKELETAL PAIN CAUSED BY SCHOOL PHOBIA

Jane is a 12-year-old girl who is brought to you by her mother for evaluation of joint pain and stiffness that has resulted in increasing absenteeism from school. Jane has complained of diffuse joint pain over the previous several months, most notable in the mornings, which cause her to stay in bed until midday. The examination was entirely normal.

Subsequently, Jane changes school, after which the problem resolves.

TYPICAL CASE: FIBROMYALGIA IN CHILDHOOD

Julia is a 13-year-old girl who is the youngest of a large family. Her father is a professor of mathematics, who is immensely proud of the success of his three eldest children, all of whom are doing well at university. He has not spent much time with Julia, who he regards as not very intelligent and who appears to be over-protected from the father's disdain by her anxious mother, who did all the talking when they first came to see you about the limb pain.

It seems that Julia had influenza about 3 months previously, ever since when she has complained of diffuse, severe aches and pains in all four limbs. She often stays in bed, has missed a lot of school recently, and frequently complains of being too ill to go out with family or friends. You note that the mother has brought Julia to see you several times in the recent past, with a variety of complaints, which include abdominal pains and dysmenorrhea.

Examination is entirely normal apart from multiple tender spots in the typical distribution of adult fibromyalgia (see Chapter 28), but because of the severity of anxiety in the mother you obtain a full blood count and erythrocyte sedimentation rate (ESR), each of which is normal. You reassure Julia (and her mother), without suggesting that there is nothing wrong with her, tell her that it is vital that she gradually becomes more active, even if it hurts, and arrange for a program of graded physical therapy to help her do that.

She improves gradually, and a year later her talent as an artist is recognized at school, to her father's great pleasure. After that, life is much improved for Julia.

⚠ POINTS TO LOOK OUT FOR

Nonorganic musculoskeletal problems in childhood can lead to protracted physical and psychologic problems if mismanaged. Factors to be particularly wary of include:

- *Rest and immobilization* – this always makes things worse and can result in the development of flexion contractures and family problems.
- *Psychopathology and family problems* – it is important to look out for psychologic stress factors and to address them; they may include domestic strife or abuse, as well as factors such as undue expectations of children, bullying, or even depression.
- *Dismissal of the problem* – it is important that the problem is taken seriously, and that neither the child nor his or her parents become too involved in the deliberation of organic or psychosomatic causes.

INVESTIGATIONS

If the examination is normal, and no clues to a serious disorder are found (see below), investigations are not warranted. However, the concerns of the parents or child may in themselves warrant the extra reassurance that can be gained by showing that the blood count and ESR are both normal (which helps to exclude many of the possible organic causes).

If pain is confined to a single region and is persistent, a radiograph may also be warranted.

DIFFERENTIAL DIAGNOSIS

The main concern is to exclude the organic causes, which are listed in Figure 37.2.

It is obviously vital to take a full history from the child and the parents, and to undertake a full examination to help exclude these disorders. The particular things to take note that might indicate an organic cause include:

- Rashes, especially if accompanied by a fever, which may suggest a viral illness.
- Lyme disease;
- Systemic onset juvenile chronic arthritis (less common).
- A swollen joint in a child – this indicates significant pathology, as does any weight loss.

 MANAGEMENT

The problems presented by nonorganic musculoskeletal pain in childhood have to be approached with sensitivity and tact. The physician must avoid saying that nothing is wrong, but also needs to avoid reinforcement of concerns about serious organic illness.

The child needs to be given an optimistic outlook.

The cornerstones of therapy are a combination of graded physical therapy to return the child to normal activities, and a sensitive search for and treatment of any stress factors that may be contributing to the problem.

DIFFERENTIAL DIAGNOSIS OF THE MAJOR ORGANIC CAUSES OF MUSCULOSKELETAL PAIN IN CHILDHOOD
Infections
Viral (rubella, adenovirus, parvovirus) Bacterial (rheumatic fever, and other) Borrelia (Lyme disease) Mechanical trauma Regional disorders and overuse syndromes Hypermobility
Inflammatory
Juvenile chronic arthritis and related disorders Systemic rheumatic disorders
Blood dyscrasias
Hemophilias Sickle cell disease and other hemoglobinopathies
Neoplasia
Preleukemic leukemia and others
Genetic/congenital
Variety of unusual disorders

Fig. 37.2 Differential diagnosis of the major organic causes of musculoskeletal pains in childhood.

CHILDHOOD RHEUMATIC DISORDERS

38

JUVENILE CHRONIC ARTHRITIS

INTRODUCTION

Although an uncommon disease, juvenile chronic arthritis (JCA; synonym juvenile rheumatoid arthritis, JRA) is the most frequently diagnosed rheumatic disorder in childhood, and an important cause of physical disability, as well as blindness, in children.

The condition can only be considered after arthritis (clear evidence of inflammation of one or more joints) has been present for at least 6 weeks; other diagnostic criteria include onset under 16 years of age and exclusion of other forms of juvenile arthritis. After 6 months of disease, the condition can generally be subtyped into one of three main categories, as shown in Figure 38.1.

Systemic onset JCA is the least common form, but is the type that carries the highest short- and long-term morbidity, as well as having a significant mortality. It can also present in adults. In this chapter, the two more common forms of the childhood condition, in which joint disease predominates, are considered.

PAUCIARTICULAR AND POLYARTICULAR JUVENILE CHRONIC ARTHRITIS

KEY POINTS

- An uncommon condition, but the most frequent cause of inflammatory joint disease in children.
- Diagnostic criteria include arthritis in at least one joint for at least 6 weeks in someone who is under 16 years of age and in whom other causes of arthritis have been excluded.
- There are three main subtypes – pauciarticular (1–4 joints involved), polyarticular (>4 joints involved), and systemic (with fevers and rash) – each of which has different clinical features and carries a different prognosis.
- The more common nonsystemic forms of the disease – pauciarticular and polyarticular juvenile chronic arthritis (JCA) – tend to present with a limp, loss of use of a limb, or because parents notice swelling or some abnormal function; pain is relatively uncommon at presentation.
- Diagnosis and differential diagnosis can be difficult, particularly as a number of other rare disorders can also cause arthritis in children.
- Special problems include the risk of silent eye disease (which can blind children), growth abnormalities, and serious joint deformities or joint destruction.
- All children with JCA are referred for diagnostic work-up and management in specialist centers.

DIAGNOSTIC CRITERIA AND SUBTYPES OF JCA/JRA

Diagnostic criteria

Onset <16 years
Duration >6 weeks
Arthritis present (joint swelling or effusion)
Exclusion of other forms of juvenile arthritis

Main subtypes

Pauciarticular (only 1–4 joints involved) – 55–75% of cases
Polyarticular (>4 joints involved) – 15–25% of cases
Systemic onset (with fever and rash) – <20% cases

Fig. 38.1 Diagnostic criteria and subtypes of juvenile chronic arthritis.

CHILDHOOD RHEUMATIC DISORDERS

FEATURES OF PAUCIARTICULAR JUVENILE CHRONIC ARTHRITIS

- Largest subtype of juvenile chronic arthritis.
- Most common presentation is in young girls aged 1–5 years.
- Frequently presents with a limp or because parents have noticed joint swelling.
- Pain is uncommon and no systemic features are present.
- Knees, ankles, and wrists are the most commonly affected joints.
- Local growth abnormalities commonly develop (Figs 38.2–38.4).
- Some 40% of cases have antinuclear antibodies, and it is this group which is at risk of the development of painless anterior uveitis that can lead to blindness (Fig. 38.5).
- In the majority of those cases with the most common onset of lower limb disease before 5 years of age, the arthritis has resolved by the time the child is 15 years old.
- About 10% of this group have some residual eye problems.

1 TYPICAL CASE: PAUCIARTICULAR JUVENILE CHRONIC ARTHRITIS

Renata is a 4-year-old girl who was very active until some 6 weeks before her mother first brought her to see you, which was when the parents first noticed that she was limping. No other problems have occurred with Renata or in the family.

On examination you find a swollen, warm right knee and left ankle. Nothing else in the history or examination suggests any other form of juvenile arthritis, so you make a diagnosis of pauciarticular JCA by exclusion, and refer Renata to the local pediatric rheumatology clinic.

Renata is found to have a positive antinuclear factor, and is followed carefully at the hospital clinic, including regular eye checks. She is treated with anti-inflammatory drugs and physical therapy, and does well. She has very little time off school, and by the time she reaches the seventh grade has improved enough to be allowed to take part in gym classes for the first time in her life, in spite of the fact that she has one leg longer than the other.

JUVENILE SPONDYLITIS AND PSORIATIC ARTHRITIS

Juvenile onset ankylosing spondylitis presents like pauciarticular JCA: older boys with arthritis of a few lower limb joints and periarticular pain (usually around the heels, patellae, or hips), often with a positive family history (see Fig. 38.6). The antinuclear antibody (ANA) test is negative and

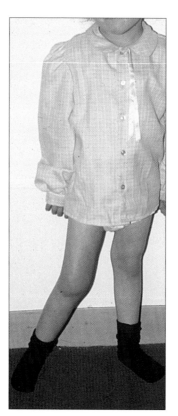

Fig. 38.2 A 6-year-old girl with pauciarticular juvenile chronic arthritis that is affecting her right knee. Her right leg is 3 cm longer than her left leg.

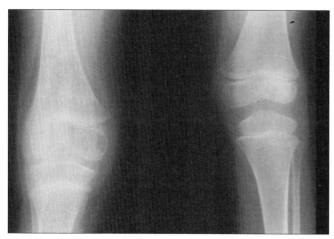

Fig. 38.3 Pauciarticular juvenile chronic arthritis that involves the right knee. Overgrowth of the leg and widening of the epiphysis is shown.

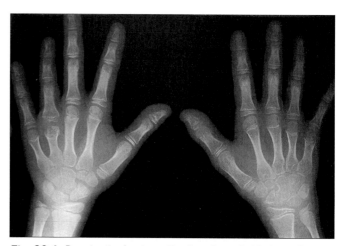

Fig. 38.4 Pauciarticular juvenile chronic arthritis in an 8-year-old girl. Epiphyseal destruction and undergrowth of the third metacarpophalangeal joint of the left hand are seen, as well as overgrowth of the carpal bones of the right wrist compared to the left wrist. Also note the widened appearance of the third phalanges because of periosteal new bone formation.

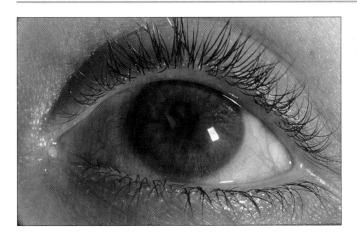

Fig. 38.5 Iritis that demonstrates cataract and irregular pupil secondary to posterior synechiae. (Courtesy of JJ Kanski.)

chronic eye disease is not a risk. Back pain may follow in late adolescence, but sacroiliitis is not detectable on radiographs until after the age of 20 years.

Psoriatic arthritis can occur in children, and usually presents with involvement of a few joints (as in pauciarticular JCA), a personal family history of psoriasis, and psoriatic nail changes (thimble pitting or separation of the finger nail from the nail bed). Most children do well, but multiple joints become involved in some; this typically affects the hands asymmetrically, with involvement of the end finger joints and a sausage finger (swelling of all the joints and the flexor tendon in one finger).

2 TYPICAL CASE: POLYARTICULAR ONSET JUVENILE CHRONIC ARTHRITIS

Carla is a 7-year-old girl who had abundant energy and was very active until about 2 months ago when she started to complain of aches and pains and feeling unwell. At first her parents dismissed this as a symptom of school worries (Carla's elder sister had developed school phobia a few years earlier), but about 2 weeks ago they noticed that Carla seemed stiff and to be limping in the mornings, and a few days ago her mother noticed that her knees were swollen.

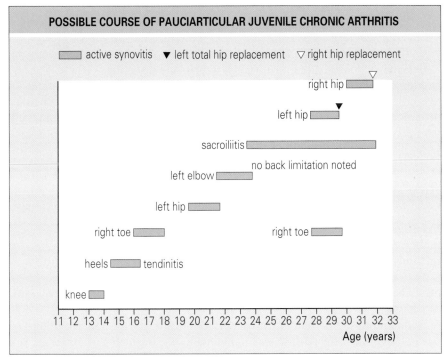

Fig. 38.6 Pauciarticular onset juvenile chronic arthritis with evolution into juvenile spondyloarthropathy.

FEATURES OF POLYARTICULAR JUVENILE CHRONIC ARTHRITIS

- Occurs at any time in childhood, and more commonly in girls over 7 years of age.
- Symmetric polyarthritis, with the knees, wrists, and ankles most commonly affected.
- Neck, shoulder, and hip disease, as well as small joint involvement, can occur.
- Mild malaise, low-grade fevers, and anemia may occur, but other systemic complications or problems are uncommon.
- The majority of patients have a favorable prognosis, but symmetric joint damage and overall growth retardation are frequent sequelae (Fig. 38.6).
- In a few children (particularly adolescent girls), polyarticular juvenile chronic arthritis is associated with a positive rheumatoid factor and follows a clinical pattern and course identical to severe adult rheumatoid arthritis – these children often develop both severe joint disease (Fig. 38.7) and systemic complications of rheumatoid arthritis.

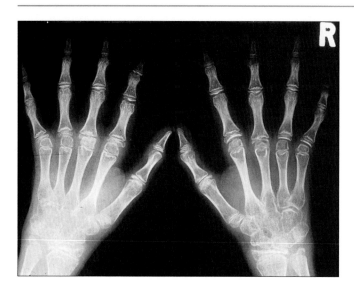

Fig. 38.7 Seropositive juvenile chronic arthritis in an 11-year-old girl. Erosions are seen at several metacarpophalangeal joints and there is carpal bone fusion in the wrist.

On examination you find swelling, warmth, and tenderness of the knees, ankles, and wrists, and possibly of the interphalangeal joints. Blood tests show a high erythrocyte sedimentation rate (ESR) and a mild anemia, but the rheumatoid factor is negative. You prescribe NSAIDs (which help) and refer her to the local pediatric rheumatology clinic.

! POINTS TO LOOK OUT FOR

The major concerns to be aware of in any child with arthritis include the risk of serious eye disease, growth abnormalities, and severe joint damage.

- *Eye disease* – occurs predominantly in the pauciarticular onset type of JCA and is strongly associated with ANAs. The uveitis does not cause pain or redness, so it is mandatory that these children have regular checks by an ophthalmologist.
- *Growth abnormalities* – these are of two kinds: local, which is associated with an inflamed joint and causes asymmetry of limb sizes, and general, which causes overall growth retardation, related to active arthritis and corticosteroid treatment.
- *Local growth abnormalities* – occur in some 50% of those with pauciarticular JCA. In young children arthritis leads to local overgrowth of bone, whereas arthritis in an older child can lead to premature fusion of the epiphyses and shortening of a limb. The common sites involved include the knee (leading to leg length inequalities, which can also cause scoliosis) and wrist (which results in a smaller hand).
- *General growth abnormalities* – involve an overall slowing of growth, which is caused either by prolonged active inflammatory disease or by corticosteroids.
- *Severe joint deformity or damage* – in a minority of children, severe joint damage develops. This commonly affects the hips, and diagnosis can be delayed in stoical children who adapt to pain and disability.

In addition, any child with JCA of any type can develop insidious deformities or loss of joint motion, which can affect function and autonomy and lead to permanent damage. It is a crucial part of management to make sure that children and their parents are on the lookout for this, and that, with the help of a therapist, they know how to avoid and treat such problems.

INVESTIGATIONS

Investigations are of little or no value in diagnosis, except as an aid to differentiating inflammatory arthritis (in which the ESR and other serum markers of inflammation are raised) from nonorganic musculoskeletal pains in children.

In those with established JCA, rheumatoid factor and ANA tests are carried out to help differentiate those at risk of severe joint disease or eye problems, respectively.

Radiographs are normal in the early stages of the disease and should not be taken, but in late disease they may help diagnose growth abnormalities as well as the development of severe joint damage.

DIFFERENTIAL DIAGNOSIS

Arthritis in young children can be difficult to diagnose. Complaints of pain are relatively rare, and common presentations are with a limp, because a child is not using a limb, or with swelling, deformity, or growth abnormalities that arise from prolonged 'silent' joint disease.

The key to the diagnosis of an arthritis, as opposed to the more common non-organic musculoskeletal problems in children and regional orthopedic disorders, is to recognize signs of local articular inflammation (warmth, swelling, effusion, joint line tenderness) and a raised acute phase response (raised ESR and C-reactive protein).

If an arthritis is present, the main differential diagnosis is between infectious and postinfectious conditions (such as Lyme arthritis or rheumatic fever), connective tissue disorders (such as systemic lupus erythematosus) that develop in childhood, or hematologic and malignant disorders, such as hemophilia or leukemia. The diagnosis of JCA is one of exclusion.

 ## MANAGEMENT

DRUGS AND LOCAL INJECTION THERAPY

Drug treatment is somewhat different for the two main categories of disease.

In pauciarticular disease, nonsteroidal anti-inflammatory drugs (NSAIDs) – either aspirin at doses of around 60–80mg/kg/day, or others in doses licensed for use in children (Fig. 38.8) – are used, along with local intra-articular cortico-steroid injections to treat pain or limb overgrowth. Disease-modifying drugs are not generally needed.

In polyarticular disease, aspirin is rarely used, but other NSAIDs are indicated. In addition, these children are often treated with methotrexate. Low-dose cortico-steroids may be used in refractory cases and intra-articular corticosteroids are reserved for individual joints. Systemic corticosteroids can have serious side effects in children (Figs 38.9 & 38.10).

RECOMMENDED AND MAXIMUM DOSES OF NONSTEROIDAL ANTI-INFLAMMATORY DRUGS (NSAIDs) IN CHILDREN			
	NSAID	Recommended (mg/kg/day)	Maximum/day (mg)
	Acetylsalicylic acid	60–80 *or* 100–120	4000
Propionic acid derivatives	Naproxen	15–20	1500
	Ibuprofen	40–50	2400
	Ketoprofen	3–5	300
	Flurbiprofen	3–4	300
	Fenoprofen	40–50	3200
Indoleacetic acids	Sulindac	4–6	400
	Indomethacin	1.5–3	200
	Tolmetin	20–30	1800
Phenylacetic acids	Diclofenac	2–3	150
Oxicams	Piroxicam	0.2–0.3	20

Fig. 38.8 Recommended and maximum doses of NSAIDs in children.

RECOMMENDATIONS FOR REFERRAL

- The management of juvenile chronic arthritis requires a team approach, coordinated with care by a pediatric rheumatologist.
- The team includes experienced physicians, physical therapists, and surgeons, along with other specialists such as psychologists and ophthalmologists.
- All patients with this condition must be referred to a specialist center.

TOXIC EFFECTS OF CORTICOSTEROID THERAPY IN CHILDREN	
Endocrine, metabolic	Cushingoid features
	Growth failure
	Glucose intolerance
	Adrenal insufficiency
	Menstrual irregularities
Musculoskeletal	Osteoporosis
	Osteonecrosis
	Vertebral collapse
	Myopathy
Cutaneous	Striae
	Acne
	Hirsutism
	Thin, fragile skin
	Alopecia
Gastrointestinal	Gastritis
	Pancreatitis
Ocular	Cataracts
	Glaucoma
Neurologic	Mood disturbances
	Pseudotumor cerebri
Immuno-suppression	Reduced resistance to infection

Fig. 38.9 Main adverse reactions of systemic corticosteroid therapy in children.

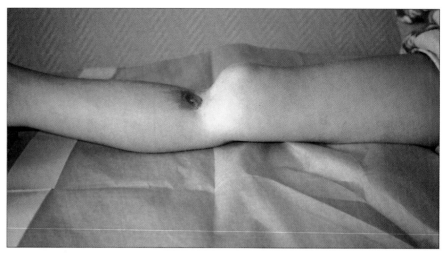

Fig. 38.10 Severe skin atrophy after intra-articular injection of triamcinolone hexacetonide in oligoarticular disease. (Courtesy of Professor Phillipe Touzet.)

SURGERY

Surgery can be of value in different stages of JCA. Flexion contractures of the hips may require soft-tissue release. With serious joint destruction, reconstructive surgery may be indicated.

EDUCATION

Education of the child and the parents is of crucial importance to the management of JCA. They need to understand the condition, and have a realistic view of the likely outcome. Disease in children often causes a great deal of stress for the family, and may have adverse effects on siblings. Family counseling may be appropriate in some cases.

PHYSICAL THERAPY

One of the main reasons for the improved prognosis in recent years for children with JCA is the better use of physical therapy to prevent and treat any joint deformities during the period of active disease. Physical therapists must be involved in the management of all cases, even if only one joint is involved. The aims of therapy are to preserve functional capacity of the joint and the autonomy of the child. Preservation of full joint motion is crucial, and may be aided by hot or cold packs to relieve discomfort and relax muscles, heated pools, and hot baths.

Active and passive joint stretching may also be necessary.

Splinting of joints, particularly at night, is often necessary, both to rest inflamed joints and to help prevent the development of contractures.

Further help from occupational therapists to circumvent functional problems may be necessary, and various technical aids, such as writing aids for school, or special tricycles, may be needed.

Physical therapy needs to be geared to the age of the child, and the central role of the therapist in management requires him or her to be able to establish a good rapport with both the child and the parents, who need to be taught how best to help preserve joint function at home.

COMPLEMENTARY THERAPY

Children with arthritis, and their parents, can be prey to any number of suggested 'miracle cures' for disease, most of which have no proved efficacy; these patients need protection from ineffective or expensive treatments that do not work.

CHILDHOOD RHEUMATIC DISORDERS

39

ACUTE RHEUMATIC FEVER

Acute rheumatic fever is a sequela of pharyngeal infection with group A β-hemolytic *Streptococcus* spp. Rheumatic symptoms typically develop 2–4 weeks after the pharyngitis; onset is usually with an acute febrile illness associated with migratory polyarthritis. The peak incidence is in children between 5 and 9 years of age; however, teenagers and adults may develop the disease. The disease is self-limited, but may cause damage to heart valves, which can lead to chronic, progressive cardiac dysfunction.

 TYPICAL CASE: RHEUMATIC FEVER

Mark is a 9-year-old boy with a 1-week history of high fevers, pains in his knees, and shortness of breath. His mother indicates that both he and his younger sister have complained of sore throats several times over the winter. On physical examination he appears listless with a temperature of 39.1°C and a pulse rate of 120 beats per minute. Both knees are swollen and markedly tender to palpation. An irregular-shaped erythematous rash is noted on his trunk and arms (Fig. 39.1). His heart sounds are difficult to hear and a chest radiograph reveals prominent cardiomegaly (Fig. 39.2).

DEFINITION

- An acute, systemic inflammatory illness that usually occurs 2–4 weeks after group A β-hemolytic streptococcal infection of the pharynx.
- It appears to be related to a series of immunologic reactions to antigenic components of the Streptococcus spp., which also cross-react with various human tissues, including heart muscle, valvular structures, articular tissues, and neuronal antigens.

Clinical features
- Characterized by fever, migrating arthritis, and destructive inflammatory lesions within the myocardium, endocardium, pericardium, heart valves, joints, periarticular regions, lungs, and subcutaneous tissues.
- Can be associated with chorea that may be transient or persistent.

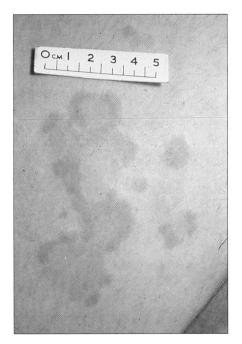

Fig. 39.1 Typical rash of erythema marginatum in a child with acute rheumatic fever. The varying border and tendency to clear in the central zones of the lesions are typical.

FEATURES OF RHEUMATIC FEVER

- Fever.
- Polyarthritis, typical pattern of migration from one joint to another.
- Subcutaneous nodules over elbows, occiput, and ankles.
- Rash ('erythema marginatum') on trunk and upper arms, often accentuated by a warm bath.
- Chorea ('Sydenham's chorea').
- Pancarditis, and valvulitis with mitral or aortic regurgitation are the most common abnormalities.
- Evidence of an antecedent group A streptococcal infection.
- Marked elevation of erythrocyte sedimentation rate.

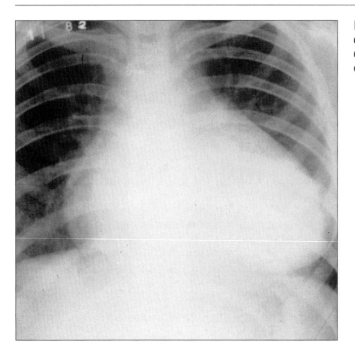

Fig. 39.2 Chest radiograph of a 9-year-old boy with sudden onset of shortness of breath and orthopnea preceded by 1 week of transitory and mild arthralgias. Marked cardiac enlargement associated with active carditis is present.

NATURAL HISTORY AND OTHER CLINICAL FEATURES

Antecedent group A streptococcal pharyngitis is present in virtually all patients, typically 2–4 weeks before the onset of rheumatic symptoms. In some children, a severe sore throat with fever and malaise usher in the disease, and in others actual streptococcal pharyngitis occurs followed by scarlet fever. The usual episode of acute rheumatic fever lasts from a few days to 4–6 weeks; however, repeated attacks over a period of several years may occur. Long-term outcome depends on the presence and severity of carditis. Patients who do not have carditis recover completely without complications, whereas those with carditis may develop chronic, progressive valvular heart disease.

 POINTS TO LOOK OUT FOR

- Congestive heart failure – a sign of severe valvular insufficiency or myocarditis.

INVESTIGATIONS

LABORATORY TESTS

It is important to document exposure to group A β-hemolytic *Streptococcus* spp. Throat cultures are obtained, but typically are negative by the time rheumatic manifestations are present. Serum antibodies against extracellular products of streptococci are present in nearly all patients. Antistreptolysin O (ASO) is elevated in the vast majority of patients; in those few patients with a negative ASO, antiDNAse B, antistreptokinase, or antihyaluronidase may be elevated. In patients with cardiac murmurs, blood cultures are obtained to rule out bacterial endocarditis (see differential diagnosis below). Blood cultures are negative in patients with acute rheumatic fever.

Acute phase reactants such as the erythrocyte sedimentation rate (ESR) and C-reactive protein (CRP) are invariably increased and often remain elevated well after clinical signs have resolved. Leukocytosis and a mild normochromic, normocytic anemia are often present.

CARDIAC STUDIES

An electrocardiogram is obtained to detect conduction abnormalities; common findings include a slight or moderate lengthening of the P–R interval and, on occasion, second-degree or even complete heart block. In patients with cardiac murmurs or evidence of heart failure, a two-dimensional echocardiogram is obtained to detect abnormalities of myocardial function and define the anatomy of cardiac valve leaflets.

DIFFERENTIAL DIAGNOSIS

Establishing a diagnosis of rheumatic fever is often difficult, but is aided by the Jones criteria (Fig. 39.3). A firm diagnosis requires that two major, or one major and two minor, criteria are satisfied, along with clear evidence of a recent antecedent streptococcal infection.

In children, the principal diseases that may cause diagnostic confusion are viral infections (rubella, hepatitis B, adenovirus), systemic onset juvenile chronic arthritis, systemic lupus erythematosus, and bacterial endocarditis. The patterns and course of arthritis, nature of the rashes, and serologic abnormalities help to make the correct diagnosis.

 ## MANAGEMENT

The objectives of treatment of acute rheumatic fever are symptomatic treatment of the arthritis with anti-inflammatory drugs and antibiotic treatment of any residual β-hemolytic streptococcal, pharyngeal infection.

DRUG THERAPY

Salicylates given in adequate doses suppress fever and arthritis highly effectively and a dramatic response is usually observed 12–24 hours after therapeutic blood levels (20–30mg/dl) have been attained. Initial dosages are usually 80–100mg/kg/day in children. Other nonsteroidal anti-inflammatory agents are probably equally effective, but have not been well studied. Anti-inflammatories are maintained until the patient is completely asymptomatic, and ESR or CRP has

Major manifestations	Minor manifestations	Supporting evidence of antecedent group A streptococcal infection
Carditis	Clinical findings:	Positive throat culture
	Arthralgia	or rapid streptococcal
Polyarthritis	Fever	infection test
Chorea	Laboratory findings:	Elevated or rising
	Elevated acute phase reactants	streptococcal
Erythema marginatum	Erythrocyte sedimentation rate	antibody titer
	C-reactive protein	
Subcutaneous nodules		
	Prolonged P–R interval	

GUIDELINES FOR THE DIAGNOSIS OF INITIAL ATTACK OF RHEUMATIC FEVER*

* If supported by evidence of preceding group A streptococcal infection, the presence of two major manifestations or of one major and two minor manifestations indicates a high probability of acute rheumatic fever.

Fig. 39.3 Guidelines for the diagnosis of initial attack of rheumatic fever. (Jones criteria, updated 1992.)

returned to normal levels. Typically, 6–8 weeks of therapy are needed.

Patients with carditis are generally treated with 1–2mg/kg of prednisone daily along with bed rest or restricted physical activity until signs of active carditis have resolved.

If streptococcal pharyngitis has been documented at the time of diagnosis, a course of antibiotics is indicated. Oral penicillin V (250,000 units, 3–4 times daily) is given for 10 days; erythromycin (maximum 1g/day) is a suitable alternative for patients allergic to penicillin. If compliance is a problem, a single intramuscular injection of benzathine penicillin G (600,000 units for children) may be given.

Antibiotic prophylaxis is started immediately after successful treatment of the acute episode of rheumatic fever. The optimal regimen consists of oral penicillin V, 250,000 units twice daily, or injection of benzathine penicillin (1.2 million units) intramuscularly every 4 weeks. Erythromycin (250mg/day) can be substituted in penicillin-sensitive patients. Prophylaxis is maintained for a minimum of 5 years after the most recent attack for all patients and indefinitely for patients with established, clinically confirmed rheumatic heart disease.

RECOMMENDATIONS FOR REFERRAL

- Patients with acute rheumatic fever complicated by carditis should be referred to a cardiologist for evaluation and assistance with acute and chronic management.

SURGERY AND OTHER TREATMENT MODALITIES

Rheumatic fever may have chronic cardiac sequelae that require surgical procedures such as mitral valve replacement.

MONITORING PROGRESSION AND OUTCOME

Most attacks of acute rheumatic fever subside within 6–12 weeks. Recurrences are most common within 2 years of the original attack, but can happen any time; the risk of recurrence decreases with age.

LESS COMMON CHILDHOOD RHEUMATIC DISORDERS

SPINAL PROBLEMS IN CHILDREN

WHEN IS BACK PAIN IN CHILDREN OF PARTICULAR CONCERN?

Back pain in children should always raise suspicion. Particular warning features of a serious disorder include presentation before 4 years of age; symptoms that persist beyond 4 weeks; interference with school, play, or sports; systemic features such as sweats or fevers; increasing pain; sleep disturbance; and any neurologic changes. On examination it is important to seek any midline skin lesion, such as a dimple or pigmented, or hairy nevus, which might indicate a congenital anomaly.

DIAGNOSIS AND MANAGEMENT

Any child with back pain or with a developing deformity must be referred for a full diagnostic work-up and management. Most deformities develop during the growth spurt and do not need intervention, but if severe deformities develop they can impair pulmonary function and have other consequences that require splinting or surgical correction. The treatment of back pain obviously depends upon the cause.

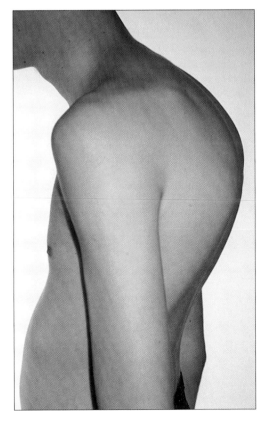

Fig. 40.1 Exaggerated thoracic kyphosis in Scheuermann's disease. (Courtesy of Peter Hollingworth.)

KEY POINTS

Definition
• Children can present with either deformity (often painless) or back pain.

Main clinical features
• Deformities are of two main types – scoliosis and kyphosis.
• Scoliosis is generally idiopathic and must be closely observed as rapid deterioration can occur, but this can be treated surgically.
• Kyphosis (round shoulders) can develop in teenage boys because of Scheuermann's disease; it may be painful, but requires no treatment (Fig. 40.1).
• Back pain is uncommon, but must be taken seriously as some 50% of cases have significant pathology.
• Infection and tumors can occur at any age, and the symptoms and signs may be misleadingly mild.
• Spondylosis and spondylolisthesis usually present in athletic children, with low back pain after exercise.
• Other causes include disk herniation and ankylosing spondylitis, as well as conversion hysteria.

Diagnosis
• A full history and examination are necessary in any child with back pain, and radiographs need to be taken.
• Scintigraphy is the most useful investigation in those in whom the level of suspicion is high but in whom the radiograph is normal.

OSTEOMYELITIS

KEY POINTS

Definition

- Osteomyelitis is an acute bacterial infection of bone ends in children.
- Haemophilus influenzae, Escherichia coli, Staphylococcus aureus, and Streptococcus spp. are the most common organisms responsible.

Main clinical features

- High fevers and septicemia are present in most cases.
- The knee area and humerus are the sites most affected.
- The pelvis can also be affected, especially in athletic youngsters.
- The child is unwilling to move the limb.
- The affected area is tender and warm; it may be swollen.
- Infection may spread into the adjacent joint.

Diagnosis

- Urgent specialist management is mandatory.
- Cultures are taken from the blood and from any possible septic focus.
- Needle aspiration or surgical exploration of the area may be necessary.

WHEN SHOULD ACUTE OSTEOMYELITIS BE SUSPECTED?

Any child with a high fever and other signs of septicemia must be urgently investigated and could have osteomyelitis – it occurs in children of all ages, including those below 1 year old (Fig. 40.2).

Unwillingness to move a limb as well as local signs (warmth, tenderness, and swelling) should also alert you to the possibility of osteomyelitis (Fig. 40.3).

DIAGNOSIS AND MANAGEMENT

The organism responsible needs to be isolated, cultured, and examined for antibiotic sensitivity as quickly as possible, via blood cultures and, if necessary, aspiration or surgical exploration of the lesion. Treatment needs to be prompt to

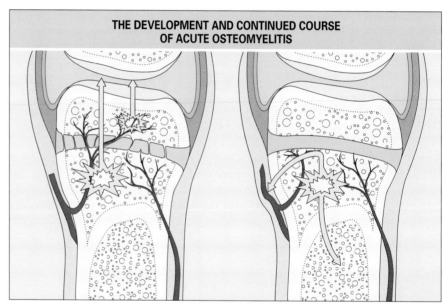

THE DEVELOPMENT AND CONTINUED COURSE OF ACUTE OSTEOMYELITIS

Fig. 40.2 **The development and continued course of acute osteomyelitis differs with age.** In infants below 1 year of age the epiphysis is nourished by arteries penetrating through the physis, which allows development of the condition within the epiphysis. In children up to 15 years of age, the infection is restricted to below the physis because of interruption of the vessels.

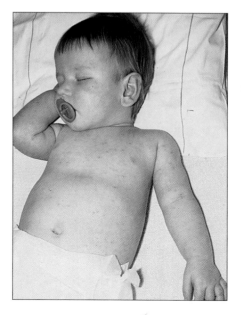

Fig. 40.3 **An acute osteomyelitis in the proximal metaphysis of the left humerus.** The child is not willing to move the affected limb. The roseola is consistent with a salmonellal infection, which was confirmed by fecal cultures.

avoid chronic osteomyelitis and other dangerous sequelae, and parenteral antibiotics need to be given as soon as possible. In view of the likely organisms responsible, high doses of benzylpenicillin and isoxazolyl penicillin are recommended prior to cultures and sensitivities becoming available. Surgical decompression of any abscess is carried out.

SYSTEMIC JUVENILE ARTHRITIS

IN WHAT CIRCUMSTANCES SHOULD SYSTEMIC JUVENILE ARTHRITIS BE SUSPECTED?

Systemic juvenile arthritis is considered in children with persistent, high-spiking fevers for which no cause can be found. The fever usually occurs late in the afternoon or evening, and is often accompanied by shaking chills, but the child's temperature returns to normal or below normal in the morning. Classically, the child appears toxic with the fever, but is entirely normal when the fever subsides.

The majority of patients develop a salmon-colored rash on the trunk and thighs which is most prominent when the fever is present (Fig. 40.4). The rash can often be brought out by scratching the skin (Koebner's phenomenon) and is occasionally pruritic. Systemic involvement varies, but includes generalized lymph node enlargement, hepatosplenomegaly, and polyserositis (Fig. 40.5). Polyarthritis occurs within 3–12 months of the onset of fever and most commonly involves the wrists, knees, and ankles.

HOW IS SYSTEMIC JUVENILE ARTHRITIS MANAGED?

Systemic juvenile arthritis is a serious disease with short- and long-term morbidity and the risk of mortality. Prompt early referral of patients with suspected systemic juvenile arthritis to a pediatric rheumatologist for diagnosis and development of a plan of treatment is essential. In most patients, care is often provided by a multidisciplinary team, which is coordinated by the pediatric rheumatologist.

KEY POINTS

Definition
- Systemic juvenile arthritis is a rheumatic syndrome of children with high-spiking fever and rash accompanied by systemic manifestations, which include polyarthritis.

Main clinical features
- Fever, rash, lymphadenopathy, polyserositis, and hepatosplenomegaly.
- The majority of patients develop a symmetric polyarthritis, typically involving the upper and lower extremity joints.

Diagnosis
- Clinical diagnosis, based on characteristic clinical features.

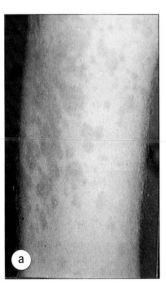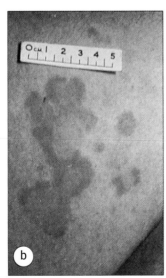

Fig. 40.4 The rash of systemic-onset juvenile chronic arthritis. (a) Larger lesions becoming confluent. (b) This condition must be differentiated from erythema marginatum, of which the rash seen in rheumatic fever is characteristic. (Courtesy of Barbara Ansell.)

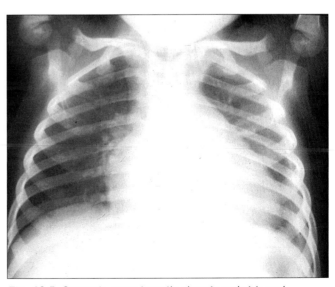

Fig. 40.5 Systemic onset juvenile chronic arthritis and pericardial effusion in a 3-year-old.

CONNECTIVE TISSUE DISEASE IN CHILDREN

KEY POINTS

Definition
- Connective tissue diseases are rare, systemic, rheumatic syndromes usually associated with vasculitis and major organ [kidney, central nervous system (CNS), etc.] disease.

Main clinical features
- Vary by specific syndrome, but include fever, polyarthritis, rashes or skin changes, pleurisy, muscle weakness, Raynaud's phenomenon, nephropathy (edema, abnormal sediment, renal failure), or CNS disorders (seizures, cranial neuropathies, psychiatric disorder).
- Antinuclear antibody is positive in the majority of patients.

Diagnosis
- Clinical syndromes with characteristic features (see text).

IN WHAT CIRCUMSTANCES IS CONNECTIVE TISSUE DISEASE SUSPECTED?

These children typically present with perplexing, multisystem illness and are often quite sick with high fevers and weight loss, and do not want to move or get out of bed. Connective tissue diseases are often first ascribed to a viral illness, but then fail to resolve. Signs and symptoms usually settle into a pattern which allows a specialist (pediatric rheumatologist) to make a diagnosis (see below). The other major group of disorders that falls into this group are the systemic vasculitis syndromes, of which Henoch–Schönlein purpura is the most common in children.

WHAT ARE THE MOST COMMON CONNECTIVE TISSUE DISEASES SEEN IN CHILDREN?

SYSTEMIC LUPUS ERYTHEMATOSUS

Systemic lupus erythematosus (SLE) usually occurs with fever, polyarthritis, malar rash, and pleurisy. Nephritis and central nervous system diseases (seizures, psychiatric illness, etc.) are more common and severe than in adults. Neonates born to mothers with SLE may develop a transient skin rash (Fig. 40.6), hematologic abnormalities, and heart block (neonatal lupus syndrome).

JUVENILE DERMATOMYOSITIS

Juvenile dermatomyositis shows proximal muscle weakness with elevation of serum muscle enzymes (creatine kinase, aldolase, and transaminases) and unique rashes over the eyelids (heliotrope) and extensor surfaces of the knuckles, knees, and elbows (Gottron's papules). Rare serious problems include pulmonary fibrosis, heart failure, or abdominal vasculitis.

SCLERODERMA

Localized (morphea) or linear scleroderma is much more common than progressive systemic sclerosis. Scleroderma typically begins as erythematous lesions that progress to patches on firm, white, fibrotic skin; linear lesions usually follow a dermatomal pattern. Extensive disease may affect the tendons, joints, and bones, and result in severe growth abnormalities.

HOW ARE CONNECTIVE TISSUE DISEASES MANAGED?

Connective tissue diseases in children are potentially serious and life-threatening, and so demand prompt referral to a pediatric rheumatologist for diagnosis and management.

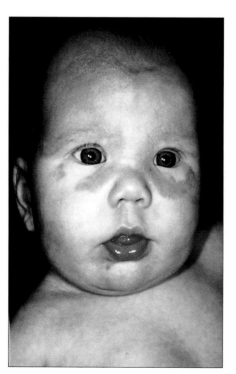

Fig. 40.6 Typical skin rash in neonatal lupus, showing the predilection for the periorbital area. This rash resolved completely without scarring. (Courtesy of Dr Susan Manzi.)

HENOCH–SCHÖNLEIN PURPURA

IN WHAT CIRCUMSTANCES IS HENOCH–SCHÖNLEIN PURPURA SUSPECTED?

Henoch–Schönlein purpura is considered in any child who presents with purpura, a normal platelet count, and signs of systemic illness. In the differential diagnosis, SLE, hypersensitivity vasculitis, and a rare syndrome termed acute hemorrhagic edema of infancy (AHEI) must be considered.

HOW IS HENOCH–SCHÖNLEIN PURPURA MANAGED?

Henoch–Schönlein purpura is a self-limited disease and treatment is largely supportive with adequate hydration, analgesics, and nonsteroidal anti-inflammatory drugs for arthritis. Corticosteroids are widely used in patients with severe or persistent abdominal pain or nephritis.

CLINICAL MANIFESTATIONS OF HENOCH–SCHÖNLEIN PURPURA		
	At onset (% of cases)	During course (% of cases)
Purpura	50	100
Subcutaneous edema	10–20	20–50
Arthritis (large joints)	25	60–85
Gastrointestinal	30	85
Renal	?	10–50
Genitourinary (scrotal swelling)	?	2–35
Pulmonary	?	95
Pulmonary hemorrhage	?	Rare, may be fatal
Central nervous system (headache, organic brain syndrome, seizures)	?	Rare, may be fatal

Fig. 40.7 Frequency of clinical manifestations of Henoch–Schönlein purpura.

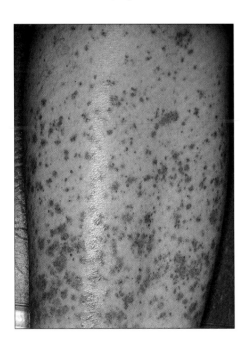

Fig. 40.8 Palpable purpura in a patient with Henoch–Schönlein purpura.

KEY POINTS

Definition
- Henoch–Schönlein purpura is the most common form of vasculitis seen in children.
- Typically, it occurs from September to April and is preceded by upper respiratory syndrome in most patients.

Main clinical features
- Classic disease triad of palpable purpura, colicky abdominal pain, and arthritis is seen in the majority of patients (Fig. 40.7).
- Purpura typically occurs on the lower extremities (Fig. 40.8) and on the buttocks.
- The majority of patients have marked, colicky abdominal pain; gastrointestinal bleeding, intussusception, or bowel infarction may occur.
- Arthritis most commonly occurs in the knees and ankles.
- Rare complications include nephritis, scrotal swelling, central nervous system signs, and pulmonary hemorrhage.

Diagnosis
- Diagnosis is based on the characteristic clinical picture
- No distinguishing laboratory abnormalities are found.
- Thrombocytopenia is not a feature of Henoch–Schönlein purpura and its presence suggests sepsis (particularly meningococcemia), a hematologic disorder (i.e. leukemia, idiopathic thrombocytopenic purpura, or TTP), or an autoimmune syndrome such as systemic lupus erythematosus.
- Serum levels of IgA may be elevated.
- Skin biopsy may be helpful in difficult cases and shows leukocytoclastic vasculitis with granulocytes in the walls of arterioles and veins and IgA staining on immunofluorescence sections.

FAMILIAL MEDITERRANEAN FEVER

KEY POINTS

Definition
- Familial Mediterranean fever is a rare, inherited syndrome with periodic fevers, seen in ethnic groups of Mediterranean and Middle Eastern ancestry, especially non-Ashkenazi Jews, Armenians, Turks, and Levantine Arabs.

Main clinical features
- Intermittent attacks of high fevers, peritonitis, pleurisy, erysipelas-like rashes, and arthritis (knees and hips).
- Attacks last 24–72 hours with patient entirely well between episodes.
- Major, serious, long-term complications are amyloid nephropathy and renal failure.

Diagnosis
- Presence of diagnostic riteria (Fig. 40.9) and consideration of ethnic background of the patient.
- The gene responsible for the disease is now identified (short arm of chromosome 16) and genetic testing is now possible.

IN WHAT CIRCUMSTANCES IS FAMILIAL MEDITERRANEAN FEVER SUSPECTED?

Familial Mediterranean fever (FMF) is considered in children with attacks of unexplained fevers, particularly when accompanied by arthritis and serositis. The principal differential diagnoses include systemic juvenile chronic polyarthritis, hyperimmunoglobulin D syndrome, and familial Hibernian fever.

HOW IS FAMILIAL MEDITERRANEAN FEVER MANAGED?

Attacks of FMF resolve spontaneously. Prophylactic colchicine 1–2mg daily decreases the frequency and severity of attacks and, most importantly, prevents the development of amyloidosis.

TEL-HASHOMER CRITERIA FOR THE DIAGNOSIS OF FAMILIAL MEDITERRANEAN FEVER

Major criteria
1. Recurrent febrile episodes accompanied by peritonitis, synovitis, or pleuritis.
2. Amyloidosis of the AA type without predisposing disease.
3. Favorable response to continuous colchicine treatment.

Minor criteria
1. Recurrent febrile episodes.
2. Erysipelas-like erythema.
3. Familial Mediterranean fever in a first degree relative.

Definitive diagnosis: 2 major or 1 major and 2 minor.
Probable diagnosis: 1 major and 1 minor.

Fig. 40.9 Tel-Hashomer criteria for the diagnosis of familial Mediterranean fever.

KAWASAKI DISEASE

KEY POINTS

Definition
- Kawasaki disease is a rare, acute febrile disease of children under 5 years of age.

Main clinical features
- Fever (>38°C for 10–14 days), cervical lymphadenopathy, conjunctival congestion, redness and fissuring of the lips, rash, and desquamation of the skin of the fingertips.
- Coronary artery aneurysms are the most serious long-term complication.

Diagnosis
- Presence of diagnostic criteria(Fig. 40.10).

IN WHAT CIRCUMSTANCES IS KAWASAKI DISEASE SUSPECTED?

Although a rare disorder, it is important to recognize Kawasaki disease early since it is potentially fatal and coronary artery aneurysms can be prevented with early, aggressive treatment. The major clinical clues to suggest the disease include bilateral conjunctival congestion with crusting of the lips (Fig. 40.11), polymorphous exanthema of the trunk or extremities (Fig. 40.12), and a desquamation of the skin of the fingertips (Fig. 40.13). Two-dimensional echocardiography is carried out weekly for the first month of the disease to detect involvement of the coronary arteries.

HOW IS KAWASAKI DISEASE TREATED?

Kawasaki disease is typically a self-limited illness that lasts 10–14 days. Hydration with intravenous fluids and aspirin in doses of 30–50mg/kg/day generally helps to suppress the fever and make the child more comfortable. Antibiotics are of no value in treatment of the disease. If aneurysms are detected on echocardiography, treatment with immunoglobulin is indicated; anticoagulants are used in children with evidence of large aneurysm formation.

THE SIX PRINCIPAL SYMPTOMS OF KAWASAKI DISEASE

Fever persisting 5 days or more

Bilateral conjunctival congestion

Changes in lips and oral cavity:
 Reddening of lips, strawberry tongue, diffuse injection of oral and pharyngeal mucosa

Acute nonpurulent cervical lymphadenopathy

Polymorphous exanthem

Changes in peripheral extremities:
 Reddening of palms and soles, indurative edema in acute phase
 Membranous desquamation later

Diagnosis
5/6 symptoms present or
4/6 plus coronary aneurysm visualized by two-dimensional
 echocardiography or coronary angiography

Fig. 40.10 The six principal symptoms of Kawasaki disease.

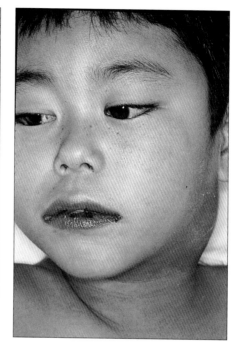

Fig. 40.11 Conjunctival congestion, bleeding, and crust formation on the lips and left cervical adenopathy, in Kawasaki disease.

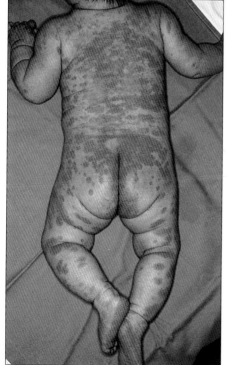

Fig. 40.12 Polymorphous exanthema on the limbs and trunk of an infant with Kawasaki disease.

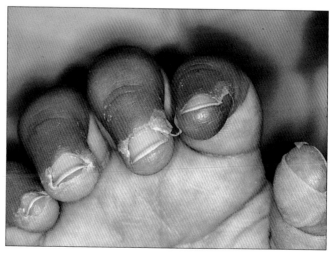

Fig. 40.13 Desquamation of the fingertips in a child with Kawasaki disease.

OLDER PEOPLE

MUSCULOSKELETAL PROBLEMS IN OLDER PEOPLE

INTRODUCTION

Musculoskeletal disorders are one of the most frequent and important healthcare problems of older people, being responsible for a huge burden of pain and disability.

Given the increasing numbers of older people in Western countries, with the associated increase in their demands for fitness in the latter part of their lives, these problems have started to assume huge importance, and will do so to an even greater degree in the future.

AGING AND THE MUSCULOSKELETAL SYSTEM

As people age, a decrease in function of many tissues occurs; however, this varies in effect on different organs, and in different individuals. Some examples of the types of changes in organ structure and function are shown in Figure 41.1; less is known about the individual variations in different people.

Special features of relevance to aging of the musculoskeletal system include its exposure to physical trauma throughout people's lives, and the general paucity of repair capacity in many musculoskeletal tissues.

Muscle power decreases markedly with age (Fig. 41.2), but it can be retained by training and physical therapy at any age. This is very important, as it may be that the age-related loss of muscle power tips the balance between someone being able to get on a toilet seat and off it, for example, when they have an osteoarthritic knee – and the muscle power can be improved.

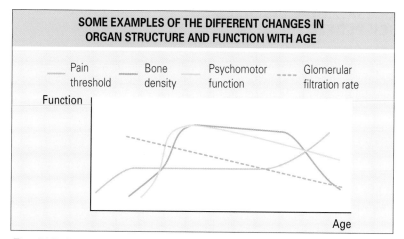

SOME EXAMPLES OF THE DIFFERENT CHANGES IN ORGAN STRUCTURE AND FUNCTION WITH AGE

Pain threshold   Bone density   Psychomotor function   Glomerular filtration rate

Function

Age

Fig. 41.1 Examples of the different age-related changes in organ structure and function. Note the increase in pain threshold, and the different rates and times of decrease in function of different organs.

THE MUSCULOSKELETAL SYSTEM IN OLDER PEOPLE

- Age-related changes in musculoskeletal tissues reduce functional ability – e.g. the normal loss of muscle power in older people.
- The accumulated burden of rheumatic disorders that arise at any time in life and cause age-related increases in disability without shortening life span – eg. the increasing problems of long-standing rheumatoid arthritis in an older patient.
- The existence of a number of rheumatic diseases that are confined largely to older people – such as polymyalgia rheumatica.
- The high prevalence of osteoporosis, falls, and fractures in older people.
- Co-morbidities in older people, which increase the impact of any rheumatic disorder – eg. the combination of Parkinson's disease and osteoarthritis in an older person can be devastating to function.
- Changes in the immune system that lead to false-positive tests for autoantibodies and changed expression of rheumatic diseases in older people.
- The altered expression of rheumatic diseases in older people, which can lead to delays in diagnosis and treatment – for example, the presentation of gout in older women is quite different from that in middle-aged men.
- Other age-related disorders can present with a syndrome that mimics a rheumatic disease – for example, tumors and thyroid disease may present with musculoskeletal pain.
- The susceptibility of older people to drug toxicities – eg. the high prevalence of problems with nonsteroidal anti-inflammatory drugs in older people.
- The increasing importance of psychosocial factors that interact with impairments in older people.

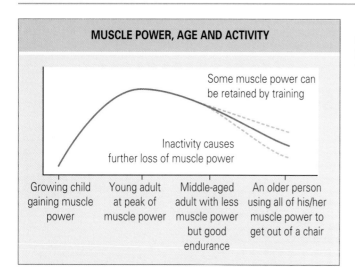

MUSCLE POWER, AGE AND ACTIVITY

Some muscle power can be retained by training

Inactivity causes further loss of muscle power

Growing child gaining muscle power

Young adult at peak of muscle power

Middle-aged adult with less muscle power but good endurance

An older person using all of his/her muscle power to get out of a chair

Fig. 41.2 Muscle power, age, and activity. Note the decrease in muscle power with age, which can be made worse by loss of activity, but is improved by training at any age.

Bone mass also decreases with age, which is a major factor in the high prevalence of problems related to osteoporosis in older people.

Tendons, ligaments, and cartilage also age, which contributes to the alterations in function associated with older people.

Dramatic age-related changes in the immune system also have a major impact on rheumatic disease expression and diagnosis. As people age they produce more autoantibodies, so 'false-positive' tests for rheumatoid and antinuclear factors, among others, are particularly common in older people; the alteration in immune reactions also contributes to the altered expression of some inflammatory rheumatic diseases in old people. In very old people, defense to infections is impaired, which results in an increased prevalence of bone and joint sepsis.

Pain thresholds change with age, as does the interpretation and response to pain. Pain thresholds tend to increase in older people, and pain behavior may be less overt, which leads to confusion between pain and depression for example.

Locomotor function changes with age, with a gradual decrease in the range of motion of many joints as people age, and decreases in aspects of function, such as dexterity, also occur.

Spontaneous tendon ruptures and collapse of the arches of the feet are also common age-related problems.

MUSCULOSKELETAL DISEASES IN OLDER PEOPLE

The special problems of older people can be categorized as:
- Diseases that cause a huge burden of pain and disability in older people.
- Diseases that usually have their onset in older people.
- Diseases that have an altered expression when the onset is in older people.
- Age-related disorders that can mimic a rheumatic disease.
- Age-related hazards to the musculoskeletal system.

DISEASES THAT CAUSE A HUGE BURDEN OF PAIN AND DISABILITY IN OLDER PEOPLE
- Osteoporosis.
- Osteoarthritis.

Osteoporosis and osteoarthritis both have their peak of incidence in middle age. However, they tend to progress with age, without shortening life span, so the accumulated burden of disease is largely in the older population.

DISEASES THAT USUALLY HAVE THEIR ONSET IN OLDER PEOPLE
- Polymyalgia rheumatica and giant cell arteritis.
- Pseudogout.
- Paget's disease.
- Spinal stenosis.
- Large-joint destructive arthropathies.

These conditions are all largely confined to people over the age of 60 years, and are rare in anyone under 50 years of age.

DISEASES THAT HAVE AN ALTERED EXPRESSION WHEN THE ONSET IS IN OLDER PEOPLE
- Rheumatoid arthritis.
- Systemic lupus erythematosus.
- Gout.

The altered expression of these conditions in older people leads to both delayed diagnosis and misdiagnosis.

AGE-RELATED DISORDERS THAT CAN MIMIC A RHEUMATIC DISEASE
- Thyroid and parathyroid disorders.
- Malignant diseases, which include multiple myeloma.
- Parkinson's disease.
- Pernicious anemia.
- Peripheral neuropathies.
- Depression.

Each of these conditions can present with symptoms and signs that mimic a rheumatic disease, which results in diagnostic problems.

AGE-RELATED HAZARDS TO THE MUSCULOSKELETAL SYSTEM
- Increased prevalence of falls,
- Increased susceptibility to infections of bones and joints.
- Co-morbidities – especially those that affect cognitive or neuromuscular function.
- Nutritional problems, which include osteomalacia.
- The hazards of excessive rest (particularly bed rest) in older people.

These extra hazards, which affect the very old in particular, result in an increased burden of damage to the musculoskeletal system, and also contribute to the impact of any musculoskeletal problem on an older individual.

DIAGNOSIS
Diagnosis obviously presents special problems in an older individual. Combinations of co-morbidities, variable responses to pain and disability, altered disease expression, and altered blood tests (such as the high prevalence of raised erythrocyte sedimentation rates or of autoantibodies) make the physician's job much more difficult than for younger patients. A high level of awareness of the range of age-related problems of older people is essential.

Particularly common problems that arise include the presentation of occult carcinoma, masked depression, or hypothyroidism as arthritis in an older person.

THREE IMPORTANT ISSUES IN THE MANAGEMENT OF OLDER PEOPLE	
Issue	Main Aspects
Drugs	Increased susceptibility to drug toxicity Polypharmacy
Rehabilitation	The hazards of rest and benefits of activity Increasing problems with activities and participation Changing needs and aspirations
Psychosocial isolation	Cognitive and psychologic problems Poverty Social isolation The importance of caregivers

Fig. 41.3 Three important issues in the management of older people.

DRUG USE FOR MUSCULOSKELETAL DISORDERS IN OLDER PEOPLE

- Beware polypharmacy and drug interactions.
- Beware the use of over-the-counter medications that may interact with prescribed drugs.
- Consider simple analgesics before using nonsteroidal anti-inflammatory drugs (NSAIDs).
- Consider the use of intra-articular corticosteroids in acute situations, and rubefacients in chronic pain as alternatives to NSAIDs.
- Beware reduced renal or hepatic function – doses of any drug may need to be reduced because of these changes.

Fig. 41.4 Drug use for musculoskeletal disorders in older people

 MANAGEMENT OF MUSCULOSKELETAL DISORDERS IN OLDER PEOPLE

The special problems of disease management in older people revolve around three separate issues that have to be considered (Fig. 41.3):
- drug problems (Fig. 41.4);
- rehabilitation of older people who have musculoskeletal problems; and
- psychosocial issues.

DRUG PROBLEMS IN OLDER PEOPLE

Changes in renal and hepatic function with age mean that drugs are metabolized and excreted less well in older people, and thus their susceptibility to drug toxicity is increased. The 'hidden' reduction in renal function (Fig. 41.5) is particularly important, as many drugs are also potentially toxic to the kidney.

Nonsteroidal anti-inflammatory drugs (NSAIDs) present special problems, as older people are more susceptible to gastric ulceration, bleeding, and perforation; also, NSAIDs often cause renal problems in older people, which can lead to renal failure. They should be used with extreme caution, and renal function must be checked frequently before and after an NSAID is started in an older individual.

Intra-articular corticosteroids and percutaneous drugs (rubefacients) present reasonable alternatives to systemic agents like NSAIDs in older people.

The dose of several drugs used in rheumatic diseases needs to be reduced in older people because of reduced renal and hepatic function.

Polypharmacy in older people is a common problem; the average ambulatory elderly patient in the USA is taking seven prescribed medicines, as well as three over-the-counter medications.

REHABILITATION OF OLDER PEOPLE WHO HAVE MUSCULOSKELETAL PROBLEMS

As people age, their needs and aspirations change. In addition, many older people adapt remarkably well to musculoskeletal problems. Both factors result in changing perceptions of the nature of the remedial input that is required. The physician must always be sensitive to the needs and wishes of the older patient, and (where appropriate) the family and caregivers.

In the management of the older patient, the emphasis often needs to be on the consequences of a disease, rather than its cause or activity.

Comprehensive assessment of the issues of importance to the patient and caregivers is the first step – it often helps to list the problems. It may also be helpful to categorize the problems in terms of the impairment, restricted activities (or disability), and any issues that relate to participation (or handicap).

Goal setting is the next step in the process. Simple, attainable goals should be set and agreed between patient, caregivers, and health-care professionals. Regular review is appropriate, and a team approach may be necessary, and may involve a variety of professionals such as physical therapists and occupational therapists.

It is important to try to avoid excessive rest in older people – bed rest can result in a number of disastrous complications, which include skin ulceration, deep vein thrombosis, and infections. Immobilization of individual joints can lead to stiffness and severe muscle wasting, with further loss of function.

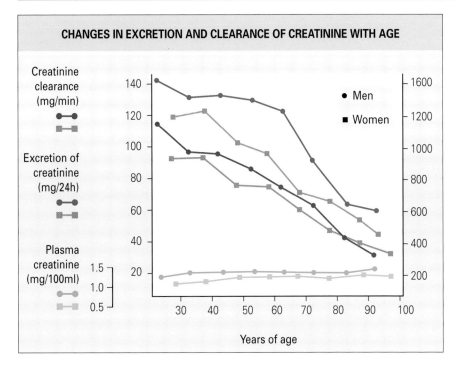

CHANGES IN EXCRETION AND CLEARANCE OF CREATININE WITH AGE

Creatinine clearance (mg/min)

Excretion of creatinine (mg/24h)

Plasma creatinine (mg/100ml)

Years of age

Fig. 41.5 The 'hidden' reduction in renal function with age. Although the normal creatinine clearance decreases dramatically with age to a mean of only 40ml/min in the very elderly, the plasma creatinine remains constant up to 100 years of age because of a concomitant reduction in excretion (and by inference, production) of creatinine as a result of reduction in muscle mass. (Data from Kampmann J, Siersbaek-Nielsen K, Kristensen K, Moholm-Hamnsen J. Rapid evaluation of creatinine clearance. Acta Med Scand. 1974;196:517–20.)

PSYCHOSOCIAL ISSUES

The psychosocial circumstances must be assessed carefully. In many older people, the family and financial situations, cultural and ethnic background, religious beliefs, and personality traits are of greater significance to the development of an appropriate management plan than any specific rheumatic condition or its treatment with a drug or operation.

The history must include cognizance of the observations and views of family and caregivers as well as the patient. Cognitive and mood problems are common and color the development of a management plan. Poverty and social isolation are often major issues that need to be addressed.`

OLDER PEOPLE

GENERALIZED OSTEOARTHRITIS

Osteoarthritis can present in single joints (particularly the knee or hip) in relatively young people, most commonly as a result of previous congenital abnormalities, disease, or injury in that joint (see Chapters 13 and 14 on the knee and hip, respectively). In addition, the condition sometimes presents as a polyarthritis of the hands in middle-aged women.

However, generalized osteoarthritis is largely a problem of older people, for two reasons. First, the onset of the common form of 'primary' osteoarthritis peaks in the sixth and seventh decades. Second, as people who have any form of osteoarthritis grow older the number of joint sites affected by the condition tends to accumulate, which leads to a pattern in place of a previous pattern of just one or two joints being involved (Fig. 42.1).

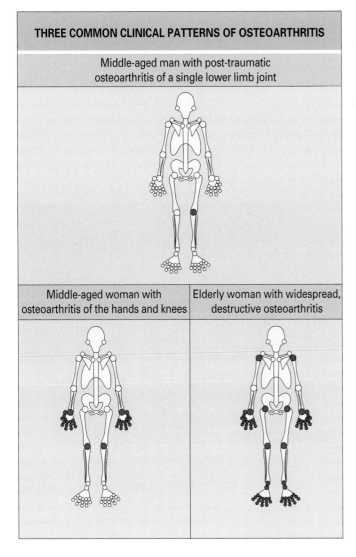

THREE COMMON CLINICAL PATTERNS OF OSTEOARTHRITIS

Middle-aged man with post-traumatic osteoarthritis of a single lower limb joint

Middle-aged woman with osteoarthritis of the hands and knees

Elderly woman with widespread, destructive osteoarthritis

Fig. 42.1 Different patterns of osteoarthritis occur at different ages. In younger groups a single joint is often affected, whereas in older people the condition is more likely to be generalized.

KEY POINTS

- Osteoarthritis that affects several different joints in an older person.
- The most common peripheral joint sites affected include the distal interphalangeal joints and thumb base in the hands, the hips and knees, and the first metatarsophalangeal joints.
- Spinal osteoarthritis (spondylosis) frequently coexists with this peripheral joint pattern.
- Affected joints develop use-related pain, inactivity gelling, and a reduced range of joint motion.
- Physical signs include bony swelling, crepitus, and pain on movement.
- The outcome for the individual is often dominated by the degree of pain and impairment that arises from peripheral large-joint damage.
- Spinal stenosis can complicate spondylosis.
- Patients of any age should be encouraged to be more active, and may respond well to simple physical interventions.
- Drug treatment is hazardous.
- Patients who suffer advanced hip or knee involvement may benefit greatly from a joint replacement.

FEATURES OF ESTABLISHED GENERALIZED OSTEOARTHRITIS

- An extremely common problem, especially in older women.
- Risk factors include a family history and previous or current obesity, as well as increasing age.
- Heberden's nodes on the fingers are usually present and are a marker of the tendency to generalized osteoarthritis (GOA) – they rarely cause clinical problems in older patients.
- Thumb base disease is also present in most cases, and can cause a great deal of problems with hand function.
- Bilateral hip or knee disease is usually present, although severe disease in both the hips and knees of the same patient is uncommon.
- One or both hips or knees may become damaged, which can cause severe pain, including night pain, and great disability.
- Most patients have spondylosis of both the cervical and lumbar spine, which results in pain and stiffness.
- Root and cord compression (especially spinal stenosis) occasionally complicate GOA.

1 TYPICAL CASE: ESTABLISHED GENERALIZED OSTEOARTHRITIS

Fiona is a 79-year-old woman who has a long history of joint problems. Problems began when she was a somewhat overweight but otherwise fit and active 61-year-old; her knees slowly became stiff and painful, which made it difficult for her to walk as far as she had been able to previously. A few years later, as her knees deteriorated, she noticed the development of pain at the base of her right thumb, which made it difficult to grip things and to sew clothes. She has also developed pain and stiffness in her neck, which sometimes flares up badly for a week or two, and has much discomfort in the lower part of her back, particularly if she sits or stands in one position for any length of time.

Her main problem when she consults you is the increasingly severe pain in her right knee joint, which now keeps her awake at night, and prevents her from walking to such a degree that she has become dependent on others for the first time in her life.

On examination she is generally well for her age. You notice Heberden's nodes on her fingers (Fig. 42.2) and squaring of the base of the thumbs. A great deal of stiffness of both the cervical and lumbar spine is present, but you find no neurologic symptoms or signs to suggest any root or cord complications. Her knees both have advanced osteoarthritis, but you are particularly worried about the right knee, which has a large varus deformity and appears unstable. She can hardly stand up because of the knee problem.

You refer her to an orthopedic surgeon who performs a successful knee replacement. She is grateful, as she can now be independent again, in spite of the continuing problems with the back and other joints.

NATURAL HISTORY AND OTHER CLINICAL FEATURES

Established generalized osteoarthritis (GOA) tends to be slowly progressive, although patients may go through periods of many months or years when things do not change a great deal, and the combination of adaptation to the condition,

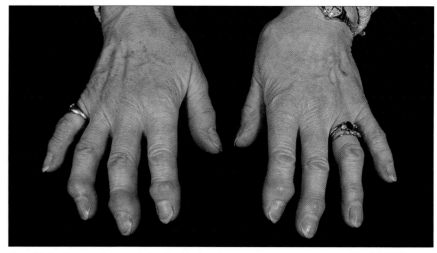

Fig. 42.2 Osteoarthritis of the distal interphalangeal (DIP) joints. This patient has the typical clinical findings of advanced osteoarthritis of the DIP joints, including large, firm swellings (Heberden's nodes), some of which are tender and red because of associated inflammation of the periarticular tissues as well as of the joint.

increased pain thresholds in older people, and changing needs and aspirations lead to apparent improvements.

Severe destruction of one or both hips or knees can occur relatively rapidly (over a period of about a year) at any time in patients who have established GOA, and leads to very severe pain and disability (Fig. 42.3).

Some patients develop spinal stenosis (see Chapter 44); cervical myelopathy is much less common (Chapter 25), but root compression can occur in either the neck or lumbar spine.

Other complications that can occur include attacks of pseudogout (Chapter 44) and osteonecrosis.

 ## POINTS TO LOOK OUT FOR

The severity of the problems experienced by this group of patients is often underestimated in primary care. The main problems to be aware of in older people who have GOA include the development of severe large joint or spinal damage, and increasing disability or psychosocial problems – either of which can happen without the patient complaining unduly. Drug toxicity is another issue.

- Spinal stenosis can develop insidiously, which leads to increasing functional problems and neurologic complications that are mistaken for age-related changes.
- Severe hip or knee destruction can occur either relatively quickly or relatively slowly, and leads to severe pain and/or disability; too many older people are denied joint replacements on the basis of age or because the severity of their problem is not understood by doctors.
- Isolation and depression are common complications of generalized osteoarthritis (GOA); as pain on walking worsens, older people venture out less and become socially isolated; the combination of pain and reduced function is also a potent cause of anxiety and depression.
- Drug toxicity is common in older people who suffer from GOA, as they frequently use over-the-counter medications in addition to prescribed ones, co-morbidities leading to polypharmacy and drug interactions.

INVESTIGATIONS

No investigations are indicated in the majority of people who have GOA. Radiographic evidence of osteoarthritis in affected joints is of no interest, as decision making is based on the clinical assessment of the severity and impact of the condition, and the correlation between radiographic damage and clinical features is poor. Also, blood tests are not abnormal in osteoarthritis. There are limited indications for the use of investigations.

INDICATIONS FOR INVESTIGATING PATIENTS WHO HAVE GENERALIZED OSTEOARTHRITIS

CONCERNS WITH DRUG TOXICITY
Hepatic and renal function may need to be assessed; for example, renal function should be checked frequently after the initiation of nonsteroidal anti-inflammatory drug (NSAID) therapy.

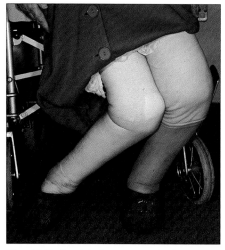

Fig. 42.3 An elderly woman who has advanced, destructive osteoarthritis of the knees, leading to total instability. This patient may have benefited from earlier referral for total knee replacements.

SUDDEN WORSENING

Some patients undergo a sudden deterioration of pain or function, which may be caused by a complication such as osteonecrosis or a concomitant fracture around a joint, or by the development of another co-morbid condition. Investigations, which include radiographs, may be appropriate.

CONSIDERATION OF REFERRAL FOR SURGERY

If surgery is considered, radiographs are needed by the surgeon as part of his/her assessment, but special views (such as weight-bearing radiographs) may be required; depending on circumstances, the radiography may be best done in primary care, or left to the surgeon.

CONCERN ABOUT COMPLICATIONS, PARTICULARLY NERVE ROOT OR SPINAL CORD COMPRESSION

Such concerns warrant radiography, the most useful being lateral views of either the cervical or lumbar spine, from which spinal canal width can be assessed – referral for further investigations and treatment may also be needed.

DIFFERENTIAL DIAGNOSIS

No significant diagnostic issue arises (another reason not to investigate patients). Other types of joint damage that can occur in older people include those associated with neurologic disease (neuropathic arthritis, Chapter 18), with pyrophosphate crystal deposition (pseudogout,), and with large-joint atrophic, destructive arthritis (Chapter 44) – but these are best viewed as variants within the spectrum of GOA, and management is essentially the same whether these conditions are present or not.

 ## MANAGEMENT OF GENERALIZED OSTEOARTHRITIS

OBJECTIVES OF THERAPY
The main objectives of therapy are:
- To reduce pain and stiffness as much as possible with minimum risk.
- To treat any associated psychologic problems such as anxiety or depression.
- To improve function and general activity as much as possible, thus increasing participation (reducing disability and handicap).
- To empower people, through education and support, to live as fulfilling a life as possible.
- To look out for any complications, such as severe joint destruction, spinal stenosis, sudden worsening, or drug toxicity, and to treat these promptly.

EDUCATION AND SUPPORT
Education of both patients and caregivers is important. A positive approach is appropriate, as only a minority of GOA patients come to surgery or become severely disabled. It is clear that increased activity and exercise, at any age, is advantageous to both body and mind, and patients may need reassurance that, contrary to their expectations, joints do not wear out through use.

Psychosocial issues and drugs need to be considered, and a very careful assessment of the degree of impairment disability and handicap needs to be made, so that clear, simple goals can be set for the patient – such as a gradual improvement in a certain task – which can be agreed upon and reviewed between the patient and all concerned.

Evidence indicates that simple, regular contact can help people greatly.

SUMMARY OF MANAGEMENT

- Use a 'pyramidal' approach – start with education and empowerment, as well as simple physical modalities and life-style modifications, before drugs and/or surgery are considered.
- Reduce joint pain and excess loading by weight loss and, use of a cane, shock-absorbing insoles, heel wedges, and other simple measures.
- Improve function of affected joints by maintaining the range of movement, increasing muscle strength and stability, and correcting abnormal biomechanics.
- Maintain and increase general activity levels and advise a moderate, regular exercise program.
- Consider intermittent use of local rubefacients and simple analgesics for pain relief.
- Reserve nonsteroidal anti-inflammatory drugs, intra-articular therapy, and other drugs for symptom flares, and use as an adjunct to physical therapy.
- A wide variety of surgical options are available for patients who suffer persistent, severe symptoms.
- Several new therapeutic approaches are being developed. These should not be used outside trials until their benefits and safety are proved.

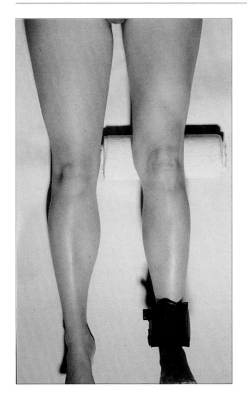

Fig. 42.4 Quadriceps exercises for knee osteoarthritis. Quadriceps exercises are of proved value for pain relief and improvement in function, and everyone with knee osteoarthritis must be taught the correct techniques and encouraged to make these exercises a lifetime habit. This patient is being shown how to fully straighten the knee, with the ankle dorsiflexed, and then practice straight-leg raising, as well as the extension exercises, with a weight on the ankle.

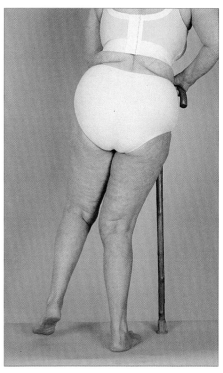

Fig. 42.5 Use of a cane, stick, or other walking aid. This patient, who has hip osteoarthritis, has found that she can reduce the pain in her damaged left hip by leaning on the stick in the right hand as she walks. The reduction in loading can be huge, and the effect on symptoms and confidence with walking can be very beneficial.

PHYSICAL THERAPY

Physical therapy can help with education and support. An increase in simple activities such as walking can help if patients are able to tolerate it. For those who have access to it, exercise in warm water can be very beneficial (such as 'aqua-jogging'). Local heat packs can help relieve pain. Specific exercise therapy may help for a specific joint site, such as the spine or knee (Fig. 42.4).

In addition, much help can be obtained by alterations to footwear, walking and other aids, and orthoses. All patients who have GOA must be advised to use footwear with good, shock-absorbing properties (such as 'jogging' shoes); walking sticks can help enormously; and the very disabled may need walkers or chairs to increase independence (Fig. 42.5). The need for aids to steps, stairs, showers, or baths must be considered. Bandages around knees can provide a sense of security, and orthoses for knees or thumb bases may reduce disability and pain (see also knee osteoarthritis management, Chapter 14).

DRUGS

The reduced renal function in older people demands great care in the context of NSAIDs, which are more likely to cause gastrointestinal toxicity in this age group and which can also lead to fluid retention, cardiac failure, and renal failure in older people. Simple analgesics and local rubefacients are preferred to NSAIDs.

The thumb base and knee (if an effusion is present) may benefit from local injection therapy.

SURGERY

Joint replacements are probably underutilized in older people who have GOA. The combination of the tendency to underestimate the severity of patient problems and a prejudice against using surgery in older people can mean that they are denied operations that could result in a huge improvement (Figs 42.6 & 42.7). Recent evidence suggests that the consideration of joint replacement should not be ruled out on the basis of advanced age.

In addition to total joint replacement, simpler measures, such as joint lavage, can be useful.

DIET AND COMPLEMENTARY TECHNIQUES

A large number of products for joints are available over the counter, and these are very widely used by patients who suffer from GOA.

Several dietary supplements are recommended, including glucosamine, avocado products, and vitamins – although the amount of benefit achieved by these sorts of product appears to be generally either small or (in some cases) no greater than that of a placebo.

Transcutaneous electrical nerve stimulation, acupuncture, and a variety of heat, light, magnetic, or filing therapies are also popular, although very little evidence of efficacy is available.

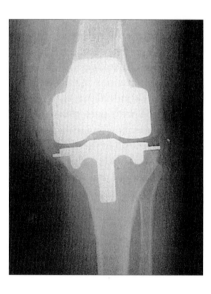

Fig. 42.6 Radiograph showing a modern (Kinemase) knee replacement for knee osteoarthritis. (Courtesy of I Learmonth.)

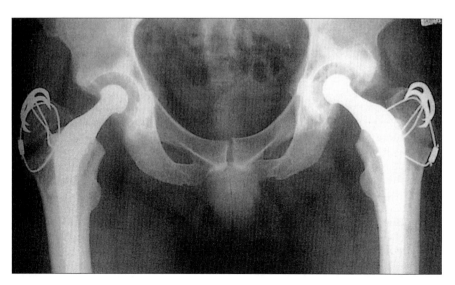

Fig. 42.7 Radiograph showing bilateral, low-friction arthroplasties for hip osteoarthritis. (Courtesy of I Learmonth.)

POLYMYALGIA RHEUMATICA AND GIANT CELL ARTERITIS

Polymyalgia rheumatica and giant cell (temporal) arteritis are related systemic disorders seen in older (>50 years) patients often of North European descent. Both diseases are more common in women than in men. Patients typically present with prominent constitutional signs (fever, weight loss, and fatigue), unexplained anemia and musculoskeletal symptoms localized to the shoulders and hips. The clinical response to corticosteroids is often dramatic.

TYPICAL CASE:
POLYMYALGIA RHEUMATICA

Mary is a 64-year-old retired librarian seen with a 3-week history of low-grade fevers, and severe pain and stiffness in her shoulders. Her symptoms seem to be much worse in the mornings and over the past week she has had great trouble dressing. Her appetite has been poor and she notes a 4.5kg (10lb) weight loss.

On examination, palpation or movement of both shoulders produces marked pain. Her muscle strength, however, appears to be normal. Mild swelling is noted in both wrists. Laboratory studies show a hematocrit of 23%, a negative rheumatoid factor and the erythrocyte sedimentation rate (ESR) is 120mm/h Westergren.

FEATURES OF POLYMYALGIA RHEUMATICA

- Constitutional signs – fever, fatigue, anorexia, weight loss, depression.
- Pain and stiffness in the neck, proximal shoulder, and hip girdle muscles.
- Muscles tender on examination, with normal muscle strength.
- Morning stiffness common – patients are often unable to rise out of bed or dress themselves.
- Mild arthritis of wrists and hands, knees, and feet.
- Marked elevation of erythrocyte sedimentation rate.
- Normochromic, normocytic anemia

KEY POINTS

Polymyalgia rheumatica
Definition
- A clinical syndrome of the middle-aged and elderly characterized by pain and stiffness in the neck, proximal shoulder, and hip girdle muscles.
- The clinical response to small doses of corticosteroids can be dramatic.

Clinical features
- The musculoskeletal symptoms are usually bilateral and symmetric.
- Stiffness is the predominant feature; it is particularly severe after rest and may prevent the patient from rising out of bed in the morning.
- Muscular pain is often diffuse and is accentuated by movement; pain at night is common.
- Corticosteroid treatment is usually required for at least 2 years. Most patients should be able to stop taking corticosteroids after 4–5 years.
- Systemic features include low-grade fever, fatigue, weight loss, and an elevated erythrocyte sedimentation rate.

Giant cell arteritis
Definition
- A vasculitis that commonly accompanies polymyalgia rheumatica. Other terms used include temporal arteritis, cranial arteritis, and granulomatous arteritis.
- Early recognition and treatment can prevent blindness and other complications caused by occlusion or rupture of involved arteries.

Clinical features
- A wide range of symptoms are seen, but most patients have clinical findings related to involved arteries.
- Frequent features include fatigue, headaches, jaw claudication, loss of vision, scalp tenderness, polymyalgia rheumatica, and aortic arch syndrome.

FEATURES OF GIANT CELL ARTERITIS

- Signs and symptoms of polymyalgia rheumatica in the majority of patients.
- Scalp tenderness with pain on combing or brushing hair.
- Claudication of jaw muscles with pain on chewing.
- Severe headache, mostly commonly localized to temporal regions.
- Transient or persistent visual disturbances, including blindness.

2 TYPICAL CASE: GIANT CELL ARTERITIS

Mr Svensson is a 74-year-old widower who has lived in a Lutheran nursing home since the death of his wife 6 months ago. He has shown increasing signs of depression over the past several months and for the past week has spent most of the time in bed claiming he hurts all over. He complains of a severe headache that began 2 days ago, which has not been relieved by aspirin, and he states that the vision in his right eye has been blurred since early this morning.

On physical examination the right temporal artery is dilated and very tender to palpation (Fig. 43.1). Funduscopic evaluation of the right eye reveals a pale optic disc with blurring of the disc margins (Fig. 43.2).

NATURAL HISTORY AND OTHER CLINICAL FEATURES

Most studies suggest that polymyalgia rheumatica and giant cell arteritis are self-limited disorders that last for approximately 2–4 years. The majority of patients become completely free of symptoms and are taken off drug therapy. Relapses are most likely in the first 18 months of treatment and, at present, it is not possible to predict which patients are at risk of relapse.

Less common features include:
- Depression and confusion.
- Aortic regurgitation and congestive heart failure.
- Peripheral neuropathy.
- Abnormalities of liver function.

! POINTS TO LOOK OUT FOR

- Visual symptoms – blurring of vision indicates ischemia of optic nerve, retina, choroid, or cerebral vascular involvement.
- Rising erythrocyte sedimentation rate – generally indicates a relapse of the disease.
- Extracranial vasculitis – rarely giant cell arteritis affects extracranial arteries to cause strokes, aortic aneurysms or dissection, coronary artery disease, or renal artery stenosis (Fig. 43.3).

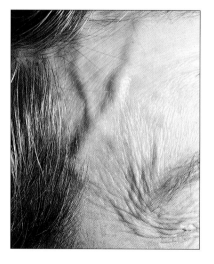

Fig. 43.1 Dilated temporal arteries in a patient who has giant cell arteritis.

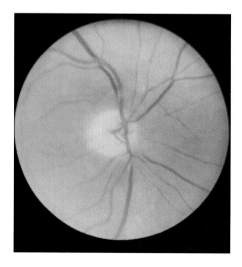

Fig. 43.2 A fundus photograph showing optic atrophy secondary to giant cell arteritis.

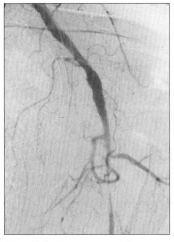

Fig. 43.3 Arteriogram showing an area of marked narrowing of the axillary artery caused by giant cell arteritis inflammation in the vessel wall.

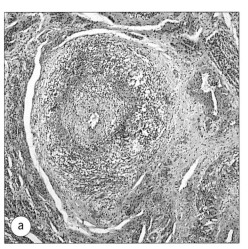

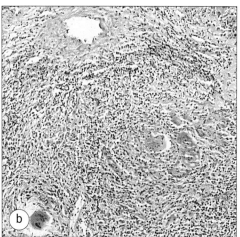

Fig. 43.4 Histology of giant cell arteritis. (a) Low-powered view of arterial wall showing infiltration by lymphocytes and plasma cells. (b) High-powered view showing giant cells in close relationship to elastic lamina.

INVESTIGATIONS

Laboratory tests. Marked elevation of ESR is present in almost all patients. Anemia, typically with microchromic, microcytic indices, is common. Increased levels of alkaline phosphatase are often present.

Biopsy of temporal artery. Indicated in patients who have suspected giant cell arteritis. The arteritis is histologically a panarteritis with giant-cell granuloma formation, often in close proximity to a disrupted, internal elastic lamina (Fig. 43.4) with narrowing of the lumen. Up to one-third of patients who have signs and symptoms of giant cell arteritis have a negative temporal artery biopsy, presumably because of the localized nature of the pathology. Conversely, pathologic abnormalities on temporal artery biopsy are detected in 10–15% of patients who have polymyalgia rheumatica but who demonstrate no symptoms suggestive of giant cell arteritis.

Imaging. Angiography of the temporal arteries is not helpful. However, in patients who have symptoms that suggest involvement of large, extracranial arteries (aorta, renal, etc.), angiography is indicated.

DIFFERENTIAL DIAGNOSIS OF POLYMYALGIA RHEUMATICA	
Neoplastic disease	Muscle disease:
Joint disease:	Polymyositis
Osteoarthritis, particularly of cervical spine	Myopathy
Rheumatoid arthritis	Infections, e.g. bacterial endocarditis
Connective tissue disease	Bone disease, particularly osteomyelitis
Multiple myeloma	Hypothyroidism
Leukemia	Parkinsonism
Lymphoma	Functional

Fig. 43.5 Differential diagnosis of polymyalgia rheumatica.

DIFFERENTIAL DIAGNOSIS

The differential diagnosis of polymyalgia rheumatica is extensive (Fig. 43.5) and typically a delay of several months, or more, occurs before diagnosis. Patients who present with fever or weight loss generally undergo evaluations for infection or malignancy that are unrevealing. The principal rheumatic diseases that need to be considered are rheumatoid arthritis and inflammatory muscle diseases such as polymyositis. Polymyalgia rheumatica can usually be differentiated from late-onset rheumatoid arthritis by the absence of prominent peripheral joint pain and swelling and by a negative or low-titer rheumatoid factor. Patients who have inflammatory muscle diseases typically complain of muscle weakness, as opposed to the muscle pain seen in polymyalgia rheumatica, and show elevations of serum muscle enzymes (creatine phosphokinase or aldolase), which are normal in polymyalgia rheumatica.

The diagnosis of giant cell arteritis should be considered in any patient over the age of 50 years who has severe headaches of recent onset, transient or sudden loss of vision, musculoskeletal complaints localized to the neck and shoulders, unexplained fever or anemia, or an elevated ESR.

R_x MANAGEMENT

The objectives of treatment of polymyalgia rheumatica and giant cell arteritis are to relieve musculoskeletal signs and symptoms, normalize the ESR, and prevent vascular complications developing from an underlying vasculitis. No objective means are available that determine the prognosis in any individual patient and treatment decisions are essentially empiric.

DRUG THERAPY

Corticosteroids are the drug of choice for both polymyalgia rheumatica and giant cell arteritis. Prompt treatment with high-dose corticosteroids is mandatory in patients who have giant cell arteritis to reduce the frequency of vascular complications such as blindness. In polymyalgia rheumatica, the response to corticosteroids is often dramatic with complete resolution of symptoms in a matter of days. Corticosteroid doses are adjusted based on the needs of the individual patient (Fig. 43.6). The overall strategy is to use an adequate dose of prednisolone for the first month to obtain good symptomatic control with a fall in ESR, after which the aim is maintenance doses of <10mg after 6 months. Patients must be advised to expect treatment with corticosteroids for at least 2 years, but most should be able to stop corticosteroid treatment after 4–5 years.

Nonsteroidal anti-inflammatory drugs may provide partial relief of musculoskeletal symptoms, but do not prevent arteritic complications. They have little or no role in primary disease management, but may be used along with corticosteroids.

Immunosuppressive drugs such as azathioprine or methotrexate are used in patients resistant to treatment with corticosteroids.

RECOMMENDATIONS FOR SPECIALIST REFERRAL

- Patients who are suspected of having polymyalgia rheumatica or giant cell arteritis should be referred to a rheumatologist to determine the need for temporal artery biopsy and plan corticosteroid therapy.
- Primary disease management by a rheumatologist is indicated in patients who relapse during reductions of corticosteroid dosages, who develop new signs or symptoms of arteritic involvement, or who still require corticosteroid treatment after 12 months.

MONITORING PROGRESSION AND OUTCOME

In most patients, ESR is a useful monitor of the disease, along with clinical signs and symptoms. No objective measures predict outcome and patients need to be carefully followed for signs that indicate vasculitis, such as headaches, visual changes, scalp tenderness, jaw claudication, or (rarely) involvement of thoracic or abdominal organs.

TREATMENT OF POLYMYALGIA RHEUMATICA AND GIANT CELL ARTERITIS	
For polymyalgia rheumatica*	**Initial dosage** Prednisolone 10–20mg initially for 1 month, reduced by 2.5mg every 2–4 weeks to 10mg daily, then 1mg daily every 4–6 weeks (or until symptoms return).
	Maintenance dosage Prednisolone 5–7mg daily for 6–12 months. Final reduction of 1mg every 6–8 weeks. Most patients require treatment for 3–4 years, but withdrawal after 2 years is worth attempting.
	Special points In patients who cannot reduce prednisolone dosage because of recurring symptoms or who develop serious corticosteroid-related side effects, azathioprine has been shown to have a modest corticosteroid sparing effect, and methotrexate may be more effective.
	Main side effects Weight gain, skin atrophy, edema, increased intraocular pressure, cataracts, gastrointestinal disturbances, diabetes, osteoporosis.
	Risk of side effects Increased risk with high initial doses (>30mg) of prednisolone, maintenance doses of 10mg, and high cumulative doses. Maintenance doses of 5mg are relatively safe.
Giant cell arteritis without visual symptoms	Prednisolone 20–40mg daily initially for 8 weeks reduced by 5mg every 3–4 weeks until dose is 10mg daily; then as for polymyalgia rheumatica.
Giant cell arteritis with possible or definite ocular involvement	Prednisolone 40–80mg daily initially for 8 weeks reduced to 20mg daily over next 4 weeks; then as for giant cell arteritis without visual symptoms.
*Recurrence of symptoms requires an increase in prednisolone dose.	

Fig. 43.6 Treatment of polymyalgia rheumatica and giant cell arteritis.

OTHER DISEASES OF OLDER PEOPLE

PSEUDOGOUT

IN WHAT CIRCUMSTANCES SHOULD PSEUDOGOUT BE SUSPECTED?

Any acute arthritis in older people is regarded as pseudogout until proved otherwise. The most important differential diagnosis is septic arthritis, which is made difficult because pseudogout may cause mild fevers and other evidence of systemic inflammation, and because pseudogout and sepsis occasionally coexist. Ideally, joint fluid should be aspirated and examined for both crystals (by polarized light microscopy) and organisms (by Gram stain and culture).

 MANAGEMENT

Distinction between pseudogout and sepsis by synovial fluid analysis is an essential part of the management. If the patient is very ill and the presence of sepsis is likely, it is reasonable to treat on this assumption while awaiting culture results, by admission for intravenous antibiotics. However, in the majority of cases the patient is not that ill, and the likelihood is that the diagnosis is pseudogout alone, in which case the most effective treatment is intra-articular corticosteroid injections to suppress the inflammation, accompanied by early mobilization to prevent the problems of resting a joint in an elderly person.

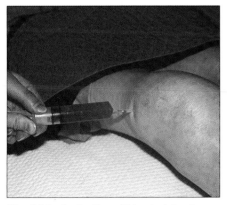

Fig. 44.1 Aspiration of blood-stained synovial fluid in a case of pseudogout. Pseudogout most commonly affects the knee and causes a painful effusion, which is sometimes blood stained.

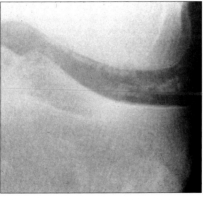

Fig. 44.2 Knee radiograph showing chondrocalcinosis of both fibrocartilage (meniscus) and hyaline cartilage.

KEY POINTS

Definition
- An acute arthritis caused by calcium pyrophosphate crystals.

Main clinical features
- The most common cause of acute arthritis in the elderly.
- Usually affects the knee, but many other joints may be involved, including wrists, shoulders, ankles and elbows.
- Acute, painful swelling of the joint, which develops over 1–3 days, sometimes after trauma, surgery, or in association with some other illness.
- The joint is usually very swollen and painful, and redness of overlying skin and fever may be present.
- Synovial fluid is frequently blood stained (Fig. 44.1), and contains calcium pyrophosphate dihydrate crystals.

Diagnosis
- Radiographs may show chondrocalcinosis (Fig. 44.2), but confirmation of the diagnosis requires identification of the synovial fluid crystals by polarized light microscopy .

PAGET'S DISEASE OF BONE

KEY POINTS

Definition
- A localized disorder of bone remodeling.

Main clinical features
- Rare before 40 years of age and doubles in prevalence with each decade of age thereafter; some 4% of people over 55 years of age have Paget's disease, which is slightly more common in men than in women.
- Bones most frequently affected are, in order – the pelvis, lumbar spine, femur, thoracic spine, sacrum, skull, tibia, and humerus.
- Only some 30% of lesions are symptomatic.
- When symptomatic, pain is the major feature.
- May cause severe deformities because of bone remodeling (Fig. 44.3).
- May result in arthritis of the adjacent joints.
- Pagetic bones may fracture and may develop osteosarcoma.
- Spinal Paget's disease can cause cord compression.

Diagnosis
- Radiographs show the characteristic features (Figs 44.4 & 43.5), and Paget's disease is frequently a chance finding on radiographs.
- Serum alkaline phosphatase is raised, and levels provide a guide to disease activity.

IN WHAT CIRCUMSTANCES SHOULD PAGET'S DISEASE BE SUSPECTED?

Any older person who has bone pain (pain in the bones not relieved by rest) should be suspected of having Paget's disease, as should anyone who complains of bony swelling, such as enlargement of the head (Fig. 44.6).

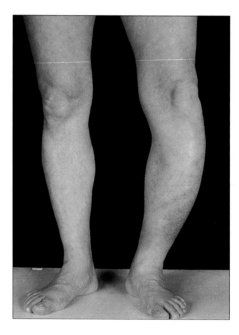

Fig. 44.3 The leg of a patient who has advanced Paget's disease of the tibia. Shown are the marked bowing deformity and the associated varus deformity of the knee caused by the secondary osteoarthritis of this joint.

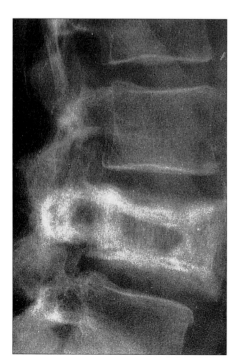

Fig. 44.4 Paget's disease of the lumbar spine. Shown is an expanded vertebral body and involvement of the neural arches with marked bony sclerosis, which results in the 'picture frame' appearance.

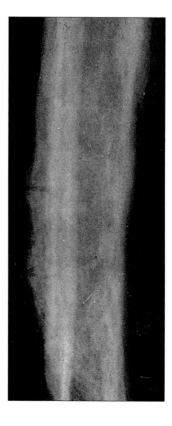

Fig. 44.5 Anteroposterior radiograph of the leg. Shown are characteristic features of advanced Paget's disease of the tibia with disorganized architecture, mixed osteosclerosis, an osteolysis, bowing, and fractures on the convex surface.

Paget's disease of bone is often a chance finding through radiographs or the discovery of a high alkaline phosphatase in an older person.

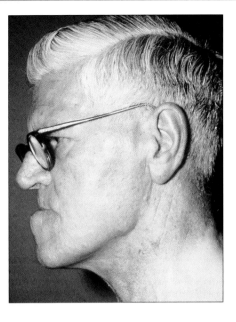

Fig. 44.6 Paget's disease of the jaw, showing the bony expansion.

 MANAGEMENT

Paget's disease of bone is now treatable, either with calcitonin or second-generation bisphosphonates, which are currently the preferred treatment. For example, doses of pamidronate disodium 600mg orally for 6–9 months normalize the alkaline phosphatase in some 80% of patients, and also completely relieve pain in the majority. If gastrointestinal problems arise with oral therapy, intravenous therapy is considered.

LUMBAR SPINAL STENOSIS

IN WHAT CIRCUMSTANCES SHOULD LUMBAR SPINAL STENOSIS BE SUSPECTED?

Spinal stenosis is a relatively common complication in older people who have spondylosis or other disorders of the lumbar spine. It is under-recognized.

The main differential diagnosis is with peripheral vascular disease, that causes claudication, although tumors in the spine or central lumbar disc herniation in older people may also produce a similar problem.

The key feature of 'pseudoclaudication' is characteristic – the production of atypical symptoms in the buttocks and legs on standing and walking, and the relief produced by flexion of the spine, as can be achieved by bending forward, sitting, or when cycling (it also means that it is easier to go downhill than uphill). However, careful direct questioning may be needed to elicit this characteristic story.

If the condition is suspected, plain lateral radiographs are taken. If these are negative and the suspicion is low no further tests are required, but if they are positive or when suspicion is high further investigations using computed tomography or magnetic resonance imaging are recommended (Fig. 44.9).

 MANAGEMENT

The condition does not always progress, and many people can cope with it once its significance is explained to them. Physical therapy or back bracing may help. If symptoms are severe or disability is present, or if significant neurologic involvement is found, such as sphincter abnormality, surgical decompression is indicated.

KEY POINTS

Definition
- A condition in which narrowing of the spinal canal results in compromise of the neural elements (Fig. 44.7).

Main clinical features
- A strongly age-related, common condition of older people, and rare below the age of 50 years.
- Associated with midsagittal narrowing of the spinal canal to 10mm or less.
- Can be caused by almost any disorder of the lumbar spine in people who have a congenitally narrow spinal canal.
- Described in association with spondylosis, spondylitis, Paget's disease, diffuse skeletal idiopathic hyperostosis, and osteoporotic fractures.
- The main clinical feature is 'pseudoclaudication' – any discomfort around the buttocks, thighs, or legs produced by standing or walking and relieved by rest and by flexion of the spine.
- A variety of symptoms such as paresthesia or numbness may be described and several dermatomes are affected.
- Spinal stiffness and discomfort are common.
- Symptoms of sciatica may occur.
- Occasionally bowel or bladder problems develop.

Diagnosis
- Radiographs provide suggestive evidence for lumbar spinal stenosis; confirmation requires computed tomography or magnetic resonance imaging (Fig. 44.8).

THE LUMBAR SPINAL CANAL IN HEALTH AND DISEASE

Normal lumbar spinal canal	Lumbar spinal stenosis in neutral position	Lumbar spinal stenosis in extension

Normal lumbar spinal canal: disc; nerve root canal; facet joint; spinal canal; ligamentum flavum

Lumbar spinal stenosis in neutral position: disc with posterior bulge; nerve root canal stenosis; hypertrophic change; ligamentum flavum thickened; spinal canal dimensions mildly reduced

Lumbar spinal stenosis in extension: disc with marked posterior bulge; hypertrophic change; spinal canal dimensions further reduced; ligamentum flavum thickened and bulging anteriorly

Fig. 44.7 Normal spinal canal, spinal canal in central spinal and nerve root canal stenosis in the neutral position, and the effect of lumbar extension on the spinal canal.

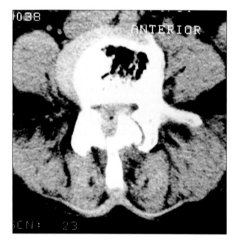

Fig. 44.8 Computed tomography scan of the lumbar spine in spinal stenosis. Shown is the characteristic trefoil deformity of the lumbar spinal canal, which is associated with facet joint hypertrophy and posterior disc bulging.

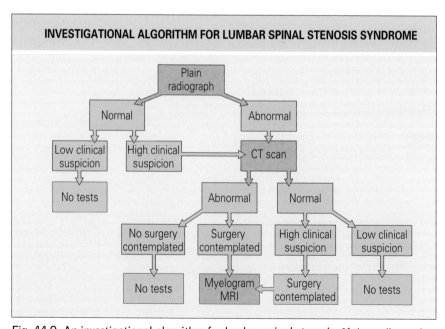

Fig. 44.9 An investigational algorithm for lumbar spinal stenosis. If the radiograph is normal no other investigations are undertaken, unless there is a very high clinical index of suspicion, or a suspected need for surgery, in which case computed tomography scanning and/or magnetic resonance imaging are indicated to obtain a better view of the anatomy.

RHEUMATOID ARTHRITIS IN OLDER PEOPLE

 ## MANAGEMENT

In established rheumatoid arthritis (RA) in older people, the physician needs to concentrate on the needs and wishes of the patient and his or her caregivers, and to concentrate on the consequences of the disease and its treatment, rather than on trying to treat the arthritis (Figs 44.10 & 44.11).

In recent-onset RA in older people, it is important to try to suppress disease activity, and low-dose corticosteroids are particularly useful in this group (although concerns about making worse any coexistent osteoporosis need to be considered).

In both established and recent-onset RA, it is important to try to keep patients active and to avoid the further damaging consequences of immobility. A team approach may be needed.

KEY POINTS

Definition
- Established or recent onset rheumatoid arthritis (RA) in older people.

Main clinical features
- Established RA in older people is characterized by the consequences of joint damage, any coexistent osteoporosis, any longstanding damage from drug toxicity, and other complications such as joint or bone sepsis.
- Recent-onset RA in older people can present in a variety of ways, which include an acute, self-limiting form, and a form that mimics polymyalgia rheumatica.
- When RA starts in older people the relative tendency is for more large-joint involvement and less small-joint disease or nodules.

Diagnosis
- Rheumatoid factor is commonly elevated in normal older people, and the presentation may be so atypical as to make diagnosis extremely difficult – regular clinical review and a high degree of suspicion in any older person who has recent onset arthritis is warranted.

POTENTIAL PROBLEMS FACED BY THE ELDERLY PERSON WITH RA		
Impairment (pathology, symptoms, signs)	Disability (functional limitation – task oriented)	Handicap (social context – role oriented)
Pain	Difficulty walking	Financial problems
Stiffness	Difficulty washing and dressing	Inadequate or inappropriate housing
Diminished renal function		
Confounding illnesses	Difficulty making snack/meal	Death of spouse/care-giver
Multiple drug therapy		Isolation
Predisposition to adverse drug reactions and interactions	Difficulty keeping house	Social support limited (family scattered)
Diminishing vision and hearing	Difficulty engaging in leisure activities	Housebound
Decline in cognitive function		
Incontinence		
Poor diet		
Poor skin		
Senile osteoporosis		
Depression		

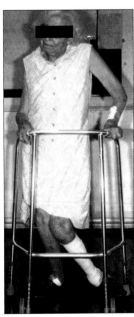

Fig. 44.11 Typical findings in an elderly woman who has long-standing rheumatoid arthritis. Note the multiple joint deformities, poor muscle bulk, and poor skin, with ulceration on the left leg and right ankles.

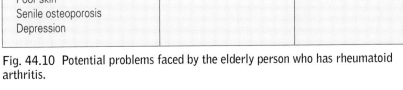

Fig. 44.10 Potential problems faced by the elderly person who has rheumatoid arthritis.

TOPHACEOUS GOUT IN OLDER PEOPLE

KEY POINTS

Definition
- A distinctive form of tophaceous gout only seen in older people; more common in women than in men.

Main clinical features
- Predisposing factors include renal disease and diuretics, in addition to age.
- Acute attacks of classic gout are uncommon.
- Tophi form, particularly over the interphalangeal joints of the hands.
- The tophi sometimes become infected (Fig. 44.12).
- Management is very difficult because of problems of drug toxicity in older people who have renal disease (Fig. 44.13).

Diagnosis
- The diagnosis may need to be confirmed by examining material from the tophi, using polarized light microscopy to identify the urate crystals.

IN WHAT CIRCUMSTANCES SHOULD TOPHACEOUS GOUT IN OLDER PEOPLE BE SUSPECTED?

Any older person who develops white nodules in the hands is likely to have tophaceous gout, particularly if he or she has renal disease or is taking diuretics.

The condition is confused with calcific deposits and other nodules (such as hyperlipidemia), and with infections.

Rx MANAGEMENT

Management of these patients is difficult because of the coexistent renal disease and because tophaceous gout occurs in frail, elderly people who often have co-morbidities. Drug toxicity can be a major problem with NSAIDs, colchicine, and allopurinol. NSAIDs need to be used with care in older people, with frequent monitoring of renal function.

Where possible, any predisposing factors are removed – if the patient is on diuretics and these can be stopped, this is done and other factors that might contribute to hyperuricemia, such as salicylates, obesity, or alcohol must be attended to.

Low-dose colchicine (0.5mg q12h) may be useful; and corticosteroids may be the best treatment for any acute attacks of gout.

Other drugs are avoided if possible; if NSAIDs or allopurinol are considered, they must be used in low doses with extreme caution.

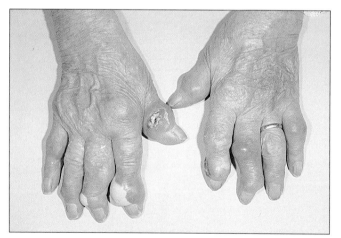

Fig. 44.12 Gouty tophi in an elderly woman who has pre-existing osteoarthritis of the hands. Note the typical, shiny white deposits, most of which are painless. However, the ulcerated lesions cause her considerable pain and are at risk of secondary infection.

AN APPROACH TO THE MANAGEMENT OF TOPHACEOUS GOUT IN OLDER PEOPLE

- Confirm the diagnosis by crystal identification
  Beware of coexistent infections

- Check serum uric acid, renal function and blood count
  Further investigations usually unnecessary

- Consider current drug therapy
  Is the patient on unnecessary diuretics or salicylates?

- Ask if any treatment is needed for the gout
  These patients may not need any intervention

- Consider systemic corticosteroids or low-dose colchicine (if creatinine clearance is <50ml/min) These are the drugs of first choice for painful inflammatory episodes

- Beware of NSAIDs
  There may be a high risk of gastrointestinal problems and renal failure

- Beware of allopurinol, uricosuric drugs and colchicine
  The risk of serious toxicity is high; if used the doses may need to be very low

Fig. 44.13 The management of tophaceous gout in older people.

FALLS AND FRACTURES IN OLDER PEOPLE

IN WHAT CIRCUMSTANCES SHOULD FALLS AND FRACTURES BE A CONCERN?

Older people who have osteoporosis are at risk of fractures from falls. Those at most risk of osteoporosis include thin people who are not very active, those who smoke or drink, and those on a poor diet.

Poor diets in the elderly contribute to the development of osteomalacia, rather than osteoporosis, in some. Other risk factors include a dark skin, genetic susceptibility, and anticonvulsant therapy. Investigations may be necessary to exclude osteomalacia (radiography and calcium, phosphate, and alkaline phosphatase levels).

Those people at most risk of falls are those who have cardiovascular disorders, particularly postural hypotension, strokes, or cognitive impairment, as well as people who are on any sedative drugs or who have balance problems. Patients with abnormal vestibular function, visual problems, those with Parkinsonism and people taking are also at high risk of falls.

Sideways falls are more likely to result in hip fractures than other forms of fall, and falls on the outstretched hand can cause wrist fractures.

KEY POINTS

Definition
- Accidental falls in older people that cause fractures.

Main clinical features
- Falls are common in older people, and one of the most important causes of osteoporotic fractures (Fig. 44.14).
- Over a third of the elderly fall at least once a year, but only some 5% of falls result in a fracture (Fig. 44.15).
- The many possible causes of falls include gait problems, balance impairment, muscle weakness, dizziness, vision impairment, hypotension, sedative use, and hazards in the environment such as slippery floors.
- The force of the fall, combined with the strength of the bone determine whether a fracture occurs.

Diagnosis
- From the history given by the patient, family, and caregivers.

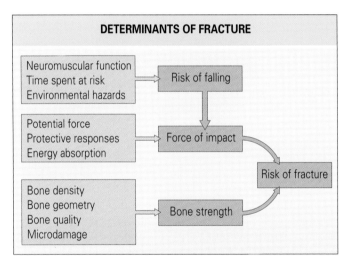

Fig. 44.14 Conceptual model of determinants of age-related fractures. (Adapted with permission from Melton LJ, Cummings SR. Heterogeneity of age-related fractures: implications for epidemiology. Bone Miner. 1987;2:321–31.)

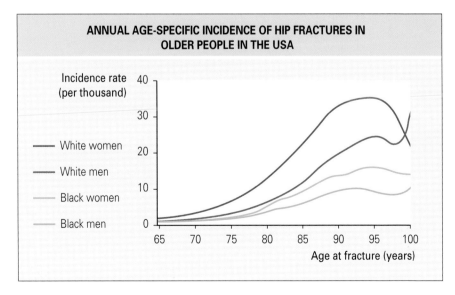

Fig. 44.15 Annual age-specific incidence of hip fracture in older people, by race and sex, United States, 1984–1987 (Medicare and Veterans Administration discharge records). (Adapted with permission from Jacobsen S, Goldberg J, Miles T, et al. Hip fracture incidence among the old and very old: a population-based study of 745,435 cases. Am J Public Health. 1990;80:871–3.)

MANAGEMENT

Hip protectors can reduce the risk of hip fracture. Attention should be given to any potential environmental hazards that might make it more likely that the patient falls, and any treatable cause of falls, such as reduction of sedative drugs, should be considered.

If osteomalacia is present the patient should be treated with calcium and vitamin D. The management of osteoporosis is considered in Chapter 33.

If fractures occur they need prompt orthopedic attention, followed by early mobilization and further attention to risk factors for thin bones and falls (Fig. 44.16).

LARGE JOINT DESTRUCTIVE ARTHRITIS

KEY POINTS

Definition
- A severe destructive arthritis of large joints in older people (90% women, 90% of all patients >70 years of age).

Main clinical features
- Most commonly affects the shoulder ('Milwaukee' shoulder), but can also affect the knees, hips, ankles and elbows.
- Painful, swollen joint, with severe instability.
- Effusions are usually blood stained (Fig. 44.17), and contain large amounts of bone dust.
- Radiographs show extensive bony damage, with extensive loss of bone on both sides of the joint (Fig. 44.18).
- May complicate previous osteoarthritis, follow injury, or occur spontaneously.
- Joint destruction occurs relatively rapidly (over a few months) when large effusions are present, but the condition often stabilizes after a year or two.

Diagnosis
- Clinical evidence of a severely unstable joint with the radiographic evidence of bone destruction is characteristic.

IN WHAT CIRCUMSTANCES SHOULD LARGE JOINT DESTRUCTIVE ARTHRITIS BE SUSPECTED?

Any older woman who has a large joint effusion, particularly of the shoulder, may have this condition.

The main differential diagnoses are neuropathic arthritis (Chapter 18), osteonecrosis (Chapter 35), rapidly progressive osteoarthritis, but the radiographic features of the condition are distinctive.

 MANAGEMENT

Management is the same as for osteoarthritis. Joint lavage may help during the active phase of the condition and should be considered earlier than would be the case in simple osteoarthritis.

AN APPROACH TO THE MANAGEMENT OF HIP FRACTURES IN OLDER PEOPLE

Unless there are contraindications the patient should undergo the operation as soon as possible

Rehabilitation should start as soon as possible, since these patients are prone to complications when bedridden

Check vision, muscle strength and coordination of the patient

Check the medication the patient is using

Let somebody (a nurse practitioner or rehabilitation specialist) check the situation at home

Try to find out whether osteoporosis or osteomalacia is involved

In cases of osteomalacia, start treatment with calcium and vitamin D

In cases of osteoporosis, start physical therapy and activities such as walking; consider dietary advice. Control pain. The benefit of other treatment modalities in elderly patients is limited

Fig. 44.16 An approach to the management of hip fractures in the elderly.

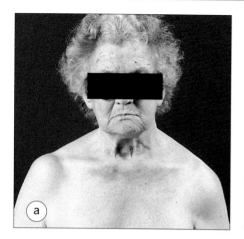

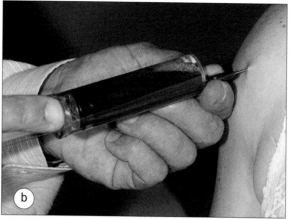

Fig. 44.17 Apatite-associated destructive arthritis ('Milwaukee shoulder'). (a) This elderly patient has visible swellings of both shoulders. (b) Aspiration revealed a large amount of blood-stained fluid, which contained numerous particles of basic calcium phosphates.

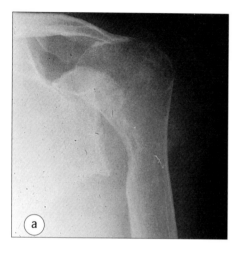

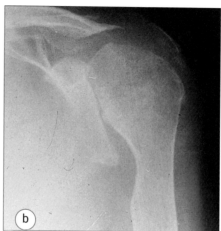

Fig. 44.18 Anteroposterior radiographs of a shoulder joint affected by apatite-associated destructive arthritis ('Milwaukee shoulder'). The extensive destruction of periarticular tissues, including the rotator cuff, has led to instability of the shoulder. (a) The upward subluxation of the humerus can be overcome by traction on the shoulder. (b) Note the extensive atrophic destruction and loss of bone in both the acromion and the glenohumeral joint.

CONNECTIVE TISSUE DISEASE IN OLDER PEOPLE

IN WHAT CIRCUMSTANCES SHOULD CONNECTIVE TISSUE DISEASES BE SUSPECTED IN OLDER PEOPLE?

In most instances the possibility of connective tissue disease (CTD) in older people arises with the finding of a positive antinuclear antibody test, usually unexpected, in a patient who has a poorly defined illness. Constitutional signs, particularly fever or weight loss, often suggest a malignancy or occult infection. Clues to the diagnosis include intermittent arthritis, muscle weakness, chest pain or dyspnea, rashes or skin changes, and sicca (Fig. 44.19). Patterns of disease typical of CTDs in older people are given in Figure 44.20.

 MANAGEMENT

Drug management of CTD in older people is complicated by co-morbid conditions and risks of drug toxicities. Musculoskeletal complaints are often helped by NSAIDs, but these days must be used with extreme caution to avoid fluid retention and gastrointestinal complications.Hydroxychloroquine is valuable for persistent inflammatory arthritis, and particularly useful in lupus and dermatomyositis. Fluid replacement with artificial tears or frequent sips of water help in the management of sicca symptoms. Corticosteroids

> **KEY POINTS**
>
> **Definition**
> - Systemic inflammatory syndromes with a positive antinuclear antibody (ANA) test.
>
> **Main clinical features**
> - Most patients have constitutional signs of illness, which include fever, weight loss, anorexia, and fatigue. Musculoskeletal complaints are often vague and poorly localized.
> - Dryness (sicca) of the mouth or eyes is common.
> - Organ involvement is similar to that with conventional connective tissue diseases (see below), yet generally less severe.
>
> **Diagnosis**
> - Diagnosis is difficult and a major dilemma is to differentiate connective tissue disease in older people from other conditions associated with positive ANA.
> - Generally requires consultation from an experienced rheumatologist to establish a clear diagnosis.

PATTERNS OF DISEASE TYPICAL OF CONNECTIVE TISSUE DISEASES IN OLDER PEOPLE

Disease	Comments
Systemic lupus erythematosus	Fever, photosensitivity, arthralgias, lymphadenopathy, and pleuropulmonary complaints are common Renal or central nervous system involvement is generally absent or mild Important to exclude drug-induced lupus syndromes (Fig. 44.20)
Inflammatory myopathies	Weakness of shoulder and hip girdle muscles – difficulty climbing stairs, climbing out of the bathtub, or reaching for high shelf Serum muscle enzymes (creatine kinase and aldolase) invariably elevated May be associated with unique rashes (see Chapter 33))
Scleroderma	Raynaud's phenomenon, skin thickening, gastrointestinal dysmotility, and dyspnea
Sjögren's syndrome	Severe dryness of the mouth and eyes; commonly seen with most forms of connective tissue disease that occur in older people (Fig. 44.21)

Fig. 44.19 Patterns of disease typical of connective tissue diseases in older people.

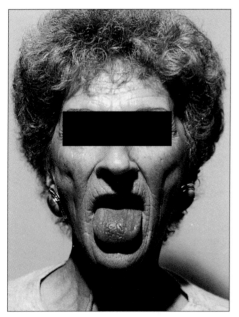

Fig. 44.21 Severe mouth dryness in an older person who has sicca syndrome. The tongue is parched and hypopapillated.

may be indicated in patients who have lupus or myositis, but should only be begun after a clear diagnosis has been made and a plan for disease monitoring and dose adjustments established.

DRUGS IMPLICATED IN DRUG-INDUCED LUPUS

Drugs with good evidence of association

Carbamazepine	Hydralazine	Procainamide
Chlorpromazine	Isoniazid	Quinidine
Diphenylhydantoin	Methyldopa	Sulfasalazine
Ethosuximide	Penicillamine	

Case reports

Acebutolol	Interferon (α,γ)	Phenylethylacetyl urea
Allopurinol	Labetalol	Pindolol
Aminoglutethimide	Leuprolide acetate	Practolol
Amoproxan	Levodopa	Prazosin
Anthiomaline	Levomepromazine	Primidone
Atenolol	Lithium carbonate	Promethazine
Benoxaprofen	Lovastatin	Propranolol
Canavanine (L-)	Mephenytoin	Propylthiouracil
Captopril	Methimazole	Psoralens
Chlorprothixene	Methysergide	Pyrathiazine
Chlorthalidone	Metoprolol	Pyrithoxine
Cimetidine	Minoxidil	Reserpine
Cinnarizine	Nalidixic acid	Spironolactone
Clonidine	Nitrofurantoin	Streptomycin
Danazol	Nomifensine	Sulfadimethoxine
Dapsone	Oral contraceptives	Sulfamethoxypyridazine
Debrisoquine	Oxprenolol	Sulfonamides
Diclofenac	Oxyphenisatin	Sulindac
1,2-Dimethyl-3-hydroxypyride-41 (L1)	Para-aminosalicylic acid	Tetracyclines
	Penicillin	Tetrazine
Disopyramide	Perazine	Thionamide
Ethylphenacemide	Perphenazine	Thioridazine
Gold salts	Phenelzine	Timolol
Griseofulvin	Phenopyrazone	Tolazamide
Hydrazines	Phenylbutazone	Tolmetin
Ibuprofen		Trimethadione

Fig. 44.20 Drugs implicated in drug-induced lupus.

APPENDIX:
PATIENT SELF-HELP PAGES

A SELF HELP FOR SHOULDER PAIN

UNDERSTANDING YOUR CONDITION

Shoulder pain most commonly occurs as a result of injury or inflammation to the structures surrounding the shoulder, such as tendons or bursae (cushion-like sacs which allow the tendon to move freely over the bone). Shoulder pain can also originate from various forms of arthritis such as osteoarthritis or rheumatoid arthritis. In addition, disorders of the neck, heart, lungs, or abdominal organs may occasionally present with shoulder pain. Shoulder pain may result in marked limitations of shoulder movement, a condition called frozen shoulder.

EXERCISE

Exercises are *important* in the treatment of shoulder pain.

BASIC EXERCISES

1. Lie on your back holding the ends of a rod in your hands. Swing your arms up overhead, using your good arm to push the affected arm back. Bring your arms down to your side. While sitting, bring the rod above your head and then down behind your neck.
2. Lie on your back. Slide arms to the side and upward overhead, then slide them back down to your side.
3. Lie on your back with your hands clasped behind your neck. Bring elbows forward to touch each other, then push them back as far as possible.
4. Stand and face a wall. Walk the fingers of your affected arm up the wall as far as possible, keeping your elbows straight, and mark the distance you reach. Repeat this exercise ten times, trying to exceed your previous mark each time.

DO

- In most forms of shoulder pain, a combination of range of motion exercises with strengthening exercises should be performed.

DON'T

- Perform exercises that make the shoulder pain worse.

SIMPLE AIDS

- Regular use of warm packs or cold packs applied to the painful area is usually helpful.
- Use clothing that fastens in the front.

MEDICATIONS

- Analgesics (such as acetaminophen/paracetamol) or anti-inflammatory drugs may help to reduce shoulder pain.
- In the treatment of shoulder pain, injection of steroids is sometimes recommended.
- In selected patients surgery may be considered.

DIET

- Diet does not play a role in the treatment of shoulder pain.

PENDULUM EXERCISES
- Bend forward from the waist and hold onto a table with your good arm. Let the affected arm hang loosely with the shoulder relaxed. Use body movement to produce an arm swing:
- Swing the arm forwards and backwards, keeping the elbow straight.
- Swing the arm across your body, right and left. Keep the elbow straight.
- Begin to make circles with your arm. Start with two small circles, then gradually increase their size.
- Do the above exercises holding a one- or two-pound weight in your hand on the affected side.

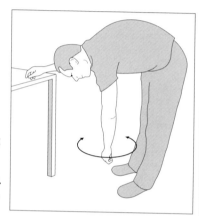

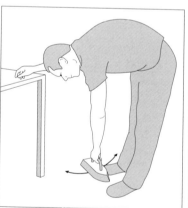

WHERE CAN YOU FIND MORE ON ARTHRITIS?

IN THE USA:
Arthritis Foundation
1330 West Peachtree Street
Atlanta, Georgia 30309, USA
Tel: +800 283 7800/+404 872 7100, or call your local chapter (listed in the telephone directory)
Web page address:
http://www.arthritis.org
This is the main voluntary organization devoted to arthritis in the USA. The Foundation publishes free pamphlets on many types of arthritis and a monthly magazine for members that provides up-to-date information on arthritis. The Foundation can also provide physician and clinic referrals.

American College of Rheumatology/Association of Rheumatology Health Professionals
1800 Century Place, Suite 250
Atlanta, Georgia 30345–4300
Tel: +404 633 3777
Fax: +404 633 1870
Web page address:
http://www.rheumatology.org
This association provides referrals to rheumatologists and physical and occupational therapists who have experience of working with people who have rheumatic diseases. The organization also provides educational materials and guidelines about many different rheumatic diseases.

IN THE UK:
Arthritis Research Campaign
Copeman House, St Mary's Court
St Mary's Gate, Chesterfield
Derbyshire S41 7TD, UK
Tel: +1246 558033
Fax: +1246 558007
E-mail address: info@arc.org.uk
Web page address: http://www.arc.org.uk

Arthritis Care
18 Stephenson Way
London NW1 2HD, UK
Tel: +171 916 1500
Fax: +171 916 1505
Web page address:
http://vois.org.uk/arthritiscare

IN CANADA:
The Arthritis Society
393 University Avenue, Suite 1700
Toronto, Ontario M5G 1E6
Canada
Tel: +800 321 1433/+416 979 7223
Fax: +416 979 8366
Web page address: http://www.arthritis.ca
This organization provides information about many types of arthritis, their treatments, management tips, programs, services and support groups.

Taken from *Primary Care Rheumatology:* Klippel, Dieppe & Ferri
© Copyright 1999 Mosby International Limited

B · SELF HELP FOR OSTEOARTHRITIS (OA) OF THE KNEE

UNDERSTAND THE CONDITION

Osteoarthritis is the most common cause of knee pain and results from thinning of the joint surfaces of the knee called cartilage. The pain is often most marked when starting to walk after resting the knee (sitting down, lying in bed, etc) and generally lessens with continued movement of the knee. Osteoarthritis can occasionally cause swelling of the knee ('water on the knee').

EXERCISE

Exercise and activity are an important part of the treatment and can help stop the condition getting worse. It is important to keep active and not to be overprotective of your knees.

DO

- Keep the joints as mobile as possible – remember to bend and straighten the knee as much as you can once or twice a day.
- Keep the thigh muscles strong by doing exercises daily.
- Keep as generally fit and active as you can – try to do a little more each day, not less; if walking is difficult think about exercises in water (such as aquajogging) or cycling.

DON'T

- Keep your leg bent in the same position for long periods or put pillows under the knees to relieve pain.
- Do things that cause a lot of excessive impact (wear and tear) on the knee joints, like jogging on hard roads.

SIMPLE AIDS

- Use footwear with good cushioning in the heel or wear shock-absorbing insoles; this reduces potentially damaging high-impact forces on the knee.
- Consider using a cane when you walk (in the hand opposite to the side of the worst knee) to reduce the load on the bad knee.
- A simple knee wrap can make the knee feel more secure and relieve the feeling that it might give way.
- Warmth will often help relieve pain. During a flare-up of pain some people also find that a cold pack on the knee helps; if so, keep a packet of frozen peas in the freezer to use in this way.
- Use a handrail on stairs or steps.

MEDICINES

- Simple pain killers such as acetaminophen (paracetamol), as well as non-steroidal anti-inflammatory drugs can help.
- Medicines that you rub on to the knee joint are very safe, may help you, and can be used when you like.

DIET

- If you are overweight you should try to get back to the weight that is right for your height. Being overweight makes the pain worse and probably makes it more likely that the knee will get worse.
- A sensible diet, with plenty of vitamins C, D and E, is advisable but there is no good evidence that any special diets make a difference. Avoid expensive diets or supplements that claim that they may cure arthritis.

EXERCISES

Choose a way of doing these exercises so that it is easy for you to do them every day. They can be done sitting or lying down.

You should be able to feel the thigh muscles working when you do these exercises, and you should aim to build them up, doing a little more each day so that the muscles get as strong as possible.

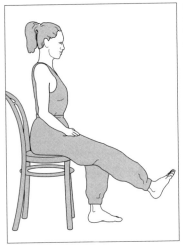

Sitting: Sit well back in the chair, straighten and raise the leg, and hold it up for a slow count of ten, and then slowly lower it again. Repeat several times.

Lying: Place a rolled-up towel under the ankle of the leg to be exercised. With one leg bent at the knee, hold the other leg straight, pull the foot up towards you, and try to push the bad knee down towards the floor. Then slowly raise the straight leg up off the floor-, hold for a slow count of five and lower it again. Repeat several times.

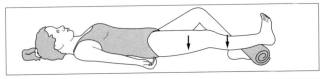

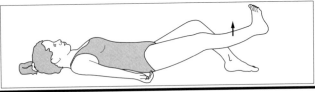

WHERE CAN YOU FIND MORE ON ARTHRITIS?

IN THE USA:

Arthritis Foundation
1330 West Peachtree Street
Atlanta, Georgia 30309, USA
Tel: +800 283 7800/+404 872 7100, or
call your local chapter (listed in the
telephone directory)
Web page address:
http://www.arthritis.org
This is the main voluntary organization devoted to arthritis in the USA. The Foundation publishes free pamphlets on many types of arthritis and a monthly magazine for members that provides up-to-date information on arthritis. The Foundation can also provide physician and clinic referrals.

American College of
Rheumatology/Association of
Rheumatology Health Professionals
1800 Century Place, Suite 250
Atlanta, Georgia 30345–4300
Tel: +404 633 3777
Fax: +404 633 1870
Web page address:
http://www.rheumatology.org
This association provides referrals to rheumatologists and physical and occupational therapists who have experience of working with people who have rheumatic diseases. The organization also provides educational materials and guidelines about many different rheumatic diseases.

IIN THE UK:

Arthritis Research Campaign
Copeman House, St Mary's Court
St Mary's Gate, Chesterfield
Derbyshire S41 7TD, UK
Tel: +1246 558033
Fax: +1246 558007
E-mail address: info@arc.org.uk
Web page address: http://www.arc.org.uk

Arthritis Care
18 Stephenson Way
London NW1 2HD, UK
Tel: +171 916 1500
Fax: +171 916 1505
Web page address:
http://vois.org.uk/arthritiscare

IN CANADA:

The Arthritis Society
393 University Avenue, Suite 1700
Toronto, Ontario M5G 1E6
Canada
Tel: +800 321 1433/+416 979 7223
Fax: +416 979 8366
Web page address: http://www.arthritis.ca
This organization provides information about many types of arthritis, their treatments, management tips, programs, services and support groups.

Taken from *Primary Care Rheumatology:* Klippel, Dieppe & Ferri
© Copyright 1999 Mosby International Limited

C SELF HELP FOR GOUT

UNDERSTAND THE CONDITION

Gout is an abrupt and painful form of arthritis. It usually affects only one joint at a time (typically the big toe, foot, ankle, knee, wrist or elbow); it affects men more commonly than women. The most accurate way to diagnose gout is through removal of fluid from the joint and examination of the fluid under a microscope for the crystals that cause gout. Gout is a very treatable disease but untreated it can cause permanent damage to the joints.

EXERCISE

You will not be able to exercise while your joint is inflamed and you must only resume normal activity when the inflammation has gone down.

DO

- Watch out for early signs of an acute attack. The earlier you start treatment the better.
- Be alert for attacks of gout following minor injury to a joint, other illnesses, or surgery.

DON'T

- Just treat isolated attacks without consulting your physician about continuous treatment for prevention.
- Stop your medicines between attacks if you are on preventative treatment.

SIMPLE AIDS

- Rest your affected joint until the symptoms improve.
- Take your medicines as prescribed.
- Drink plenty of fluids to prevent kidney stones.

MEDICINES

Medicine is important in both the treatment and prevention of attacks. Preventative treatment is necessary in people with tophi (crystals of uric acid appearing under the skin as white pimples), kidney stones and frequent attacks.

- Attacks of gout are usually treated with non-steroidal anti-inflammatory drugs such as indomethacin. Other anti-inflammatory agents (such as colchicine, or steroids by injection or as pills) may be recommended.
- Simple pain killers such as acetaminophen (paracetamol) are sometimes added.
- Medicines that are meant to prevent gout attacks such as allopurinol and probenecid may be prescribed, but these medicines are *never* used for an acute attack of gout.
- Medicines must be taken as directed and the treatment should not be shortened unless your physician says so.
- Seek your physician's advice regarding any medicines that might interfere with the effectiveness of the ones you've been told to take.
- Lifetime treatment for prevention of gout may be necessary.

DIET

- The old belief that eating and drinking too much causes gout has now been proven wrong, but over-indulgence in alcohol can make gout attacks more likely.
- Alcohol, aspirin and certain foods (such as liver, sardines and anchovies) may make you more likely to develop gout.

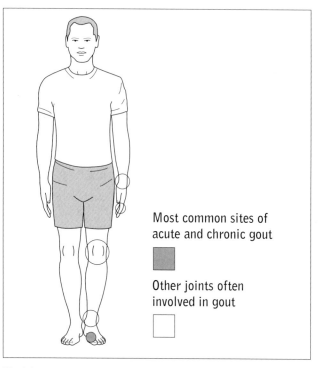

Most common sites of acute and chronic gout

Other joints often involved in gout

The joints commonly affected by or associated with gout.

WHERE CAN YOU FIND MORE ON ARTHRITIS?

IN THE USA:
Arthritis Foundation
1330 West Peachtree Street
Atlanta, Georgia 30309, USA
Tel: +800 283 7800/+404 872 7100, or
call your local chapter (listed in the
telephone directory)
Web page address:
http://www.arthritis.org
This is the main voluntary organization devoted to arthritis in the USA. The Foundation publishes free pamphlets on many types of arthritis and a monthly magazine for members that provides up-to-date information on arthritis. The Foundation can also provide physician and clinic referrals.

American College of
Rheumatology/Association of
Rheumatology Health Professionals
1800 Century Place, Suite 250
Atlanta, Georgia 30345–4300
Tel: +404 633 3777
Fax: +404 633 1870
Web page address:
http://www.rheumatology.org
This association provides referrals to rheumatologists and physical and occupational therapists who have experience of working with people who have rheumatic diseases. The organization also provides educational materials and guidelines about many different rheumatic diseases.

IN THE UK:
Arthritis Research Campaign
Copeman House, St Mary's Court
St Mary's Gate, Chesterfield
Derbyshire S41 7TD, UK
Tel: +1246 558033
Fax: +1246 558007
E-mail address: info@arc.org.uk
Web page address: http://www.arc.org.uk

Arthritis Care
18 Stephenson Way
London NW1 2HD, UK
Tel: +171 916 1500
Fax: +171 916 1505
Web page address:
http://vois.org.uk/arthritiscare

IN CANADA:
The Arthritis Society
393 University Avenue, Suite 1700
Toronto, Ontario M5G 1E6
Canada
Tel: +800 321 1433/+416 979 7223
Fax: +416 979 8366
Web page address: http://www.arthritis.ca
This organization provides information about many types of arthritis, their treatments, management tips, programs, services and support groups.

Taken from *Primary Care Rheumatology:*
Klippel, Dieppe & Ferri
© Copyright 1999 Mosby International Limited

D SELF HELP FOR RHEUMATOID ARTHRITIS (RA)

UNDERSTANDING YOUR CONDITION

RA is a disease causing inflammation in the joints of the body, leading to pain, stiffness and swelling. The joints most frequently affected are the hands, wrists, feet and knees. Fatigue can be severe in RA. Rarely, it can cause inflammation in other parts of the body including the lungs, eyes, heart, blood vessels, skin and nerves.

EXERCISE

Exercise plays an important role in the treatment of RA. It is important to strike a balance between resting inflamed joints and keeping them involved in movement so they don't stiffen.

DO

*   Take a warm shower or bath first thing in the morning to relieve stiffness.
*   Exercise to maintain range of motion and muscle strength in the joint.
*   Swim. This is an excellent exercise that places minimal stress on the joints.
*   Pace your exercises to prevent fatigue.

DON'T

*   Immobilize any joints for long periods of time.

SIMPLE AIDS

*   Wear good shoes with shock-absorbing soles.
*   Easy access, comfortable seats, automatic transmission and power steering are recommended if you are purchasing a car.
*   A cane can be a great help to decrease weight bearing on an inflamed hip or knee.
*   Temporary splinting of affected joints can help.

MEDICATIONS

*   Non-steroidal anti-inflammatory drugs are often recommended to reduce pain and swelling.
*   'Disease modifying' medications such as hydroxychloroquine, methotrexate or gold therapy may be prescribed. You might have to take these drugs for a long time, maybe even for the rest of your life.
*   Corticosteroids, such as prednisone, are sometimes prescribed and are given either by injection or as pills when inflammation is severe.
*   Multiple medications or combinations of medications may be needed.

DIET

Many diets have been published claiming to cure RA. Nearly always there is no scientific proof that these work.

*   Maintain a proper body weight so that you reduce stress on your joints.
*   Diets low in saturated fat and supplemented by fish or plant oils are often helpful.

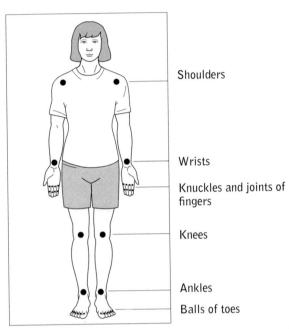

Shoulders

Wrists

Knuckles and joints of fingers

Knees

Ankles

Balls of toes

Joints frequently affected by RA; less commonly affected are the elbows, hips, and neck.

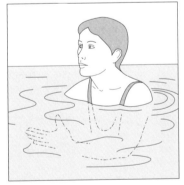

Water exercise is one of the best therapies for rheumatoid arthritis.

WHERE CAN YOU FIND MORE ON ARTHRITIS?

IN THE USA:
Arthritis Foundation
1330 West Peachtree Street
Atlanta, Georgia 30309, USA
Tel: +800 283 7800/+404 872 7100, or call your local chapter (listed in the telephone directory)
Web page address:
http://www.arthritis.org
This is the main voluntary organization devoted to arthritis in the USA. The Foundation publishes free pamphlets on many types of arthritis and a monthly magazine for members that provides up-to-date information on arthritis. The Foundation can also provide physician and clinic referrals.

American College of Rheumatology/Association of Rheumatology Health Professionals
1800 Century Place, Suite 250
Atlanta, Georgia 30345–4300
Tel: +404 633 3777
Fax: +404 633 1870
Web page address:
http://www.rheumatology.org
This association provides referrals to rheumatologists and physical and occupational therapists who have experience of working with people who have rheumatic diseases. The organization also provides educational materials and guidelines about many different rheumatic diseases.

IN THE UK:
Arthritis Research Campaign
Copeman House, St Mary's Court
St Mary's Gate, Chesterfield
Derbyshire S41 7TD, UK
Tel: +1246 558033
Fax: +1246 558007
E-mail address: info@arc.org.uk
Web page address: http://www.arc.org.uk

Arthritis Care
18 Stephenson Way
London NW1 2HD, UK
Tel: +171 916 1500
Fax: +171 916 1505
Web page address:
http://vois.org.uk/arthritiscare

IN CANADA:
The Arthritis Society
393 University Avenue, Suite 1700
Toronto, Ontario M5G 1E6
Canada
Tel: +800 321 1433/+416 979 7223
Fax: +416 979 8366
Web page address: http://www.arthritis.ca
This organization provides information about many types of arthritis, their treatments, management tips, programs, services and support groups.

Taken from *Primary Care Rheumatology:* Klippel, Dieppe & Ferri
© Copyright 1999 Mosby International Limited

E | SELF HELP FOR PSORIATIC ARTHRITIS

UNDERSTAND THE CONDITION

Psoriatic arthritis is a type of arthritis that occurs in patients with psoriasis. It can affect any joint, most commonly the tips of the fingers, and the knees and spine. The psoriasis can be variable, sometimes involving a large area of skin and sometimes a small one. Psoriatic arthritis occurs equally in men and women, usually beginning between the ages of 30 and 50 years.

EXERCISE

Exercise is important in psoriatic arthritis because it will help maintain joint range of motion and muscle strength.

DO

- Soak in warm water to help reduce morning stiffness.
- Exercise regularly.
- Seek appropriate skin care as management of the psoriasis will often help to control joint symptoms.

DON'T

- Continue to exercise if it is painful to do so.

SIMPLE AIDS

- Invest in a shopping basket on wheels.
- Try temporary splinting of inflamed joints.
- Wear low-heeled comfortable shoes.

MEDICINES

Medications help to decrease the inflammation that causes pain and swelling in psoriatic arthritis.

- Non-steroidal anti-inflammatory drugs are commonly used.
- If non-steroidals do not control the pain and swelling, then disease-modifying medications such as sulfasalazine or methotrexate may be recommended.
- Joint replacement surgery may be recommended if you have severe disease.

DIET

There are no specific diets found to be effective in psoriatic arthritis. If you are overweight, it is necessary to diet and so reduce the strain put on leg joints.

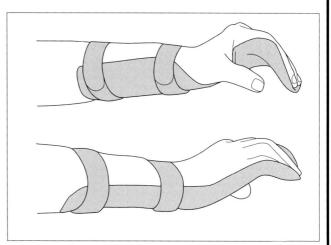

Splinting of the hand in psoriatic arthritis.

WHERE CAN YOU FIND MORE ON ARTHRITIS?

IN THE USA:
Arthritis Foundation
1330 West Peachtree Street
Atlanta, Georgia 30309, USA
Tel: +800 283 7800/+404 872 7100, or call your local chapter (listed in the telephone directory)
Web page address:
http://www.arthritis.org
This is the main voluntary organization devoted to arthritis in the USA. The Foundation publishes free pamphlets on many types of arthritis and a monthly magazine for members that provides up-to-date information on arthritis. The Foundation can also provide physician and clinic referrals.

American College of
Rheumatology/Association of
Rheumatology Health Professionals
1800 Century Place, Suite 250
Atlanta, Georgia 30345–4300
Tel: +404 633 3777
Fax: +404 633 1870
Web page address:
http://www.rheumatology.org
This association provides referrals to rheumatologists and physical and occupational therapists who have experience of working with people who have rheumatic diseases. The organization also provides educational materials and guidelines about many different rheumatic diseases.

IN THE UK:
Arthritis Research Campaign
Copeman House, St Mary's Court
St Mary's Gate, Chesterfield
Derbyshire S41 7TD, UK
Tel: +1246 558033
Fax: +1246 558007
E-mail address: info@arc.org.uk
Web page address: http://www.arc.org.uk

Arthritis Care
18 Stephenson Way
London NW1 2HD, UK
Tel: +171 916 1500
Fax: +171 916 1505
Web page address:
http://vois.org.uk/arthritiscare

IN CANADA:
The Arthritis Society
393 University Avenue, Suite 1700
Toronto, Ontario M5G 1E6
Canada
Tel: +800 321 1433/+416 979 7223
Fax: +416 979 8366
Web page address: http://www.arthritis.ca
This organization provides information about many types of arthritis, their treatments, management tips, programs, services and support groups.

Taken from *Primary Care Rheumatology:* Klippel, Dieppe & Ferri
© Copyright 1999 Mosby International Limited

F SELF HELP FOR LOW BACK PAIN

UNDERSTANDING YOUR CONDITION

The back is made up of vertebrae (back bones), disks between the vertebrae, and surrounding soft tissues such as muscles and ligaments. If the vertebrae, disks or nerves are damaged, or the muscles and ligaments are strained or torn, back pain will result.

Acute back pain usually results from an injury and lasts 1 to 7 days. Obesity, poor posture and a weak back and abdominal muscles contribute to chronic low back pain. Low back pain can also occur with diseases such as osteoarthritis, ankylosing spondylitis, Reiter's syndrome, fibromyalgia, disk problems and Paget's disease.

EXERCISE

Exercise plays an important role in the treatment of back pain. There are various types of exercises; one type may suit one back problem but not another. Your physician may recommend that exercises be carried out under the supervision of a physical therapist.

DO

- Maintain good posture while sitting and walking.
- When sitting for a long time, make a lumbar support by placing a small pillow between your lower back and the seat.
- Stand and walk frequently to reduce low back fatigue and strain.
- Lift heavy objects with the proper straight spine posture. Hold objects close to your body and use your thigh and leg muscles to lift.
- Participate in daily stretching and strengthening exercises.
- Follow a weight loss plan (if you are overweight).
- Report to your doctor if there is numbness or tingling in the legs.

DON'T

- Sit for prolonged periods.
- Lift and twist, push or pull heavy objects.
- Engage in strenuous activity until cleared by your physician.

SIMPLE AIDS

- Massage or deep heat treatments often help to relieve back pain.
- Use a firm mattress or place a board under the mattress.

MEDICINES

- Acetaminophen (paracetamol) or non-steroidal anti-inflammatory drugs are often prescribed to ease back pain.
- With severe pain, stronger narcotic-containing pain medicines may be needed for a short time.

- Muscle relaxants may be prescribed for muscle spasms.
- Injection of steroids by an anesthesiologist specializing in pain control may be recommended.

DIET

- Excessive weight will aggravate low back conditions.

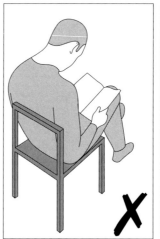 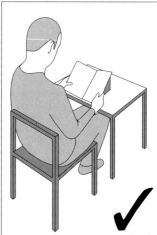

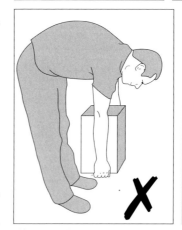 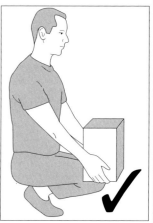

Lifting a weight with the spine bent and knees straight often makes backache worse. Bending your knees when you lift will take the strain off your back. Get as close as possible to whatever you are lifting so that you can keep your back straight.

WHERE CAN YOU FIND MORE ON ARTHRITIS?

IN THE USA:
Arthritis Foundation
1330 West Peachtree Street
Atlanta, Georgia 30309, USA
Tel: +800 283 7800/+404 872 7100, or
call your local chapter (listed in the
telephone directory)
Web page address:
http://www.arthritis.org
This is the main voluntary organization devoted to arthritis in the USA. The Foundation publishes free pamphlets on many types of arthritis and a monthly magazine for members that provides up-to-date information on arthritis. The Foundation can also provide physician and clinic referrals.

American College of
Rheumatology/Association of
Rheumatology Health Professionals
1800 Century Place, Suite 250
Atlanta, Georgia 30345–4300
Tel: +404 633 3777
Fax: +404 633 1870
Web page address:
http://www.rheumatology.org
This association provides referrals to rheumatologists and physical and occupational therapists who have experience of working with people who have rheumatic diseases. The organization also provides educational materials and guidelines about many different rheumatic diseases.

IN THE UK:
Arthritis Research Campaign
Copeman House, St Mary's Court
St Mary's Gate, Chesterfield
Derbyshire S41 7TD, UK
Tel: +1246 558033
Fax: +1246 558007
E-mail address: info@arc.org.uk
Web page address: http://www.arc.org.uk

Arthritis Care
18 Stephenson Way
London NW1 2HD, UK
Tel: +171 916 1500
Fax: +171 916 1505
Web page address:
http://vois.org.uk/arthritiscare

IN CANADA:
The Arthritis Society
393 University Avenue, Suite 1700
Toronto, Ontario M5G 1E6
Canada
Tel: +800 321 1433/+416 979 7223
Fax: +416 979 8366
Web page address: http://www.arthritis.ca
This organization provides information about many types of arthritis, their treatments, management tips, programs, services and support groups.

Taken from *Primary Care Rheumatology:*
Klippel, Dieppe & Ferri
© Copyright 1999 Mosby International Limited

G SELF HELP FOR NECK PAIN

UNDERSTANDING YOUR CONDITION

The neck is made up of the vertebrae (neck bones), disks between the vertebrae, and the surrounding soft tissues such as muscles and ligaments. Neck pain may be caused by an injury or disease process that affects any of these structures.

EXERCISE

Exercise can be an important part of the treatment of neck pain, depending on its cause.

DO

- Practice good posture when sitting and standing.
- Perform neck exercises as indicated by your physician or physical therapist.

DON'T

- Engage in strenuous activities unless cleared with your physician.

SIMPLE AIDS

- Place a pillow under your head and neck when lying in bed.
- Use a cervical collar to help relieve spasm.
- If your pain is due to injury or if you have muscle spasms, your physician may recommend the use of heat or ice on the area.
- Deep heat or traction by a physical therapist may be recommended.

MEDICATION

- Acetaminophen (paracetamol) or non-steroidal anti-inflammatory drugs may be prescribed to decrease the pain.
- In severe pain, stronger narcotic-containing medicines may be prescribed for a short time.
- If you are having muscle spasms, muscle relaxants may be prescribed.

DIET

Diet does not play a role in the management of neck pain.

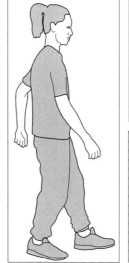
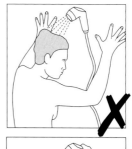
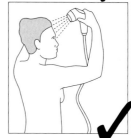
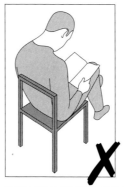
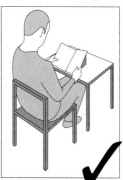
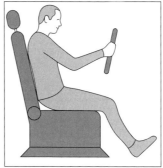

Standing. Slouching can strain your neck. When you're in the shower, bend your knees slightly to get underneath the shower head. When standing or walking, position your head squarely over your body.

Sitting. Drooping your head forward can stress the muscles in your neck. When reading, raise your reading material to eye level using a stack of books or a box.

Position your body close to the steering wheel when you drive.

WHERE CAN YOU FIND MORE ON ARTHRITIS?

IN THE USA:

Arthritis Foundation
1330 West Peachtree Street
Atlanta, Georgia 30309, USA
Tel: +800 283 7800/+404 872 7100, or
call your local chapter (listed in the
telephone directory)
Web page address:
http://www.arthritis.org
This is the main voluntary organization devoted to arthritis in the USA. The Foundation publishes free pamphlets on many types of arthritis and a monthly magazine for members that provides up-to-date information on arthritis. The Foundation can also provide physician and clinic referrals.

American College of
Rheumatology/Association of
Rheumatology Health Professionals
1800 Century Place, Suite 250
Atlanta, Georgia 30345–4300
Tel: +404 633 3777
Fax: +404 633 1870
Web page address:
http://www.rheumatology.org
This association provides referrals to rheumatologists and physical and occupational therapists who have experience of working with people who have rheumatic diseases. The organization also provides educational materials and guidelines about many different rheumatic diseases.

IN THE UK:

Arthritis Research Campaign
Copeman House, St Mary's Court
St Mary's Gate, Chesterfield
Derbyshire S41 7TD, UK
Tel: +1246 558033
Fax: +1246 558007
E-mail address: info@arc.org.uk
Web page address: http://www.arc.org.uk

Arthritis Care
18 Stephenson Way
London NW1 2HD, UK
Tel: +171 916 1500
Fax: +171 916 1505
Web page address:
http://vois.org.uk/arthritiscare

IN CANADA:

The Arthritis Society
393 University Avenue, Suite 1700
Toronto, Ontario M5G 1E6
Canada
Tel: +800 321 1433/+416 979 7223
Fax: +416 979 8366
Web page address: http://www.arthritis.ca
This organization provides information about many types of arthritis, their treatments, management tips, programs, services and support groups.

Taken from *Primary Care Rheumatology:* Klippel, Dieppe & Ferri
© Copyright 1999 Mosby International Limited

H SELF HELP FOR ANKYLOSING SPONDYLITIS

UNDERSTANDING YOUR CONDITION

Ankylosing spondylitis is a form of arthritis mainly affecting the spine, although it may involve the hips and shoulders and other peripheral joints. Ankylosing spondylitis can also produce eye irritation, heart problems and a decreased ability to expand the chest. It usually affects young men.

EXERCISE

Exercise plays a *major* role in the treatment of ankylosing spondylitis.

DO

- Perform regular non-weight-bearing exercise.
- Maintain as much motion as possible to prevent stiffness or fusion of the spine in an awkward position.
- Consult a physical therapist regarding therapy, including water therapy.
- Report any back pain following injuries (such as a fall) to your doctor.

DON'T

- Spend long periods in a poor posture, particularly with the head hanging forward.
- Ignore any symptoms of eye discomfort.

SIMPLE AIDS

- Sleep without pillows to prevent the neck from fusing in an abnormally flexed position.
- A wide rear view mirror in the car can help compensate for loss of neck motion.

MEDICATIONS

- Non-steroidal anti-inflammatory drugs are effective in managing the pain.
- Other drugs such as sulfasalazine are sometimes used if conservative treatment is not effective.
- Steroid eye-drops may be recommended if there is associated eye inflammation.

DIET

- Maintain a proper body weight as increased weight will put stress on the spine.

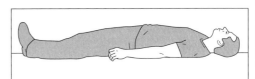

Exercise and range of motion programs will increase spine flexibility.
To maintain a straight back and neck, lie flat on the floor and relax gently so that your spine flattens out completely and your head rests on the floor.

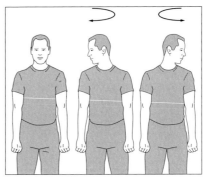

To maintain rotation of the neck, twist your neck round each side as far as you can, and repeat a few times.

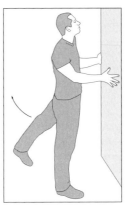

To maintain movement of your hips, stand up against a wall and then push one leg behind you as far as you can.

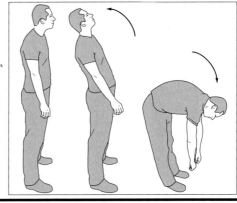

To maintain movement of your lower back, stand straight then arch your spine backwards as far as you can, and then bend forwards as far as you can.

WHERE CAN YOU FIND MORE ON ARTHRITIS?

IN THE USA:
Arthritis Foundation
1330 West Peachtree Street
Atlanta, Georgia 30309, USA
Tel: +800 283 7800/+404 872 7100, or call your local chapter (listed in the telephone directory)
Web page address:
http://www.arthritis.org
This is the main voluntary organization devoted to arthritis in the USA. The Foundation publishes free pamphlets on many types of arthritis and a monthly magazine for members that provides up-to-date information on arthritis. The Foundation can also provide physician and clinic referrals.

American College of Rheumatology/Association of Rheumatology Health Professionals
1800 Century Place, Suite 250
Atlanta, Georgia 30345–4300
Tel: +404 633 3777
Fax: +404 633 1870
Web page address:
http://www.rheumatology.org
This association provides referrals to rheumatologists and physical and occupational therapists who have experience of working with people who have rheumatic diseases. The organization also provides educational materials and guidelines about many different rheumatic diseases.

IN THE UK:
Arthritis Research Campaign
Copeman House, St Mary's Court
St Mary's Gate, Chesterfield
Derbyshire S41 7TD, UK
Tel: +1246 558033
Fax: +1246 558007
E-mail address: info@arc.org.uk
Web page address: http://www.arc.org.uk

Arthritis Care
18 Stephenson Way
London NW1 2HD, UK
Tel: +171 916 1500
Fax: +171 916 1505
Web page address:
http://vois.org.uk/arthritiscare

IN CANADA:
The Arthritis Society
393 University Avenue, Suite 1700
Toronto, Ontario M5G 1E6
Canada
Tel: +800 321 1433/+416 979 7223
Fax: +416 979 8366
Web page address: http://www.arthritis.ca
This organization provides information about many types of arthritis, their treatments, management tips, programs, services and support groups.

Taken from *Primary Care Rheumatology:* Klippel, Dieppe & Ferri
© Copyright 1999 Mosby International Limited

I   SELF HELP FOR FIBROMYALGIA

UNDERSTAND THE CONDITION

Fibromyalgia is a condition that causes widespread pain in the muscles, tendons and ligaments, and the joints. Most patients have specific areas of tenderness called trigger points. Fibromyalgia is often associated with sleep disturbance and profound fatigue.

EXERCISE

Exercise and physical activity are an *extremely important* part of the treatment of fibromyalgia.

DO

- Begin exercise slowly and increase gradually.
- Stretching exercises should be done every day.
- Endurance or aerobic exercises such as walking, cycling or swimming should be done three or four times a week.

DON'T

- Give up if exercises initially cause pain.
- Be too ambitious.

SIMPLE AIDS

There are a number of simple aids that you can use to reduce pain and decrease fatigue.

- Avoid drugs such as nasal decongestants and don't drink alcohol, tea or coffee late at night as these may disturb your sleep.
- Take time out to relax. Yoga and relaxation techniques are helpful.
- Identify the stresses in your life so that you can learn to cope with them.
- Physiotherapy and massage are sometimes helpful.
- Teach your family about fibromyalgia so that they can be supportive.

MEDICINES

Physicians prescribe medications in fibromyalgia to improve the amount and quality of sleep and to treat pain.

- Medications such as amitriptyline, nortriptyline and cyclobenzaprine in low doses are effective in helping patients sleep better, often leading to improvement in fatigue and pain.
- Pain medication, treatment of associated depression, and steroid injections into the affected area may be treatment options.

DIET

- No particular diet has been shown to help, but it is sensible to maintain your ideal body weight.
- At bedtime, avoid drinks containing caffeine.

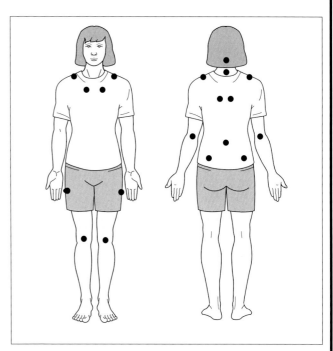

Sites of tenderness in fibromyalgia.

WHERE CAN YOU FIND MORE ON ARTHRITIS?

IN THE USA:
Arthritis Foundation
1330 West Peachtree Street
Atlanta, Georgia 30309, USA
Tel: +800 283 7800/+404 872 7100, or
call your local chapter (listed in the
telephone directory)
Web page address:
http://www.arthritis.org
This is the main voluntary organization devoted to arthritis in the USA. The Foundation publishes free pamphlets on many types of arthritis and a monthly magazine for members that provides up-to-date information on arthritis. The Foundation can also provide physician and clinic referrals.

American College of
Rheumatology/Association of
Rheumatology Health Professionals
1800 Century Place, Suite 250
Atlanta, Georgia 30345–4300
Tel: +404 633 3777
Fax: +404 633 1870
Web page address:
http://www.rheumatology.org
This association provides referrals to rheumatologists and physical and occupational therapists who have experience of working with people who have rheumatic diseases. The organization also provides educational materials and guidelines about many different rheumatic diseases.

IN THE UK:
Arthritis Research Campaign
Copeman House, St Mary's Court
St Mary's Gate, Chesterfield
Derbyshire S41 7TD, UK
Tel: +1246 558033
Fax: +1246 558007
E-mail address: info@arc.org.uk
Web page address: http://www.arc.org.uk

Arthritis Care
18 Stephenson Way
London NW1 2HD, UK
Tel: +171 916 1500
Fax: +171 916 1505
Web page address:
http://vois.org.uk/arthritiscare

IN CANADA:
The Arthritis Society
393 University Avenue, Suite 1700
Toronto, Ontario M5G 1E6
Canada
Tel: +800 321 1433/+416 979 7223
Fax: +416 979 8366
Web page address: http://www.arthritis.ca
This organization provides information about many types of arthritis, their treatments, management tips, programs, services and support groups.

Taken from *Primary Care Rheumatology:* Klippel, Dieppe & Ferri
© Copyright 1999 Mosby International Limited

J   SELF HELP FOR LUPUS

UNDERSTANDING YOUR CONDITION

Lupus is a form of arthritis that mainly affects women during their child-bearing years. Lupus usually involves joint pains, especially in the small joints of the hands and feet. Skin rashes are common and these are often made worse when exposed to sunlight. Mouth ulcers can be present and fatigue often occurs. Inflammation of the kidneys, high blood pressure and inflammation of the lining around the heart and lungs can be seen with lupus.

EXERCISE

If your joints are inflamed, exercise will help improve your mobility and help decrease fatigue. If you have lung or heart involvement, you should check with your physician before beginning an exercise program.

DO

- Use a strong sun block when going out in the sun.
- Rest as needed.
- Discuss with your physician if you are thinking about becoming pregnant.
- Get your blood pressure checked frequently.

DON'T

- Ignore headaches, fevers, coughs or abdominal pain.
- Stop your medicines without checking with your physician.

SIMPLE AIDS

- Use a hat to protect you from the sun.
- Use sunglasses to protect your eyes, which may be sensitive to light.

MEDICATIONS

- Joint pains are usually treated with anti-inflammatory drugs.
- Hydroxychloroquine may be recommended for joint and/or skin problems and fatigue.
- Corticosteroids may be prescribed if you have complications such as pleurisy or pericarditis.
- In cases of lupus involving the kidneys or blood, high doses of corticosteroids may be recommended combined with other immunosuppressive drugs (such as azathioprine or cyclophosphamide).
- Corticosteroid creams may be prescribed for rashes.

DIET

There is some evidence to suggest that a diet low in saturated fat and supplemented by fish oil may be helpful.

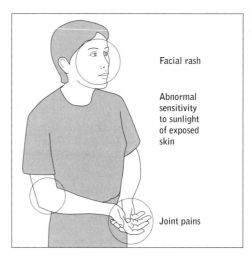

Facial rash

Abnormal sensitivity to sunlight of exposed skin

Joint pains

The main symptoms of lupus.

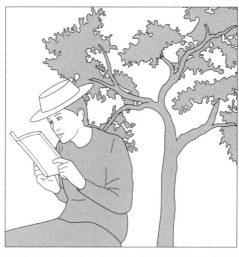

Avoid sun exposure. Too much ultraviolet radiation can flare both the skin rash and sometimes the lupus in the internal organs.

WHERE CAN YOU FIND MORE ON ARTHRITIS?

IN THE USA:
Arthritis Foundation
1330 West Peachtree Street
Atlanta, Georgia 30309, USA
Tel: +800 283 7800/+404 872 7100, or
call your local chapter (listed in the
telephone directory)
Web page address:
http://www.arthritis.org
This is the main voluntary organization devoted to arthritis in the USA. The Foundation publishes free pamphlets on many types of arthritis and a monthly magazine for members that provides up-to-date information on arthritis. The Foundation can also provide physician and clinic referrals.

American College of
Rheumatology/Association of
Rheumatology Health Professionals
1800 Century Place, Suite 250
Atlanta, Georgia 30345–4300
Tel: +404 633 3777
Fax: +404 633 1870
Web page address:
http://www.rheumatology.org
This association provides referrals to rheumatologists and physical and occupational therapists who have experience of working with people who have rheumatic diseases. The organization also provides educational materials and guidelines about many different rheumatic diseases.

IN THE UK:
Arthritis Research Campaign
Copeman House, St Mary's Court
St Mary's Gate, Chesterfield
Derbyshire S41 7TD, UK
Tel: +1246 558033
Fax: +1246 558007
E-mail address: info@arc.org.uk
Web page address: http://www.arc.org.uk

Arthritis Care
18 Stephenson Way
London NW1 2HD, UK
Tel: +171 916 1500
Fax: +171 916 1505
Web page address:
http://vois.org.uk/arthritiscare

IN CANADA:
The Arthritis Society
393 University Avenue, Suite 1700
Toronto, Ontario M5G 1E6
Canada
Tel: +800 321 1433/+416 979 7223
Fax: +416 979 8366
Web page address: http://www.arthritis.ca
This organization provides information about many types of arthritis, their treatments, management tips, programs, services and support groups.

Taken from *Primary Care Rheumatology:*
Klippel, Dieppe & Ferri
© Copyright 1999 Mosby International Limited

K · SELF HELP FOR SJÖGREN'S SYNDROME

UNDERSTAND THE CONDITION

Sjögren's syndrome is an inflammation that affects the glands, leading to dry eyes, dry mouth, dry skin and dryness of the vaginal area. It can also be associated with inflammation of the joints, lungs, kidneys, blood vessels, nerves and muscles.

EXERCISE

Exercise is not important in Sjögren's syndrome unless there is associated joint involvement.

DO

- Ask your doctor about over-the-counter eye-drops used to decrease dryness.
- Use good dental hygiene and visit your dentist frequently to avoid associated tooth decay.
- Avoid medicines like antihistamines as these have a drying effect.
- Report persistent swelling of the salivary glands or lymph nodes (found in specific areas such as the mouth, neck, lower arm, armpit and groin).

DON'T

- Ignore signs of infection.
- Eat sugary foods that will lead to tooth decay.
- Wear contact lenses.
- Use strong soaps.

SIMPLE AIDS

- Drink liquids frequently throughout the day and at night.
- Vaginal lubricants will decrease vaginal dryness and painful intercourse.
- Creams and ointments for dry skin will help seal in moisture.
- A humidifier at night will prevent dryness of the eyes, mouth and nose.
- Preservative-free eye-drops will help lubricate the eyes.
- Use sugar-free chewing gum to avoid a dry mouth.

MEDICINES

- Plugging of the tear ducts might be recommended by your eye doctor.
- Estrogen creams may be recommended to decrease vaginal dryness and painful intercourse.
- Anti-inflammatory or other medications may be recommended to control joint pain and stiffness.
- Antibiotics may be needed to treat the infections of the eye or mouth which are complications of the excessive dryness.

DIET

- Using artificial saliva or oral lubricants will ease swallowing during meals.

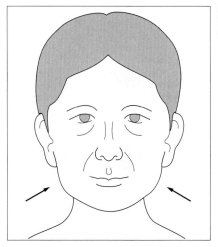

Salivary glands can become swollen in Sjögren's syndrome.

WHERE CAN YOU FIND MORE ON ARTHRITIS?

IN THE USA:
Arthritis Foundation
1330 West Peachtree Street
Atlanta, Georgia 30309, USA
Tel: +800 283 7800/+404 872 7100, or
call your local chapter (listed in the
telephone directory)
Web page address:
http://www.arthritis.org
This is the main voluntary organization devoted to arthritis in the USA. The Foundation publishes free pamphlets on many types of arthritis and a monthly magazine for members that provides up-to-date information on arthritis. The Foundation can also provide physician and clinic referrals.

American College of
Rheumatology/Association of
Rheumatology Health Professionals
1800 Century Place, Suite 250
Atlanta, Georgia 30345–4300
Tel: +404 633 3777
Fax: +404 633 1870
Web page address:
http://www.rheumatology.org
This association provides referrals to rheumatologists and physical and occupational therapists who have experience of working with people who have rheumatic diseases. The organization also provides educational materials and guidelines about many different rheumatic diseases.

IN THE UK:
Arthritis Research Campaign
Copeman House, St Mary's Court
St Mary's Gate, Chesterfield
Derbyshire S41 7TD, UK
Tel: +1246 558033
Fax: +1246 558007
E-mail address: info@arc.org.uk
Web page address: http://www.arc.org.uk

Arthritis Care
18 Stephenson Way
London NW1 2HD, UK
Tel: +171 916 1500
Fax: +171 916 1505
Web page address:
http://vois.org.uk/arthritiscare

IN CANADA:
The Arthritis Society
393 University Avenue, Suite 1700
Toronto, Ontario M5G 1E6
Canada
Tel: +800 321 1433/+416 979 7223
Fax: +416 979 8366
Web page address: http://www.arthritis.ca
This organization provides information about many types of arthritis, their treatments, management tips, programs, services and support groups.

Taken from *Primary Care Rheumatology:* Klippel, Dieppe & Ferri
© Copyright 1999 Mosby International Limited

L SELF HELP FOR RAYNAUD'S PHENOMENON

UNDERSTAND THE CONDITION

Raynaud's phenomenon results from a temporary decreased blood flow (upon exposure to cold temperatures) to one or more of the fingers, toes, ears, and occasionally the tip of the nose. Raynaud's can be associated with other diseases such as scleroderma and rheumatoid arthritis.

EXERCISE

Exercise to maintain cardiovascular fitness is recommended, but people with Raynaud's must not exercise in the cold.

DO

- Stop smoking. Smoking causes decreased blood flow to the affected areas.
- Seek medical treatment for any new sores or infections on your fingers, toes, nose or ears.
- Avoid excessive emotional stress.
- Moisturize the skin to prevent dryness and cracking.

DON'T

- Expose yourself excessively to cold.
- Treat skin infections on your extremities yourself.
- Stop prescribed medicines without checking with your physician.

SIMPLE AIDS

- Keep yourself warm by dressing in layers, mittens (rather than gloves), hat and scarf.
- If you drive then have someone else warm up your car for you.
- Wear gloves when removing food from the refrigerator and freezer.
- Warm the shower before getting in.
- Avoid second-hand cigarette smoke.
- Learn relaxation techniques.

MEDICINES

Your physician may prescribe a medication such as nifedipine for you if your condition is severe. These medicines improve blood flow to your extremities. The most common side-effects include headaches, light headedness or dizziness, swelling and rash. If medicines and other conservative measures are not successful, surgery may be suggested.

DIET

There is some evidence that a diet low in saturated fat and supplemented by fish oil may be helpful.

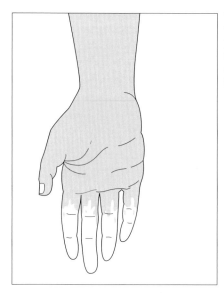

The hand of a patient with Raynaud's phenonomen, showing the typical white appearance of the fingers.

WHERE CAN YOU FIND MORE ON ARTHRITIS?

IN THE USA:

Arthritis Foundation
1330 West Peachtree Street
Atlanta, Georgia 30309, USA
Tel: +800 283 7800/+404 872 7100, or
call your local chapter (listed in the
telephone directory)
Web page address:
http://www.arthritis.org
This is the main voluntary organization devoted to arthritis in the USA. The Foundation publishes free pamphlets on many types of arthritis and a monthly magazine for members that provides up-to-date information on arthritis. The Foundation can also provide physician and clinic referrals.

American College of
Rheumatology/Association of
Rheumatology Health Professionals
1800 Century Place, Suite 250
Atlanta, Georgia 30345–4300
Tel: +404 633 3777
Fax: +404 633 1870
Web page address:
http://www.rheumatology.org
This association provides referrals to rheumatologists and physical and occupational therapists who have experience of working with people who have rheumatic diseases. The organization also provides educational materials and guidelines about many different rheumatic diseases.

IN THE UK:

Arthritis Research Campaign
Copeman House, St Mary's Court
St Mary's Gate, Chesterfield
Derbyshire S41 7TD, UK
Tel: +1246 558033
Fax: +1246 558007
E-mail address: info@arc.org.uk
Web page address: http://www.arc.org.uk

Arthritis Care
18 Stephenson Way
London NW1 2HD, UK
Tel: +171 916 1500
Fax: +171 916 1505
Web page address:
http://vois.org.uk/arthritiscare

IN CANADA:

The Arthritis Society
393 University Avenue, Suite 1700
Toronto, Ontario M5G 1E6
Canada
Tel: +800 321 1433/+416 979 7223
Fax: +416 979 8366
Web page address: http://www.arthritis.ca
This organization provides information about many types of arthritis, their treatments, management tips, programs, services and support groups.

Taken from *Primary Care Rheumatology:* Klippel, Dieppe & Ferri
© Copyright 1999 Mosby International Limited

M | SELF HELP FOR OSTEOPOROSIS

UNDERSTAND THE CONDITION

Osteoporosis is a condition where a person gradually loses bone density so that the bones become more fragile. As a result, their bones are more likely to break. There are no warning signs for osteoporosis until a fracture occurs. Osteoporosis is most common in post-menopausal women and is associated with certain risk factors such as low physical activity, smoking, alcohol and treatment with corticosteroid hormones.

EXERCISE

Exercise is an important part of the prevention and treatment of osteoporosis.

DO

- Weight-bearing exercises, such as walking, every day.
- Avoid situations that have a risk of your falling.
- Minimize alcohol intake.

DON'T

- Smoke.
- Ignore signs of loss of height or curvature of the spine as these can be indicative of osteoporosis.
- Ignore excessive pain after a fall.

SIMPLE AIDS

- Assistive devices such as canes are available if you are unsteady on your feet.
- Use a handrail on stairs.

MEDICINES

In some people, adequate calcium and vitamin D is sufficient. However, in other people medicines are needed to both prevent and treat osteoporosis.

- Post-menopausal women can be considered for estrogen, which is effective in prevention and treatment.
- Other medicines for prevention and/or treatment include calcitonin and bisphosphonates.
- Surgery may be needed to repair fractured bones.
- Drugs such as phenylhydantoin, corticosteroids or thyroid medicines may contribute to the development of osteoporosis.
- With your physician, discuss the medicines that you take now that may cause balance problems or dizziness.

DIET

- Calcium intake should be between 1000 and 1500 mg of elemental calcium a day. Dairy products are particularly rich in calcium.
- Vitamin D is necessary for the absorption of calcium from the diet, with 400 to 800 international units of vitamin D recommended daily.
- Supplemental calcium is indicated in those who do not get enough in their diet.
- Supplemental vitamin D is necessary for those who do not get it from milk or exposure to the sun.
- Avoid excess caffeine and alcohol.

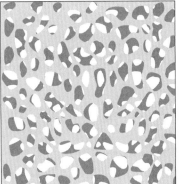

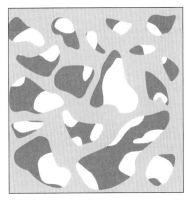

Bone is made of fibers of a material called collagen, filled in with minerals (mainly calcium salts) rather like reinforced concrete. The bones of the skeleton have a thick outer shell or 'cortex', inside which there is a meshwork of 'trabecular' bone. The drawings show (above) normal trabecular bone and (below) bone affected by osteoporosis.

WHERE CAN YOU FIND MORE ON ARTHRITIS?

IN THE USA:
Arthritis Foundation
1330 West Peachtree Street
Atlanta, Georgia 30309, USA
Tel: +800 283 7800/+404 872 7100, or call your local chapter (listed in the telephone directory)
Web page address:
http://www.arthritis.org
This is the main voluntary organization devoted to arthritis in the USA. The Foundation publishes free pamphlets on many types of arthritis and a monthly magazine for members that provides up-to-date information on arthritis. The Foundation can also provide physician and clinic referrals.

American College of Rheumatology/Association of Rheumatology Health Professionals
1800 Century Place, Suite 250
Atlanta, Georgia 30345–4300
Tel: +404 633 3777
Fax: +404 633 1870
Web page address:
http://www.rheumatology.org
This association provides referrals to rheumatologists and physical and occupational therapists who have experience of working with people who have rheumatic diseases. The organization also provides educational materials and guidelines about many different rheumatic diseases.

IN THE UK:
Arthritis Research Campaign
Copeman House, St Mary's Court
St Mary's Gate, Chesterfield
Derbyshire S41 7TD, UK
Tel: +1246 558033
Fax: +1246 558007
E-mail address: info@arc.org.uk
Web page address: http://www.arc.org.uk

Arthritis Care
18 Stephenson Way
London NW1 2HD, UK
Tel: +171 916 1500
Fax: +171 916 1505
Web page address:
http://vois.org.uk/arthritiscare

IN CANADA:
The Arthritis Society
393 University Avenue, Suite 1700
Toronto, Ontario M5G 1E6
Canada
Tel: +800 321 1433/+416 979 7223
Fax: +416 979 8366
Web page address: http://www.arthritis.ca
This organization provides information about many types of arthritis, their treatments, management tips, programs, services and support groups.

Taken from *Primary Care Rheumatology:*
Klippel, Dieppe & Ferri
© Copyright 1999 Mosby International Limited

N | SELF HELP FOR JUVENILE RHEUMATOID ARTHRITIS (JRA)

UNDERSTANDING YOUR CONDITION

JRA refers to various forms of arthritis occurring in children. It is caused by inflammation in the joints causing stiffness, warmth, swelling and pain. It is a chronic disease that may last for many months or years. There are three types of JRA: pauciarticular, polyarticular and systemic. They have different types of problems.

Pauciarticular JRA affects only a few joints, starts most commonly in the pre-school years and is more likely to occur in girls. Knees, elbows and ankles are commonly affected, and inflammation in the eyes occurs in about half the children.

Polyarticular JRA affects many joints, often the small joints of the hands and fingers. Joints commonly affected include the neck, knees, ankles, feet, wrists and hands. Girls develop this more commonly. Eye inflammation can develop, but less frequently than in pauciarticular JRA.

Systemic JRA starts with fever, rash, changes in the blood cells, and joint pain. Inflammation of the joints often develops later. Rarely, systemic JRA will involve the heart, lymph nodes, liver and lungs.

EXERCISE

Exercise is *very important* to maintain joint movement and muscle strength.

DO

• Have children participate in the same activities as other children of their age.
• Have children alternate periods of activity with periods of rest.
• Have children maintain good posture.
• Consider participation in water therapy.
• Arrange regular eye tests even if there are no symptoms.

DON'T

• Continue with an exercise program that causes increased pain.
• Put pillows under the knees as this could lead to permanently bent knees.

SIMPLE AIDS

• Use a firm mattress with one thin pillow.
• Use rest splints if recommended.
• Use a neck collar if recommended.
• Get adequate rest at night.

MEDICATIONS

• Non-steroidal anti-inflammatory drugs are frequently prescribed.
• 'Disease-modifying' medications, including gold therapy, hydroxychloroquine and methotrexate may be prescribed to slow the disease's progress.
• If your child has serious systemic JRA, prednisone may be prescribed.
• Rarely, joint replacement or synovectomy (the removal of joint lining) may be necessary.

DIET

There is no evidence that a special diet plays a part in the care of children with JRA but it is important that children have adequate caloric, protein and calcium intake.

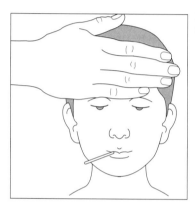

Persistent fevers may be part of JRA.

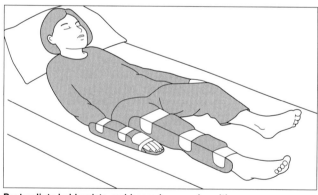

Rest splints hold wrists and knees in a good position.

WHERE CAN YOU FIND MORE ON ARTHRITIS?

IN THE USA:
Arthritis Foundation
1330 West Peachtree Street
Atlanta, Georgia 30309, USA
Tel: +800 283 7800/+404 872 7100, or
call your local chapter (listed in the
telephone directory)
Web page address:
http://www.arthritis.org
This is the main voluntary organization devoted to arthritis in the USA. The Foundation publishes free pamphlets on many types of arthritis and a monthly magazine for members that provides up-to-date information on arthritis. The Foundation can also provide physician and clinic referrals.

American College of
Rheumatology/Association of
Rheumatology Health Professionals
1800 Century Place, Suite 250
Atlanta, Georgia 30345–4300
Tel: +404 633 3777
Fax: +404 633 1870
Web page address:
http://www.rheumatology.org
This association provides referrals to rheumatologists and physical and occupational therapists who have experience of working with people who have rheumatic diseases. The organization also provides educational materials and guidelines about many different rheumatic diseases.

IN THE UK:
Arthritis Research Campaign
Copeman House, St Mary's Court
St Mary's Gate, Chesterfield
Derbyshire S41 7TD, UK
Tel: +1246 558033
Fax: +1246 558007
E-mail address: info@arc.org.uk
Web page address: http://www.arc.org.uk

Arthritis Care
18 Stephenson Way
London NW1 2HD, UK
Tel: +171 916 1500
Fax: +171 916 1505
Web page address:
http://vois.org.uk/arthritiscare

IN CANADA:
The Arthritis Society
393 University Avenue, Suite 1700
Toronto, Ontario M5G 1E6
Canada
Tel: +800 321 1433/+416 979 7223
Fax: +416 979 8366
Web page address: http://www.arthritis.ca
This organization provides information about many types of arthritis, their treatments, management tips, programs, services and support groups.

Taken from *Primary Care Rheumatology:*
Klippel, Dieppe & Ferri
© Copyright 1999 Mosby International Limited

FURTHER READING

GENERAL

RHEUMATOLOGY, SECOND EDITION
John H Klippel and Paul A Dieppe (Mosby), 1998

FERRI'S CLINICAL ADVISOR
Fred F Ferri (Mosby), 1998

PRACTICAL GUIDE TO THE CARE OF THE MEDICAL PATIENT,
FOURTH EDITION
Fred F Ferri (Mosby), 1998

TEXTBOOK OF PRIMARY CARE MEDICINE
John Noble (Mosby), 1996

EXAMINATION AND INJECTION TECHNIQUES

CLINICAL EXAMS IN RHEUMATOLOGY
Michael A Doherty (Mosby), 1992

CLINICAL EXAMINATION, SECOND EDITION
Owen Epstein, David P De Bono, G David Perkin and John Cookson
(Mosby), 1997

POCKET GUIDE TO CLINICAL EXAMINATION
Owen Epstein, David P De Bono, G David Perkin and John Cookson
(Mosby), 1997

PROCEDURES FOR PRIMARY CARE PHYSICIANS
John L Pfenninger and Grant C Fowler (Mosby), 1994

CARE OF THE ELDERLY

PRACTICAL GUIDE TO THE CARE OF THE GERIATRIC PATIENT,
SECOND EDITION
Fred F Ferri, Marsha D Fretwell and Tom J Wachtel (Mosby), 1997

REHABILITATION

EXERCISE PRESCRIPTION
Kamala Shankar (Mosby), 1998

PEDIATRICS

PRACTICAL GUIDE TO THE CARE OF THE PEDIATRIC PATIENT
Anthony J Alario (Mosby), 1997

PEDIATRIC PRIMARY CARE: A PROBLEM-ORIENTED APPROACH,
THIRD EDITION
M William Schwartz, Thomas A Curry, Albert J Sargent and
Nathan J Blum (Mosby), 1997

ADOLESCENT RHEUMATOLOGY
David A Isenberg and John J Miller (Martin Dunitz), 1998

PRIMARY PEDIATRIC CARE, THIRD EDITION
Robert A Hoekelman (Mosby), 1997

ORTHOPEDICS AND SPORTS MEDICINE

PRACTICAL ORTHOPEDICS, FOURTH EDITION
Lonnie R Mercier (Mosby), 1996

ORTHOPEDIC SECRETS
David E Brown and Randall D Neumann (Mosby), 1994

SPORTS MEDICINE: PRINCIPLES OF PRIMARY CARE
Giles R Scuderi, Peter D McCann and Peter J Bruno (Mosby), 1997

OFFICE SPORTS MEDICINE, SECOND EDITION
Morris B. Mellion (Mosby), 1995

PHYSICAL THERAPY

MANUAL OF PHYSICAL MEDICINE AND REHABILITATION
Jackson C Tan (Mosby), 1997

INDEX

INDEX

INDEX

inflammation *see* tenosynovitis
isolated swelling 131
'tennis elbow' 81, 82–83
tenosynovectomy 51
tenosynovitis 11
abductor pollicis longus 87
de Quervain's 87, 90, 91
gonococcal infection 184
villondular 131
teres minor, lesions 72
therapeutic strategies *see* management
Thompson calf-squeeze test 113
thrombocytopenia 303
thrombophlebitis 230
thumb
base, osteoarthritis 316
trigger 88, 91
thyroid acropachy 180, 181
thyroid disease 225
thyroid function tests 31
thyroiditis 180
tibia, bowing 328
tibial tuberosity, enlargement 282
tick bites 136
Tinel's sign 88, 89
tissue typing, ankylosing spondylitis 212
tophi, gouty 119, 121, 332
torticollis 206
tragus-to-wall distance 214
tramadol hydrochloride 5, 227
transcutaneous electrical nerve stimulation 208, 320
transverse ligament, laxity 207
trauma 15
elbow pain 82
reflex sympathetic dystrophy after 135
triamcinolone hexacetonide 50, 173
tricyclic antidepressants 62, 227
trigger finger (thumb) 88, 91
trochanteric 'bursa,' corticosteroid injections 97

trochanteric bursitis 95, 96–97
tuberculosis
knee 126
spinal 128, 198
tuberculous arthritis 126
tumors
bone *see* bone tumors
synovial 131–132
see also metastatic tumors

U

ulceration/ulcers
acute corneal 26
gastric 57
gouty tophi 121, 122
mouth 229, 251
necrotizing vasculitis 146, 250
pressure 134, 147, 148
rheumatoid vasculitic 25, 146, 250
ulnar nerve 89
ultrasound 34, 35, 267
therapeutic 45
uric acid
elevated 28, 119, 120
measurements 31
uricosuric agents 125
urinary tract infections 242
urticarial vasculitis 249, 250
uveitis
anterior
ankylosing spondylitis 25, 211, 212
juvenile chronic arthritis 25, 290, 291
hypopyon 221, 252
reactive arthritis 173

V

'vacuum sign' 182
vasculitis
adult Still's disease vs 248
extracranial 322
necrotizing 146, 249, 250
urticarial 249, 250

vasculitis syndromes 248–251
management 251
patterns of disease 249, 250
suspected, features 249
vasovagal attacks 77
vena caval obstruction 252
venous thromboses 252, 253
vertebrae
osteoporosis 207, 263, 264
radiolucencies 274
vertebral body, radiograph 204, 328
vertebral column 187
vertebral fractures 264
compression 197, 263, 264
viral arthritis 139, 163–167
acute/chronic 163
case history 164
differential diagnosis 166–167
management 167
natural history and features 166
referral 167
virus infections, causing arthritis 163
visual impairment, giant cell arteritis 322
vitamin A 161
vitamin D 268
deficiency 271
intake 351
supplements 61, 269, 334, 351
vitamin D2 and D3 271

W

walking aids 47–48, 98, 105, 319
'weaver's bottom' 96
Wegener's granulomatosis 31, 242, 249
weight loss 23
antinuclear antibodies (ANA) disorder 242
vasculitis syndromes 249
wheelchairs 48
whiplash injury 206, 207
Whipple's disease, polyarthritis 216

wrist
arthrography 34
de Quervain's tenosynovitis 87, 90
flexion (Phalen's maneuver) 88, 89
fractures in older people 333
injection therapy 90–92
juvenile chronic arthritis 290, 292
management 89–92
'nappy' 87
pain 85–92
case history 87, 88, 89
causes 85
periostosis in hypertrophic osteoarthropathy 178
polyarticular disorders affecting 139, 140
range of movement 86
referral recommendations 92
resisted extension test 80
splints 153

X

xerophthalmia 233
xerostomia (dry mouth) 233, 235, 236, 336

Z

zygapophyseal joints 187, 188
injections 199, 206
whiplash injury 206